Clinical Thermology

Subseries Thermotherapy

M. Gautherie (Ed.)

Thermal Dosimetry and Treatment Planning

With Contributions by
J.C. Chato · K.D. Paulsen · R.B. Roemer

With 183 Figures and 30 Tables

Springer-Verlag Berlin Heidelberg New York
London Paris Tokyo Hong Kong

Dr. Michel Gautherie
Laboratoire de Thermologie Biomédicale
Université Louis Pasteur
Institut National de la Santé
et de la Recherche Médicale
11, rue Humann
67085 Strasbourg Cedex, France

ISBN-13: 978-3-642-48714-9 e-ISBN-13: 978-3-642-48712-5
DOI: 10.1007/978-3-642-48712-5

Library of Congress Cataloging-in-Publication Data
Thermal dosimetry and treatment planning / M. Gautherie (ed.); with contributions by J.C. Chato, K.D. Paulsen, R.B. Roemer. p. cm. – (Clinical thermology. Subseries thermotherapy) Includes bibliographical references.
ISBN-13: 978-3-642-48714-9
1. Thermotherapy. 2. Thermal dosimetry. I. Gautherie, Michel. II. Paulsen, K.D. III. Roemer, R.B. (Robert B.) IV. Title. V. Series. [DNLM: 1. Hyperthermia, Induced. 2. Models, Biological. WB 469 C494t] RM865.C48 1990 615.8'32 – dc20 90-9484

Softcover reprint of the hardcover 1st edition 1990

Typesetting: K+V Fotosatz GmbH, Beerfelden

2127/3145-543210 – Printed on acid-free paper

Preface

When in the future improved and more flexible heating equipment becomes available, and when hyperthermia is applied more routinely, computerized simulations of treatments will become commonplace, as they are in radiation therapy. For hyperthermia, however, such simulations will be used not only for the traditional role of planning patient treatment, but also for three other applications not needed in radiation therapy – the comparative evaluation of equipment, feedback control during treatment, and the post-treatment evaluation of therapy. The present simulations of hyperthermia are crude and simple when compared with what is required for these future applications, a fact which indicates the nedd for considerable research and development in this area. Indeed, this research is proceeding rapidly within the hyperthermia community, whre three-dimensional power deposition and temperature calculations have just become available for realistic patient anatomies. Of equal significance are the even more rapid development in diagnostic imaging for the determination and display of patient anatomy and blood flow rates – information required for the planning of realistic hyperthermia treatment.

These simulations will be very valuable tools which can be used to great advantage when combined with data obtained from treatments of patients. This combination is a prerequisite for the optimal application of hyperthermia, and it is a particularly promising combination due to the complementary nature of the two processes: patient treatments are, in essence, poorly controlled, expensive and difficult experiments from which only sparse data can be obtained regarding the treatment conditions and results, while simulations can be easily used to reproduce such treatments in great detail, and with complete knowledge of all independent and dependent variables – once we have learned from the real treatments how to build accurate models. This combination of using the limited clinical temperature data available plus good patient treatment models has great potential usefulness in patient treatment evaluations, especially because of the present technical and practical difficulties associated with developing high-resolution, accurate, and practical noninvasive thermometry systems as outlined in the companion volume *Methods of Hyperthermia Control.* Thus, the determination, or at least estimation, of the complete temperature fields present during hyperthermia treatments, a crucial need in hyperthermia, will perhaps best be done using treatment simulation plus limited clinical thermometry.

Strasbourg, March 1990

R. B. ROEMER
M. GAUTHERIE

Preface

The [illegible] rather lengthy and [illegible] patients [illegible] and [illegible] simulations [illegible] because [illegible] complexity [illegible] therapy [illegible] hyperthermia, however, [illegible] simulations will be of [illegible] the traditional role of planning [illegible] treatment, but also [illegible] other application [illegible] not [illegible] of [illegible] feedback control during treatment [illegible] evaluation [illegible] therapy. The present [illegible] patients [illegible] the tools for considerable research and development in this area. Indeed, this is a [illegible] rapidly within the hyperthermia community, where three-dimensional power deposition and temperature calculations have just become available for realistic patient anatomies. Of equal significance are the even more rapid developments in diagnostic imaging for the determination and display of patient anatomy and blood flow rates — information required for the planning of realistic hyperthermia treatment.

These simulations will be very valuable tools which can be used to great advantage when combined with data obtained from treatments of patients. This combination is a prerequisite for the optimal application of hyperthermia, and is a particularly promising combination due to the complementary nature of the two processes: patient treatments are, in essence, poorly controlled, expensive and difficult experiments from which only sparse data can be obtained regarding the treatment conditions and results, while simulations can be easily used to reproduce such treatments in great detail, and with complete knowledge of all independent and dependent variables — once we have learned from the real treatments how to build accurate models. This combination of using the limited clinical temperature data available plus good patient treatment models has great potential usefulness in patient treatment evaluations, especially because of the present technical and practical difficulties associated with developing high-resolution, accurate, and practical noninvasive thermometry systems as outlined in the companion volume *Methods of Hyperthermia Control*. Thus, the determination, or at least estimation, of the complete temperature fields present during hyperthermia treatments, a crucial need in hyperthermia, will perhaps best be done using treatment simulation plus limited clinical thermometry.

Strasbourg, March 1990

R. B. Roemer
M. Gautherie

Contents

List of Contributors

J. C. Chato
University of Illinois at Urbana-Champaign, 1206 W. Green Street, Urbana, IL 61801, USA

K. D. Paulsen
Thayer School of Engineering, Dartmouth College, Hanover, NH 03755, USA

R. B. Roemer
Department of Radiation Oncology, Health Sciences Center, University of Arizona, Tucson, AZ 85724, USA

1 Fundamentals of Bioheat Transfer

J. C. CHATO

1.1 Introduction

It is always a difficult task to write a technical treatise which is to be understood and, what is more, to be used by professionals in widely differing fields. Bioheat transfer is a topic which is employed in the practice of biology, medicine, and engineering in a wide variety of applications. In addition, the workers in this field, i.e., the users of this treatise, will come with a variety of backgrounds and not equally strong in the scientific backgrounds involved: biology, medicine, physics, mathematics, and engineering. Thus, my task as author is to develop the topics in an orderly manner that can be followed relatively easily and to maintain a balance between the biological and physical sciences in order to show their interactions and the limitations of each. My engineering biases will undoubtedly reveal themselves but I offer no apologies since these biases are, I believe, no worse than anyone else's.

By necessity in some sections advanced mathematical techniques have to be used in describing the models. There the reader will need to have an understanding of such topics as differential calculus or partial differential equations. However, these concepts will be introduced with a qualitative description of the behavior of the system to help the reader to understand the effects of various parameters and their biological significance. Thus, I hope to help the engineer to appreciate the marvelous complexities and performance of biological systems and to help the biologically trained reader to interpret the results of the analyses properly without necessarily completely understanding the process by which they were obtained.

First, the basic thermodynamic and heat or energy transfer concepts will be introduced and developed. Next, the various modes of heat transfer will be discussed and the models for quantification will be developed with special attention to biological and medical applications. Next, heat transfer to blood vessels will be examined in detail because this constitutes the most unique and difficult problem posed by biological applications. Then, the prediction of system behavior will be studied by introducing various models of biological systems, specifically, the human body and its parts. The next section is a general introduction to numerical techniques. The final section deals with properties and measurements. There have been a few reviews written on bioheat transfer and the reader can refer to these for additional details. The most notable are by Stoll [65]; Chato [15, 18, 19, 22]; Bowman et al. [9]; Shitzer [61]; and a recent, very comprehensive set of books edited by Shitzer and Eberhart [62]. Of course, there are numerous articles dealing with various details of any of the subjects covered in several scientific journals. One of the difficulties of trying to keep up with such an interdisciplinary field is that the relevant articles occur in several engineering as well as biological or medical journals.

The units used will be primarily in modern SI, which employs the kilogram mass, kg, the meter, m, and the second, s, as the basic units. Secondary units are joules, J, for energy and watts, W = J/s, for power. Appropriate multiples of these units will also be used where convenient. A conversion table for other units is given in the Appendix.

1.2 Basic Concepts of Thermodynamics

Heat transfer is a form of energy flow which is created by a difference in the thermodynamic property called temperature between two points. It always flows from the higher temperature level toward the lower one and it cannot flow in the opposite direction. This last statement is the practical essence of the second law of thermodynamics. Thus, the study of heat transfer is only one aspect of the study of energy, its flow, and its transformation from one form to another.

In a fundamental thermodynamic sense we need to distinguish three main types of energy:

1. *Stored energy*, which is measured in terms of various energy levels or potentials such as thermal, chemical, gravitational, kinetic, electric, and magnetic
2. *Heat transfer*, which is energy in transition due to temperature differences between systems
3. *Work*, which is also energy in transition due to forces acting between systems

One of the most important fundamental concepts of thermodynamics is the conservation of energy, the so-called first law. It states that energy cannot be created or destroyed; it can only be transformed. This is true even in nuclear reactions which require consideration of the convertibility of mass into energy, i.e., mass is regarded as a form of stored energy. Thus, if we consider a *closed system* which exchanges energy with its environment but no mass crosses the system's boundaries, we can account for all the energies of the system in terms of the change in the internally stored energy, E, the heat transfer to it from the environment, Q, and the work outflow, i.e., the work done by the system on its environment, W. In mathematical terms

$$\Delta E = Q - W \ . \tag{1.1 a}$$

All terms have to be in consistent units such as joules, J. The same relation can be expressed as a rate at which these quantities change with time.

$$\frac{\partial E}{\partial t} = \frac{\partial Q}{\partial t} - \frac{\partial W}{\partial t} \ . \tag{1.1 b}$$

Or expressed with different symbols:

$$\dot{E} = \dot{Q} - \dot{W} \ . \tag{1.1 c}$$

The partial derivatives indicate that only time changes are considered. This equation is deceptively simple because the evaluation of the various terms may not be easy. As a matter of fact, it is precisely the difficulties of estimating the energy transferred by physiological means, particularly blood perfusion, which makes bioheat transfer distinctly harder to quantify than some other systems.

Let us look a typical examples of these energy forms. If the skin temperature is above that of its environment, thermal energy will flow out of the skin (heat transfer). If, however, the skin touches a hotter surface, the energy will flow into the skin. Evaporation of sweat from the skin surface will extract energy from the skin in proportion to the amount evaporated and the latent heat of vaporization of water. It is to be noted that, although heat transfer takes place in these examples in certain directions, the temperature changes depend on the overall energy balance. For example, in a hot and dry environment heat transfer is into the body by virtue of the temperature difference, but there is also sweat evaporation which removes energy from the skin. Thus the temperature patterns on the skin will depend on the relative magnitudes of these opposite energy flows as well as on the energy exchange between the skin and the inner tissues.

In the human body, work is done by the muscles exerting forces and moving various parts. The result can be either useful work done by the body, such as lifting a weight, or irreversible generation of heat due to dissipational effects, such as friction. A single muscle does positive work when it contracts. While it is stretched, however, it is doing negative work, i.e., the external forces do work on the muscle by stretching it. This negative work ends up as unrecoverable internal energy in the body because the energy of the muscle is not generated by its stretching, as a spring, but by the expenditure of chemical energy.

Energy can be stored in a system in various ways. Thermal or "internal" energy can be measured in terms of the temperature; chemical potentials represent energy sources; kinetic energy is proportional to the velocity squared; gravitational energy depends on the distance between masses, expressed usually in terms of an elevation above a reference level; and electrical and magnetic energies depend on the presence of electrical and magnetic fields. In biological and medical applications the most common forms of stored energy are thermal and chemical. In a heat transfer problem the thermal stored energy is expressed as a function of temperature and the chemical one is converted to a thermal energy source of a given strength, such as a volumetric metabolic rate, q_m.

Although with the selection of appropriate boundaries all systems could be treated as closed ones with only heat transfer and work crossing the boundaries; it is easier in many applications to define the boundaries such that mass crosses them, usually as a flowing fluid. Such systems are called *open systems* or *control volumes*. In such cases the total energy carried across the boundaries has to be accounted for. The energy content of a stream of fluid is just like any stored energy in a system, consisting of the internal, chemical, kinetic, gravitational, electric, and magnetic varieties. However, in addition, the stream has to have the energy required to push either the environment or the system out of the way as it either leaves or enters the system. Thus, in terms of a mass flow rate, m, in kg/s crossing the system's boundary the energy content can be written as:

$$m(u + pv + V^2/2 + gl + e_e + e_m)$$

where u is specific internal energy per unit mass; pv, the product of the pressure and specific volume per unit mass, is the energy (also called *flow work*) required to move a unit mass across the boundary; $V^2/2$ is the kinetic energy expressed in terms of a mean velocity; g l, the product of the gravitational acceleration and the elevation above some reference level, is the potential energy; and e_e and e_m represent electric and magnetic energies, respectively. In flow situations the first two terms always appear together and, consequently, this combination was given a special name, specific enthalpy, h, i.e.,

$$h = u + pv, \quad \text{J/kg or kJ/kg} \ . \tag{1.2}$$

Thus the first law of thermodynamics, Eq.1.1, has to be modified for an open system.

$$\Delta E_{sys} = Q - W + \sum M_{in}(h + V^2/2 + gl + e_e + e_m)_{in} - \sum M_{out}(h + V^2/2 + gl + e_e + e_m)_{out} \tag{1.3 a}$$

or in the form of a rate equation

$$\dot{E}_{sys} = \dot{Q} - \dot{W} + \sum m_{in}(h + V^2/2 + gl + e_e + e_m)_{in} - \sum m_{out}(h + V^2/2 + gl + e_e + e_m)_{out} \ . \tag{1.3 b}$$

This is then the mathematical representation of the simple statement that the net energy flow into the open system will increase its stored energy content by that amount. Let us consider as an example the amount of energy involved during the exhalation of a single breath of air from the lung. First we have to decide what should be the system. This is entirely arbitrary and the only significant criterion is to make the analysis as simple as possible. What reasonable alternatives do we have? For a closed system we could place the boundary around the air mass which is inside the body at the start of the exhalation period. During the exhalation process this boundary will expand into the surrounding atmosphere as the air is pushed out of the body. Now let us see if we can identify the various energy terms involved. Since no mass is crossing the chosen boundaries, Eq. 1.1 applies. If we consider the air mass first, we can safely assume that there is no heat transfer inside the body because the air is essentially in thermal equilibrium with the body, both being at the same temperature. However, there must be work involved in pushing the environmental air out of the way. If we assume that the internal air pressure and temperature remain approximately constant during exhalation then the work required to push out the air can be expressed as:

$$W = p_i \Delta \mathcal{V} = p_i M_e v_i \tag{1.4}$$

where p_i is internal pressure, Δ U is the volume exhaled, M_e is the mass of air which is expelled from the body, and v_i, is the specific volume per unit mass of the air at the internal conditions of the body.

So far the analysis went without much difficulty but we did have to make some assumptions (e.g., constant temperature and pressure). However, we are not finished yet because part of our system is outside the body, where conditions are not as simple. We can probably assume that the pressure is constant at the atmospheric level, p_0, which must be at least slightly below p_i to allow the air to be pushed out of the lung. There must be some heat transferred because the exhaled air is at a different temperature from the environment. As a result, the specific volume of the system as well as the internal energy will change during the process and it will change differently at different points. The exhaled air in close proximity of the environmental air, i.e., near the boundaries of our closed system, will change faster than the exhaled air near the center of the system. Thus, the complete energy equation has to be written in integral form as:

$$\int_S dQ = \int_{\mathcal{V}} dE + \int_S dW - p_i M_e v_i \ . \tag{1.5}$$

The heat transfer and work terms have to be integrated over the external surfaces which they cross, while the internal energy is integrated in the total volume. Obviously these integrals are not easy to evaluate. The heat transfer, the internal energy of the exhaled air, and the external work are all influenced by several factors. In addition, we may not even be interested in all of these anyway. Similar problems arise if we choose the entire body as the closed system and the solution may become more difficult because we have to deal with the energy content of the entire body and we still have to model the exhaled air.

Now let us consider an open system consisting of only the airways inside the body with the exhaled air crossing the boundary at the mouth and nose. Now Eq. 1.3 a applies. There is no heat transfer and the expression becomes:

$$u_i M_e = W_i + M_e h_i \ . \tag{1.6 a}$$

This can be rearranged as:

$$W_i = -M_e(h_i - u_i) = -M_e p_i v_i \tag{1.6 b}$$

which is almost the same expression as before in Eq. 1.4. However, Eq. 1.6 b represents the complete energy balance for the control volume. W_i is the work done on the air in the lung by the muscles, and is, therefore, negative; whereas Eq. 1.4 represents the work done by the exhaled air on the environment, and is, therefore, positive.

Similarly, care must be taken when selecting the control volume boundaries for heat transfer. Let us consider the energy transferred at the skin surface during sweat evaporation. First, we can locate our "boundary" right on the surface, below the sweat layer covering it. The energy transfer here consists of two parts: heat conduction across the tissue and the energy carried to the surface by liquid sweat exuded by the sweat glands. In terms of fluxes, i.e., energy flows per unit area, these quantities are:

$(q/A)_{cd,f}$ and $(m_{sweat}/A)\,h_f$.

If, however, we place the boundary just above the sweat layer, in the air, then the same quantities are: heat conduction across the air layer and the energy carried away by the vaporized sweat, i.e.,

$(q/A)_{cd,g}$ and $(m_{sweat}/A)\,h_g$.

Since $h_g \gg h_f$, hence $(q/A)_{cd,f} \gg (q/A)_{cd,g}$. Thus, the magnitudes to be calculated depend on the selection of the boundary.

The real processes occurring in the world present many difficulties to the establishment of exact magnitudes. First, we need "things" we can measure reliably and accurately, and, second, we need to establish appropriate relations among these "things", called *properties*, and the various energy quantities. *Intensive properties*, such as temperature, pressure, or density, are independent of the size of the system; whereas *extensive properties*, such as mass or stored energy, are proportional to the size. However, extensive properties can be changed to intensive ones by dividing by the volume. Thus, mass divided by the volume becomes the density.

The study of heat transfer involves primarily the evaluation of the energy balances in the system as expressed in Eqs. 1.1 for closed systems and 1.3 for open ones. Before we can use these expressions, however, we must first examine the various modes by which heat transfer occurs.

1.3 Modes of Heat Transfer

1.3.1 Introduction

We have already established that heat transfer is an energy transfer process at the boundary of a system, caused by a temperature difference between the environment and the system; and that the direction of the energy flow is always from the higher to the lower temperature level. Our next task is to establish the governing relations for heat transfer which will enable us to calculate the magnitudes. We should expect that these relations contain, in addition to temperatures, either temperature differences or gradients.

It is customary to consider three major types of heat transfer:

1. *Conduction* is the thermal energy transfer on the microscopic level from one molecule to another or by electrons. However, we are interested in its macroscopic manifestation, namely the relation between the energy flow and the temperature patterns.
2. *Convection* is the heat transfer at a boundary to a fluid which is in motion. Consequently, the energy is transferred in part by conduction and in part by the movement of the fluid. The two mechanisms can seldom be separated and they are treated most of the time as a combined phenomenon.
3. *Radiation* is the energy transferred between surfaces or bodies by electromagnetic waves through a transparent medium. All surfaces and bodies emit radiation dependent on their temperatures and other properties.

In the following sections we shall discuss the essential features of these various modes of heat transfer.

1.3.2 Conduction

For most heat transfer problems encountered, particularly in biological systems, the speed of internal energy propagation is very much faster than any other characteristic speeds associated with the thermal phenomena. Consequently, Fourier's Law applies, which states that the conductive heat transfer in a particular direction is proportional to the cross-sectional area of the flow and to the temperature gradient. In mathematical terms of heat transfer in the positive x direction of a Cartesian (x, y, z) coordinate system is

$$q_x = -A_x\left(k_{xx}\frac{\partial T}{\partial x} + k_{xy}\frac{\partial T}{\partial y} + k_{xz}\frac{\partial T}{\partial z}\right) . \tag{1.7}$$

The minus sign expresses the requirement of the second law that the direction of heat transfer is opposite to the temperature gradient. The proportionality constants, $k_{()}$, are components of the *thermal conductivity* expressed as a tensor property, i.e., it can have three components for each direction as written above. In most cases, however, only the three components in the principal directions exist, k_{xx}, k_{yy}, and k_{zz}, in which case the heat transfers in the three directions are essentially decoupled from each other, and each depends only on one temperature gradient. In addition, many materials can be considered isotropic in which the three components are the same and the thermal conductivity is a scalar constant.

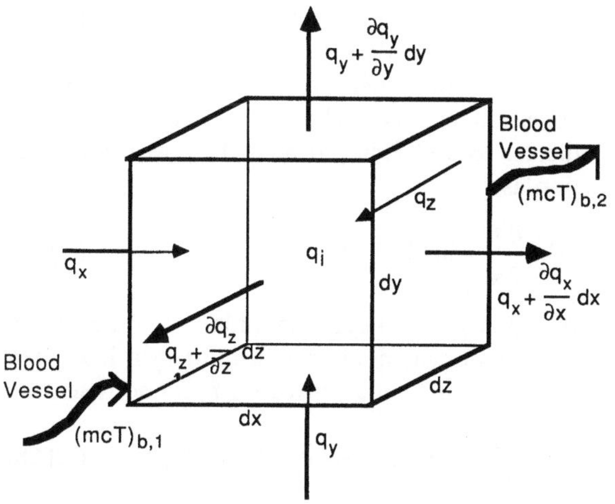

Fig. 1.1. Energy transfers in a Cartesian element

As stated previously, the working equation of heat transfer is the energy balance, i.e., the first law. In order to derive this relation for a solid body, let us consider a differential volume in Cartesian coordinates, dx dy dz, as shown in Fig. 1.1. For the sake of simplicity, we shall consider first conduction only in the x direction and an isotropic material. The following list contains the various energy terms.

At the left boundary, $x = x$:

$$q_x = -k(\partial T/\partial x)\,dy\,dz\;. \tag{1.8}$$

At the right boundary, $x = x + dx$:

$$\begin{aligned} q_{x+dx} &= q_x + \frac{\partial}{\partial x}(q_x)\,dx \\ &= \left[-k\frac{\partial T}{\partial x} + \frac{\partial}{\partial x}\left(-k\frac{\partial T}{\partial x}\right)dx\right]dy\,dz\;. \end{aligned} \tag{1.9}$$

The internal energy generation based on a volumetric rate, $q_i\,(\mathrm{W/m^3})$:

$$\bar{Q}_i = q_i\,dx\,dy\,dz\;. \tag{1.10}$$

The rate of increase of the internal energy, in terms of the specific heat at constant pressure, can be shown to be:

$$\bar{E}_{cv} = \left[\varrho c\frac{DT}{Dt} - T_{abs}\beta\frac{Dp}{Dt}\right]dx\,dy\,dz \tag{1.11}$$

where D represents the total derivative if flow is present. For example,

$$\frac{DT}{Dt} = \frac{\partial T}{\partial t} + \text{velocity terms}\;. \tag{1.12}$$

Because blood flow is treated separately, there are no velocities within the control volume, and only the first term exists in Eq. 1.12 with heat transfer in solid tissues. β is the volumetric expansion coefficient, $-(1/\varrho)(\partial\varrho/\partial T)_p = (1/v)(\partial v/\partial T)_p$. Now all these terms can be collected into the energy balance equation to yield, after dividing out the volume $dx\cdot dy\cdot dz$, in one dimension

$$\varrho c\frac{\partial T}{\partial t} = \frac{\partial}{\partial x}\left(k\frac{\partial T}{\partial x}\right) + q_i + T_{abs}\beta\frac{\partial p}{\partial t}\;. \tag{1.13}$$

If we assume that the conduction in any one of the three principal directions depends only on the temperature gradient in the same direction, then we can write the three-dimensional equation by inspection as

$$\begin{aligned} \varrho c\frac{\partial T}{\partial t} &= \frac{\partial}{\partial x}\left(k_x\frac{\partial T}{\partial x}\right) + \frac{\partial}{\partial y}\left(k_y\frac{\partial T}{\partial y}\right) \\ &\quad + \frac{\partial}{\partial z}\left(k_z\frac{\partial T}{\partial z}\right) + q_i + T_{abs}\beta\frac{\partial p}{\partial t} \end{aligned} \tag{1.14a}$$

where only single subscripts were needed for the conductivities. However, they can still vary with temperature, or with position, or with the local blood perfusion rate.

In general q_i contains several distinct energy generation terms. For biological applications one of them is the volumetric rate of metabolism, q_m. Another one can be a blood perfusion term, q_b, such as the one proposed by Pennes [58] and which is used in one form of the bioheat equation:

$$q_b = m_b c_b (T_a - T_v) \cong m_b c_b (T_a - T_t) \tag{1.15}$$

where m_b is the volumetric blood perfusion term, c_b is specific heat of blood at constant pressure and the temperature subscripts, a, v, t, refer to arterial, venous, and tissue, respectively.

Still another energy generation term could be the irreversible viscous energy dissipation. Its magnitude, however, depends on the various derivatives of the flow velocity and can be ignored in biological systems where the velocities are generally quite low. For similar reasons, the pressure derivative term, $T_{abs}\beta(\partial p/\partial t)$, can also be eliminated.

There can be artificially introduced energy generation in the tissue, such as that used in hyperthermia. The source can be, for example, electromagnetic radiation, microwave and radio frequency, or acoustic waves, particularly high-frequency ultrasound. To find the distribution of the energy deposition in these cases requires additional modeling of the interaction between the energy generating waves and the tissue (see Chap. 2 for details).

The circulatory system has various effects on the energy flows, depending on the size and arrangement of the blood vessels. A detailed discussion was given by Chen and Holmes [24]. They identified the following possible contributions to the energy equation:

1. An increase of the effective thermal conductivity, k_e. This is also the main component of the model developed by Weinbaum and Jiji, e.g. [69] for the subcutaneous muscle in which the conductivity increases with depth and with increasing blood perfusion as discussed later.
2. A scalar blood perfusion term of the Pennes type, Eq. 1.15.
3. A vectorial blood flow term depending on a definable direction of the blood perfusion

$$\varrho_b c_b \left(V_{b,x} \frac{\partial T}{\partial x} + V_{b,y} \frac{\partial T}{\partial y} + V_{b,z} \frac{\partial T}{\partial z} \right)$$

which would appear on the right-hand side of Eq. 1.14 with a negative sign. Although this type of term had been postulated before (e.g. Wulff [79]), its magnitude could not be established to date, and, consequently, has not yet been used in practice.

For the two-dimensional (r, z) cylindrical and the one-dimensional (r) spherical coordinate systems the following governing equations can be derived for heat transfer in a solid medium such as a tissue.

$$\varrho c \frac{\partial T}{\partial t} = \frac{1}{r} \frac{\partial}{\partial r} \left(k_r r \frac{\partial T}{\partial r} \right) + \frac{\partial}{\partial z} \left(k_z \frac{\partial T}{\partial z} \right) + q_i \quad (1.14b)$$

$$\varrho c \frac{\partial T}{\partial t} = \frac{1}{r^2} \frac{\partial}{\partial r} \left(k_r r^2 \frac{\partial T}{\partial r} \right) + q_i \ . \quad (1.14c)$$

The complete, three-dimensional equations are available in the literature (e.g., [12, 56]).

To solve Eq. 1.14, the appropriate number of boundary conditions must also be specified. It can be shown mathematically that the number of independent boundary conditions needed for *each variable* is equal to the order of the highest derivative with respect to that variable. Thus for the above equation two boundary conditions must be specifed with respect to each of the three spatial coordinates, x, y, and z; and one, usually an "initial condition" in terms of a temperature distribution, with respect to time.

There are four common types of boundary conditions used in heat transfer:

1. The temperature is specified on a boundary.
2. The heat flux is given which, through Fourier's law, specifies the normal first derivative of the temperature on a boundary.
3. A convective boundary condition is defined which equates the heat conduction to the surface of the body with the energy carried away by convection into the fluid flowing past the surface. With the use of the film coefficient, h_c, to be discussed in the section dealing with convection, this boundary condition can be written for a surface perpendicular to and facing toward the positive x direction as

$$-k_x \frac{\partial T}{\partial x} = h_c (T - T_\infty) \ . \quad (1.16a)$$

4. A radiative boundary condition is specified in either its exact, nonlinear form or in a linearized form similar to the convective film coefficient as

$$-k_x \frac{\partial T}{\partial x} = \sigma \varepsilon_r T_{abs}^4 - \alpha_r q_r \cong h_r (T - T_{r,env}) \ . \quad (1.16b)$$

Examples for the estimation of h_r are given later, in the section on radiation.

Let us now illustrate the methods of solution and the effects of the various terms in Eq. 1.14 by simple examples. For further information the reader should consult the comprehensive references on conduction by Ozisik [56] and by Carslaw and Jaeger [12].

Example 1.1: Steady State Conduction in One Rectangular Direction, x

Let us model a section of the outer layers of the human body as a slab shown in Fig. 1.2 with thickness, L, constant thermal conductivity, k; and no internal heat generation, blood flow, or useful work. Let us take for boundary conditions that the inner surface temperature, at x = 0, is equal to the body's core temperature, T_c; and that the skin surface temperature, at x = L, is T_s, both of which are constant. We wish to find the steady state temperature distribution and the heat transferred at the skin surface.

For this case Eq. 1.14a becomes

$$k \frac{d^2T}{dx^2} = 0 \ . \quad (1.17)$$

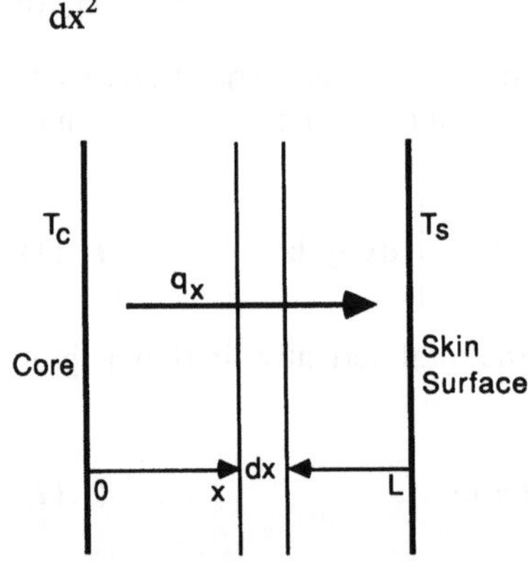

Fig. 1.2. Model for the one-dimensional conduction Examples 1.1., 1.4, 1.5, and 1.6 in Cartesian coordinates

This equation can be integrated twice directly to obtain

$$T = C_1 x + C_2 \tag{1.18a}$$

where the constants of integration, C_1 and C_2, have to be found such that the two boundary conditions are satisfied. The final result is a linear temperature distribution.

$$T = T_c - \frac{x}{L}(T_c - T_s) \ . \tag{1.18b}$$

The heat transfer rate per unit area, or heat flux, is

$$\frac{q_x}{A_x} = -k\frac{dT}{dx} = k\frac{T_c - T_s}{L} \tag{1.19a}$$

or

$$q_x = \frac{kA_x}{L}(T_c - T_s) \ . \tag{1.19b}$$

Since q_x can be considered as a flow caused by a potential difference, $(T_c - T_s)$, the group, kA_x/L, can be defined as a *conductance* and its inverse, L/kA_x, as a *resistance*. The general expressions are

Flow = conductance x potential (1.20a)

Flow x resistance = potential . (1.20b)

For typical values of $k = 0.4$ W/m-C, $(T_c - T_s) = 4$ C, and $L = 4$ cm $= 0.04$ m,

$q_x/A_x = 40 \ \mathrm{W/m^2}$.

For a person of 80 kg weight and 1.8 m height the skin area is approximately 2 m^2. With such size area the total heat transfer becomes $q_x = 80$ W and the conductance 20 W/C.

Example 1.2: Steady State Conduction in One Cylindrical Direction, r

In this model we assume that the human body is a cylinder as shown in Fig. 1.3, with the same outer surface area as in the previous example (2 m^2); with a height, i.e., length of cylinder, $H = 1.8$ m; and with the same thickness of the outer layer ($L = r_2 - r_1 = 0.04$ m). Further, we will also assume that the energy flows only in the r direction, radially symmetrically. The energy balance has to be defined in terms of this new coordinate system. Considering a cylinder of differential thickness, dr, we can write Fourier's law as

$$q_r = -k_r(2\pi H r)\frac{dT}{dr} \ . \tag{1.21}$$

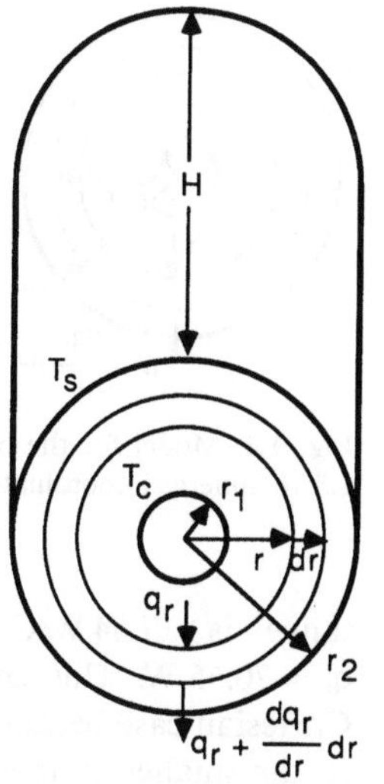

Fig. 1.3. Model for the one-dimensional conduction Example 1.2 in cylindrical coordinates

Thus the energy balance becomes

$$-\frac{dq_r}{dr} = k2\pi H\frac{d}{dr}\left(r\frac{dT}{dr}\right) = 0 \tag{1.22}$$

where the subscript r has been dropped from the conductivity. Integrating once we obtain

$$r\frac{dT}{dr} = C_1 \quad \text{or} \quad \frac{dT}{dr} = \frac{C_1}{r} \ . \tag{1.23}$$

Integrating again yields

$$T = C_1 \ln r + C_2 \ .$$

Solving for C_1 and C_2 to satisfy the two boundary conditions, at $r = r_1 : T = T_c$ and at $r = r_2 : T = T_s$, results in

$$T = T_c - \frac{\ln r/r_1}{\ln r_2/r_1}(T_c - T_s) \tag{1.24}$$

and

$$q_r = \frac{k2\pi H}{\ln r_2/r_1}(T_c - T_s) \ . \tag{1.25}$$

Thus for the cylindrical case the conductance is $k2\pi H/\ln(r_2/r_1)$. It should be noted that this solution precludes the existence of an adiabatic boundary because if $dT/dr = 0$, then $C_1 = 0$ for any finite value of r. This solution also requires an infinite heat flux at the centerline, $r = 0$, and is therefore not usable for a solid cylinder.

For the numerical values specified the outside, cylindrical surface area is $2\pi r_2 \ 1.8 = 2$, which yields $r_2 = 0.1768$ m and $r_1 = 0.1368$ m. Thus the conduc-

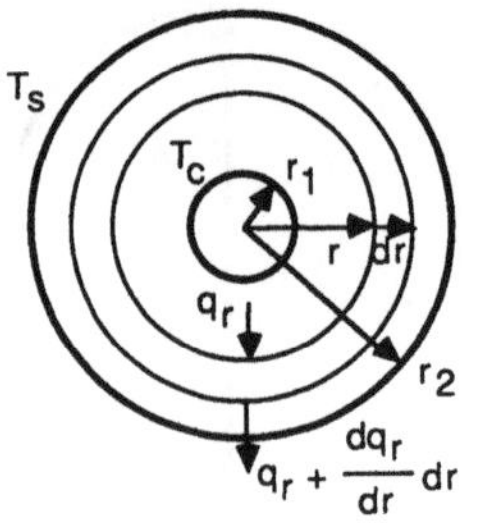

Fig. 1.4. Model for the one-dimensional conduction Example 1.3 in spherical coordinates

tance is 17.64 W/C and the total energy flow $q_r = 70.55$ W. This energy flow is less than for the Cartesian case because of the lower conductance due to the smaller average area of energy flow.

Example 1.3: Steady State Conduction in One Spherical Direction, r

Perhaps we are allowed to model a really fat person as a sphere shown in Fig. 1.4, with the same outer surface area ($2\ m^2$) and the same thickness of the outer layer ($L = 0.04$ m) as before. Again let us assume radial symmetry of heat flow and constant radial thermal conductivity. Proceeding as before, we can write Fourier's law for a spherical shell of thickness dr

$$q_r = -k(4\pi r^2)\frac{dT}{dr} . \tag{1.26}$$

The resulting energy balance is

$$-\frac{dq_r}{dr}dr = k4\pi\frac{d}{dr}\left(r^2\frac{dT}{dr}\right) = 0 . \tag{1.27}$$

Integrating once gives

$$r^2\frac{dT}{dr} = C_1 \quad \text{or} \quad \frac{dT}{dr} = \frac{C_1}{r^2} . \tag{1.28}$$

Integrating again yields

$$T = -\frac{C_1}{r} + C_2 .$$

After solving for the two constants to satisfy the two boundary conditions (T_c and T_s), we obtain the temperature distribution.

$$\begin{aligned} T &= T_c - \left[\frac{1-r_1/r}{1-r_1/r_2}\right](T_c - T_s) \\ &= T_c - \left[\frac{1/r_1 - 1/r}{1/r_1 - 1/r_2}\right](T_c - T_s) \end{aligned} \tag{1.29}$$

and

$$q_r = \frac{k4\pi r_1}{1-r_1/r_2}(T_c - T_s) = \frac{k4\pi}{1/r_1 - 1/r_2}(T_c - T_s) . \tag{1.30}$$

The conductance for this case is $k4\pi r_1/(1-r_1/r_2)$. For the given values $4\pi r_2^2 = 2$, which yields $r_2 = 0.3989$ m and $r_1 = 0.3589$ m. The resulting conductance is 17.99 W/C and the total radial energy flow is $q_r = 71.96$ W. These values are comparable to those in the cylindrical case. The comments regarding heat fluxes also apply here.

Example 1.4: Steady State Conduction in One Rectangular Direction, x, with Internal, Metabolic Heat Generation

The model is the same as shown in Fig. 1.2, but the governing equation becomes

$$\frac{d^2T}{dx^2} = -\frac{q_m}{k} . \tag{1.31}$$

Assuming constant q_m and integrating twice we obtain a parabolic temperature distribution.

$$T = -\frac{q_m}{2k}x^2 + C_1 x + C_2 .$$

Solving for the two constants to satisfy the boundary conditions yields

$$T = T_c - \frac{x}{L}(T_c - T_s) + \frac{q_m L^2}{2k}\left[\left(\frac{x}{L}\right) - \left(\frac{x}{L}\right)^2\right] . \tag{1.32}$$

Comparing this equation with Eq. 1.18 reveals that the effect of internal energy generation is given by the last term, which increases the temperatures in a parabolic fashion with the maximum increase of $q_m L^2/8k$ occurring at midpoint, $x/L = 1/2$. Intuitively we can anticipate that any energy addition will tend to drive the temperatures up.

The heat transfer now is a function of position with the maximum occurring usually at the skin surface.

$$q_x = \frac{kA_x}{L}\left[1 - \frac{q_m L^2}{2k(T_c - T_s)}\left(1 - 2\frac{x}{L}\right)\right](T_c - T_s) . \tag{1.33}$$

Obviously the conductance here is variable although we may define it in terms of the heat transmitted at the skin surface, $x = L$.

You, the reader, may derive corresponding expressions for the one-dimensional cylindrical and spherical cases. We shall look in the next example at another energy generation mode which can be used as a model for the effect of blood perfusion.

Example 1.5: Steady State Conduction in One Rectangular Direction, x, with Temperature-Dependent Energy Addition or Removal

We already discussed the problem of modeling the energy supplied by the blood flow which is at a different temperature from the tissue. Let us consider the model of Eq. 1.15 applied to a differential element, $A_x dx$, in Fig. 1.2. For this example let us assume that the blood is supplied at some fixed arterial temperature, T_a, but that it quickly equilibrates with the tissue because of the good heat exchange in the small arteries and capillaries. Thus the blood exit temperature will be taken as the tissue temperature, T. Then the energy balance for the differential element becomes

$$-\frac{dq_x}{dx}dx = m_b c_b (T-T_a) A_x dx \quad (1.34)$$

$$\frac{d}{dx}\left(kA_x\frac{dT}{dx}\right)dx - m_b c_b (T-T_a) A_x dx = 0$$

$$\frac{d^2T'}{dx^2} - \frac{m_b c_b}{k}T' = 0$$

$$\frac{d^2T'}{dx^2} - \gamma^2 T' = 0 \quad (1.35)$$

where $T' \equiv T-T_a$ and $\gamma^2 \equiv m_b c_b/k$. The boundary conditions are at $x = 0$: $T' = T_c-T_a$, and at $x = L$: $T' = T_s-T_a$.
The solution to such a second-order, ordinary differential equation is

$$T' = C_1 e^{\gamma x} + C_2 e^{-\gamma x} \ . \quad (1.36)$$

Substituting the boundary conditions and solving for the constants yields

$$T' = T-T_a = [T_s-T_a-(T_c-T_a)e^{-\gamma L}]\frac{\sinh(\gamma x)}{\sinh(\gamma L)} + (T_c-T_a)e^{-\gamma x} \ . \quad (1.37)$$

If $T_a = T_c$, a frequently made assumption, then

$$T = T_c-(T_c-T_s)\frac{\sinh(\gamma x)}{\sinh(\gamma L)} \ . \quad (1.38)$$

Figure 1.5 shows a comparison of the temperature distributions for Examples 1.1 and 1.4 with $q_m L^2/2k = T_c-T_s$ so that the maximum temperature occurs at $x = 0$, and this one with $\gamma = 2/L$ and $T_a = T_c$. The differences in the patterns are clear: according to this last model most of the energy is added near the skin surface where the tissue temperature is the lowest and, consequently, (T_a-T) is the greatest.

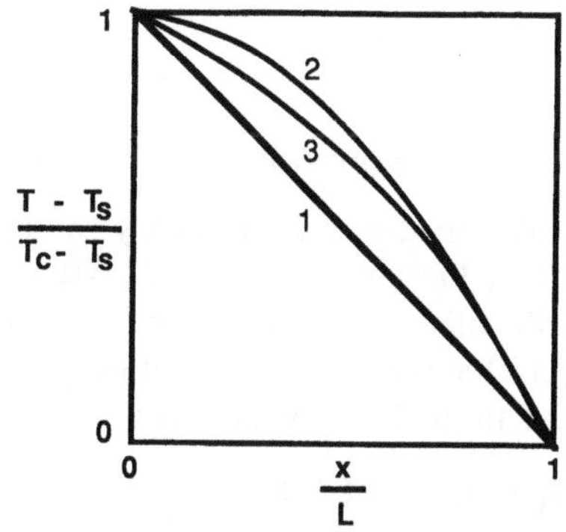

Fig. 1.5. Comparison of the temperature distributions in Examples 1.1 (*line 1*), 1.4 (*line 2*), and 1.5 (*line 3*)

Thus its temperatures deviate less from the no-source model near the core than the temperatures with constant energy input, but near the skin the two heated temperature patterns become almost identical, and the total energy transferred at the skin surface is virtually the same for both heated cases.
That heat transfer is again a function of position

$$q_x = -kA_x\gamma[T_s-T_a-(T_c-T_a)e^{-\gamma L}]\frac{\cosh(\gamma x)}{\sinh(\gamma L)} + kA_x\gamma(T_c-T_a)e^{-\gamma x} \ . \quad (1.39)$$

For Examples 1.1, 1.4, and 1.5 the dimensionless heat transfers, $q_x L/[kA_x(T_c-T_s)]$, are 1.0, 2.0, and 2.075 at the skin surface.

Example 1.6: Transient Conduction in One Rectangular Direction, x

Let us assume that the body, as modeled in Fig. 1.2, $0 \le x \le L$, has an initial temperature distribution as given by Eq. 1.18. At time $t = 0$ the skin temperature is changed suddenly to T_f. If we ignore any energy generation, then Eq. 1.14a becomes

$$k\frac{\partial^2 T}{\partial x^2} = \varrho c \frac{\partial T}{\partial t} \quad \text{or} \quad \frac{\partial^2 T}{\partial x^2} = \frac{1}{\alpha}\cdot\frac{\partial T}{\partial t} \quad (1.40)$$

where $\alpha \equiv k/\varrho c$ is the *thermal diffusivity* and will be assumed to be constant.
One method of solution for such an equation is the separation of variables. Let us assume that the solution consists of a steady state and a transient part. Further let us assume that the transient part is a product of two functions, each of which is dependent on only one of the two variables. Thus,

$$T = T_0(x) + X(x)\cdot\tau(t) \ . \quad (1.41)$$

The boundary conditions are for $T_0(x)$:

at $x = 0$ $T = T_c$ and at $x = L$ $T = T_f$

and for $X(x)\cdot\tau(t)$:

at $x=0$ and $x=L$ $X({}^{0}_{L})\cdot\tau(t)=0$ and

at $t=0$ $X(x)\cdot\tau(0)=T_c-\frac{x}{L}(T_c-T_s)-T_0(x)$.

Solutions for such boundary conditions are available in the literature (c.f. [12, pp. 102–104]). However, we will still derive the solution to illustrate the widely applicable method of separation of variables. First, we can immediately write down $T_0(x)$ from Example 1.1:

$$T_0=T_c-\frac{x}{L}(T_c-T_f)\ . \tag{1.42}$$

Thus the initial condition for the transient part becomes

at $t=0$ $X(x)\cdot\tau(0)=\frac{x}{L}(T_s-T_f)$.

Substitute $X\cdot\tau$ into the governing equation (1.40) and rearrange to obtain

$$\frac{1}{X}\frac{d^2X}{dx^2}=\frac{1}{\alpha\tau}\frac{d\tau}{dt}=-\gamma^2 \text{ a constant}\ . \tag{1.43}$$

Here it was recognized that a function of x can equal a function of t only if they are both constant. The negative sign for γ^2 was chosen in anticipation of the final form of the solution. The solution of the time-dependent part is as follows:

$$\frac{d\tau}{dt}+\alpha\gamma^2\tau=0\ . \tag{1.44}$$

This ordinary, first-order differential equation has the solution

$$\tau=C_1e^{-\alpha\gamma^2t}\ . \tag{1.45}$$

The x-dependent part is more involved.

$$\frac{d^2X}{dx^2}+\gamma^2X=0\ . \tag{1.46}$$

This ordinary, second-order differential equation has the solution

$$X=C_2\cos(\gamma x)+C_3\sin(\gamma x)\ . \tag{1.47}$$

Since the functions are periodic, we can expect an infinite number of values for γ, each of which can satisfy Eq. 1.46. However, the values will have to be chosen in such a way that all boundary conditions can be satisfied. A typical expression for one of these solutions is

$$X_n\tau_n=[A_n\cos(\gamma_nx)+B_n\sin(\gamma_nx)]e^{-\alpha\gamma_n^2t} \tag{1.48}$$

where A_n and B_n are constants to be determined. The complete solution is the sum of all these specific solutions which satisfy the boundary conditions. Consider first the initial condition. At $t=0$ the temperature is given by the boundary condition given previously and also by the sum of solutions given by Eq. 1.48. Thus

$$\frac{x}{L}(T_s-T_f)=\sum_{n=0}^{\infty}[A_n\cos(\gamma_nx)+B_n\sin(\gamma_nx)]\ . \tag{1.49}$$

Now we can apply the Fourier sine and cosine series expansion formulae to solve for the constants. Since the right-hand side of the equation must have periods corresponding to the size of the temperature field, L, let

$$\gamma_n=n\pi/L\ . \tag{1.50}$$

Now the expressions for the constants become

$$A_0=\frac{1}{2L}\int_{-L}^{L}\frac{x}{L}(T_s-T_f)\,dx=0 \tag{1.51 a}$$

$$A_n=\frac{1}{L}\int_{-L}^{L}\frac{x}{L}(T_s-T_f)\cos(n\pi x/L)\,dx=0 \tag{1.51 b}$$

$$\begin{aligned}B_n&=\frac{1}{L}\int_{-L}^{L}\frac{x}{L}(T_s-T_f)\sin(n\pi x/L)\,dx\\&=\frac{2(T_s-T_f)}{(n\pi)^2}[-n\pi\cos(n\pi)]\\&=-\frac{2(T_s-T_f)}{n\pi}(-1)^n\quad n\geq1\ .\end{aligned} \tag{1.51 c}$$

The complete solution then becomes

$$T=T_c-\frac{x}{L}(T_c-T_f)-\frac{2(T_s-T_f)}{\pi}\times\sum_{n=1}^{\infty}\frac{(-1)^n}{n}e^{-\alpha n^2\pi^2t/L^2}\sin\left(\frac{n\pi x}{L}\right)\ . \tag{1.52}$$

Figure 1.6 shows typical profiles for the transient last term in dimensionless form, i.e., divided by (T_s-T_f). The dimensionless time used was $=\alpha\pi^2t/L^2$. The

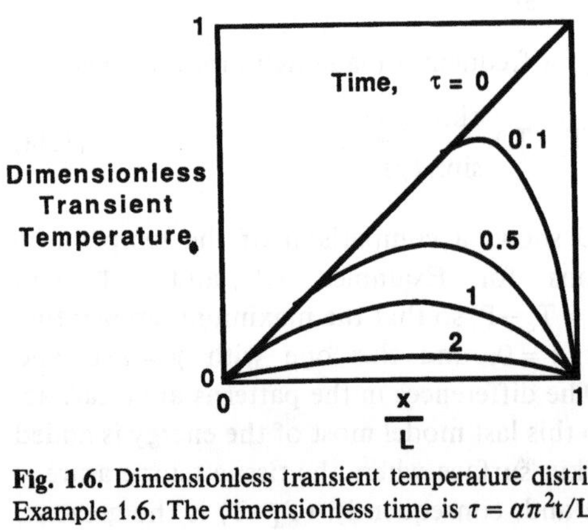

Fig. 1.6. Dimensionless transient temperature distributions for Example 1.6. The dimensionless time is $\tau=\alpha\pi^2t/L^2$

curves indicate that it takes about one unit of time for the effect of the temperature change at the skin to reach the core. In about 2.3 time units the temperature distribution reaches to within 10% of its final state. If we assume typcial values of $k = 0.4$ W/m-C, $\varrho = 10^3$ kg/m^3, and $c = 4 \times 10^3$ J/kg-C, then the unit dimensionless time corresponds to a time constant of $t = L^2/\alpha\pi^2 = 1620$ s or 27 min ($\alpha = 10^{-7}$ m^2/s). The 2.3 time units correspond to about 1 h, but it will take about twice as long to reach within 1% of the final state.

The heat transfer, of course, is a function of both position and time.

$$q_x = \frac{kA_x}{L}\left[1 + 2\,\frac{T_s - T_f}{T_c - T_f}\sum_{n=1}^{\infty}(-1)^n e^{-\alpha n^2\pi^2 t/L^2} \times \cos\frac{n\pi x}{L}\right](T_c - T_f)\ . \tag{1.53}$$

1.3.3 Convection

Convection is a combination of conduction in a fluid and the energy transport due to the motion of the fluid particles in the direction of energy flow. Thus the process is complicated by the fluid mechanics of the system, which itself can be strongly dependent on the temperature distribution in the fluid. The most common convection problems involve heat transfer between a moving fluid and a solid boundary, such as between the blood and the blood vessels or the air and the body. In the latter case, however, the situation is even further complicated by the fact that air has to be considered as a two-component mixture of dry air and water vapor. "Sensible" heat is transferred between the body and the air; and additional energy, "latent" or "insensible" heat, is transferred by the evaporation of sweat from the skin into the air.

Let us consider first ordinary convection, or "sensible" heat transfer (so called because it is caused by the sensible temperature difference), between a fluid and a solid boundary as shown in Fig. 1.7. Very close to the boundary the fluid particles flow parallel to the surface in a laminar layer. In this layer the heat transfer normal to the surface, q_n, has to be by conduction only because there are no velocity components in this direction. Outside this layer, however, the fluid particles moving partially parallel to the heat flow will transport energy in addition to conduction. This additional energy transport tends to equalize the temperatures in the nonlaminar or turbulent region, and at some distance from the wall the temperatures

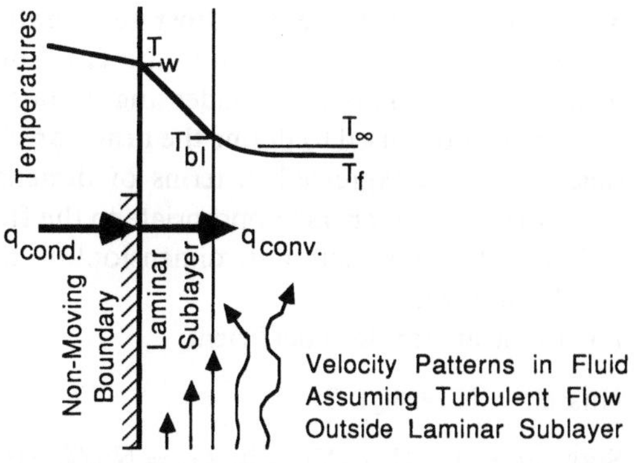

Fig. 1.7. Convective motion and heat transfer at a fluid boundary

may become constant at T_f. If the thickness of the laminar layer can be determined and if the temperatures at the wall, T_w, as well as at some known distance in the laminar layer, such as the outer edge (T_{b1}), can be established, then the "convective" heat transfer can be calculated as a conduction problem. Unfortunately, in most cases neither the thickness of the laminar layer nor its temperature distribution can be established and we are forced into empirical and semi-empirical methods of estimation. These methods are based primarily on the concept of the Newtonian heat transfer coefficient, h_c, defined as the ratio of heat flux to some temperature difference:

$$h_c \equiv (q_n/A_n)/\Delta T\ . \tag{1.54}$$

The temperature difference needs explanation because, although the wall temperature is usually well defined, the fluid temperature can be chosen with some arbitrariness. Two fluid temperatures are used most frequently. The bulk average, or mixing-cup, temperature, T_∞ is the overall average fluid temperature which, when multiplied by the mean specific heat and the total flow parallel to the wall, gives the magnitude of the enthalpy flow in the same direction. The obvious advantage of this temperature is that the heat transfer can be directly related to the energy flows due to mass movement in the energy balance equations. Thus, the bulk average temperature is particularly useful when heat transfer to flows in well-defined enclosures, such as blood vessels, is considered. The other temperature used for ΔT is the fluid temperature at some, usually long distance from the wall, T_f. This temperature is used primarily when the extent of the fluid is very large compared with the solid body; and, therefore, the energy transferred from the body has a negligible effect on this temperature. A typical example is the air temperature in a large room or outdoors when heat transfer to a human body is considered. Other temperatures are also used in special cases, such as the saturation temperature with boiling and condensing liquids.

The correlations used to define the heat transfer coefficient are best expressed in terms of dimensionless quantities, or "numbers," appropriate to the flow conditions. The most common dimensionless numbers are the following.

For the heat transfer coefficient:

$$\text{Nusselt} = \text{Nu} \equiv h_c L/k$$

$$\text{Stanton} = \text{St} \equiv h_c/\varrho V c = h_c/G c = \text{Nu}/\text{Re}\cdot\text{Pr}$$

where L is some characteristic length such as pipe diameter, k is the conductivity of the fluid, and $G = \varrho V$ is the mass flux (flow per unit cross-sectional area). Re and Pr are defined below. Note that the Stanton number can be used only in forced convection with an externally controlled flow velocity, V.

For the properties of the fluid:

$$\text{Prandtl} = \text{Pr} \equiv \mu c/k$$

where μ is the viscosity of the fluid in kg/m-s. For air at normal conditions $\text{Pr} \simeq 0.7$, for water $\text{Pr} \simeq 5$. Although blood is not a so-called Newtonian fluid with a constant viscosity, for overall estimates Pr = 25 may be used. On the low side, for liquid metals such as mercury $\text{Pr} < 0.05$.

For forced convection flow in a tube with hydraulic diameter D:

$$\text{Reynolds} = \text{Re} \equiv \varrho V D/\mu = G D/\mu = V D/\nu$$

$$\text{Graetz} = \text{Gz} \equiv \text{Re}\cdot\text{Pr}\cdot D/L$$

where L is the length of the tube, $\nu \equiv \mu/\varrho$ in m²/s, the kinematic viscosity, and the hydraulic diameter is defined as

$$D \equiv 4\,\frac{\text{cross-sectional area of flow}}{\text{wetted perimeter}}\;. \tag{1.55}$$

For a circular tube D is the actual diameter.

The completely laminar range for steady flow in tubes can be found when Re < 2000. With higher Reynold's numbers turbulence develops and increases in intensity with incresing Reynold's number. A typical correlation for laminar forced convection in nonmetallic liquids was first suggested over 50 years ago by Sieder and Tate [63].

$$\text{Nu}_D = 1.8\,\text{Gz}^{0.33}(\mu_f/\mu_w)^{0.14} \quad \text{for} \quad \text{Re} < 2100 \quad \text{and} \quad \text{Pr} > 0.7 \tag{1.56}$$

where the Nusselt number is based on D and it is an average value for the entire length of the tube. There is a lower limiting value for very long tubes ($\text{Gz} \to 0$).

With constant wall temperature:

$$\text{Nu}_{D,\min} = 3.66 \quad \text{for } T_w \text{ constant}\;. \tag{1.57}$$

For blood, Chato [17] suggested a value of 4.0 as discussed in the section on heat transfer to blood flow.

With constant heat flux:

$$\text{Nu}_{D,\min} = 4.36 \quad \text{for } q_n/A_n \text{ constant}\;. \tag{1.58}$$

For heat transfer to cylindrical bodies in a cross stream Whitaker [72] proposed the following correlation.

$$\text{Nu}_D = (0.4\,\text{Re}^{0.5} + 0.06\,\text{Re}^{0.67})\,\text{Pr}^{0.4}(\mu_w/\mu_f)^{0.25} \tag{1.59}$$

for $1 < \text{Re} < 10^5$ and $0.67 < \text{Pr} < 300$.

Specifically for the human body the following correlation is recommended in normal air environments by Winslow et al. [73] and Colin and Houdas [28].

$$h_c = 12.1\,V^{0.5} \quad \text{for} \quad V < 2.6\ \text{m/s} \tag{1.60}$$

where h_c is in W/m²-C.

In natural or free convection flows generated by temperature-dependent density variation the following parameters are in common use:

$$\text{Grashof} = \text{Gr} \equiv \varrho^2 g\beta\Delta T L^3/\mu^2 = g\beta\Delta T L^3/\nu^2$$

$$\text{Rayleigh} = \text{Ra} \equiv \text{Gr}\cdot\text{Pr} = c\varrho^2 g\beta\Delta T L^3/\mu k = g\beta\Delta T L^3/\alpha\nu$$

where g is the gravitational acceleration and β is the volumetric expansion coefficient, $(1/v)\,(\partial v/\partial T)_p$.

An accepted correlation for natural convection to a vertical cylinder or plate with height L was given by Gryzagoridis [36].

$$\text{Nu}_L = 0.555\,\text{Ra}^{1/4} \quad \text{for} \quad 10 < \text{Ra} < 10^9 \tag{1.61}$$

where the Nusselt number is based on L, as the subscript indicates. For higher Rayleigh numbers the flow is turbulent and the suggested correlation is

$$\text{Nu}_L = 0.1\,\text{Ra}^{1/3} \quad \text{for} \quad \text{Ra} > 10^9\;. \tag{1.62}$$

For air at normal conditions Eqs. 1.61 and 1.62 can be reduced to

$$h_c = 1.42(\Delta T/L)^{1/4} \quad \text{for} \quad 10^{-7} < \Delta T L^3 < 10\ \text{K-m}^3 \tag{1.61a}$$

$$h_c = 1.18(\Delta T)^{1/3} \quad \text{for} \quad \Delta T L^3 > 10\ \text{K-m}^3\;. \tag{1.62a}$$

Note that in turbulent flow the heat transfer coefficient is independent of the vertical size.

For spheres in free convection the recommended relation was developed by Yuge [80].

$$\text{Nu}_D = 2 + 0.45\,\text{Ra}_D^{1/4}\;. \tag{1.63}$$

For horizontal cylinders in air at normal conditions with free convection the average coefficient can be estimated from McAdams [50].

$$h_c = 1.32(\Delta T/D)^{1/4} \quad \text{for} \quad 10^{-5} < \Delta T D^3 < 10 \tag{1.64}$$

$$h_c = 1.24 \Delta T^{1/3} \quad \text{for} \quad 10 < \Delta T D^3 < 10^4 \ . \tag{1.65}$$

Specifically for the human body in free convection the recommended relation is from Nielsen and Pedersen [55]

$$h_c = 2.38 \Delta T^{1/4} \ . \tag{1.66}$$

Between Eqs. 1.60 and 1.66 for the human body, the larger of the two values obtained should be used.

In all of the above correlations as well as in the following text the standard SI units (kg, m, s, J, W, etc.) are to be used. Because of the dominant role of sweat evaporation in the cooling of the human body we must briefly discuss the relevant mass transfer concepts and correlations. Fortunately the diffusion of energy or mass from a surface is similar in many respects. Whereas energy is transferred in proportion to a temperature difference (or gradient), mass is transferred in proportion to a concentration difference (or gradient). For ideal gas mixtures, such as air and water vapor, the concentration of a component is directly proportional to its partial pressure. Thus water vapor will migrate from the skin surface into the surrounding air if the partial pressure of the water vapor at the skin, taken as the saturated water pressure at the temperature of the skin, is greater than the partial pressure of the water vapor in the air. The evaporation rate can be expressed as

$$m_{evap} = a A_{evap} (p_{w,skin} - p_{w,air}) \tag{1.67}$$

where "a" is constant. The energy required to evaporate this amount of sweat can be written as an evaporative heat term

$$q_{evap} = m_{evap} h_{fg} = h_{evap} A_{evap} (p_{w,skin} - p_{w,air}) \tag{1.68}$$

where h_{fg} is the enthalpy of evaporation and h_{evap} is an energy transfer coefficient, similar to a heat transfer coefficient, in units of W/m^2-unit pressure. In standard SI units the pressure is N/m^2(Pa), which yields W/N as the dimension for the coefficient. In practice, however, gas pressures are most commonly measured in mmHg, which makes the dimension W/m^2-mmHg.

It has been proposed theoretically by Woodcock et al. [77], and shown experimentally by Brebner et al. [10], that for normal air environments with moderate wind speeds a simple relation exists between the convective heat transfer coefficient, h_c, and the evaporative energy transfer coefficient, h_{evap}

$$h_{evap}(\text{in mmHg}) = 2 h_c(\text{in } ^\circ\text{C}) \ . \tag{1.69}$$

Direct measurements of the maximum evaporative capacity from human beings yielded for Clifford et al. [27]

$$\frac{q_{evap}}{A} = 14.6 \, V_{air}^{0.63} (p_{w,skin} - p_{w,air}) \tag{1.70a}$$

where q_{evap}/A is in W/m^2 and the pressures in mmHg. In order to convert to more consistent units, we could use the atm $\simeq 10^5$ N/m^2 = 761 mmHg

$$\frac{q_{evap}}{A} = 1.11 \times 10^4 \, V_{air}^{0.63} (p_{w,skin} - p_{w,air}) \tag{1.70b}$$

where the pressures are in atmospheres. However, since most direct pressure measuring instruments use either mercury or water, the practical advantage of this conversion is questionable.

A very convenient approximation to make is to convert the vapor pressure at the skin surface, $p_{w,skin}$, to a linear temperature scale using the saturated vapor pressure data. In the temperature range of 30 °–40 °C the following saturated pressure-temperature relation is accurate to within 2.2%.

$$p(\text{mmHg}) = -39.4 + 2.364 \, T(C) \quad \text{for} \quad 30 \leq T \leq 40 \ . \tag{1.71}$$

Thus Eq. 1.70a can be written in terms of the skin temperature, T_s, as

$$\frac{q_{evap}}{A} = 34.5 \, V_{air}^{0.63} \, [T_s - (16.67 + 0.423 \, p_{w,air})] \tag{1.70c}$$

where $p_{w,air}$ is in mmHg (to be determined from psychrometric measurements, such as dry-bulb and wet-bulb temperatures) and the two terms in parentheses represent a constant pseudo-temperature of the fluid. Thus, the terms in front of the left bracket can be considered as a convective film coefficient due to vaporization, h_{evap}. It is important to note that the pseudo-fluid temperature is different from the actual fluid temperature to be used with the convective heat transfer at the skin surface.

The convective heat transfer in many cases provides the boundary conditions to another, e.g., conduction, problem. Thus, instead of specifying a surface temperature or heat flux for a body, we can specify the energy balance between the heat conducted internally normal to the surface and the heat transferred externally. Referring to Fig. 1.7 and Eq. 1.16

$$-k_n \left(\frac{\partial T}{\partial n}\right) = h_f(T_w - T_f) = h_\infty (T_w - T_\infty) \tag{1.72}$$

where the subscripts for the heat transfer coefficients were used to emphasize the dependence on the selection of the reference fluid temperatures. Note also that the signs must agree with the direction of heat flow (second law again!).

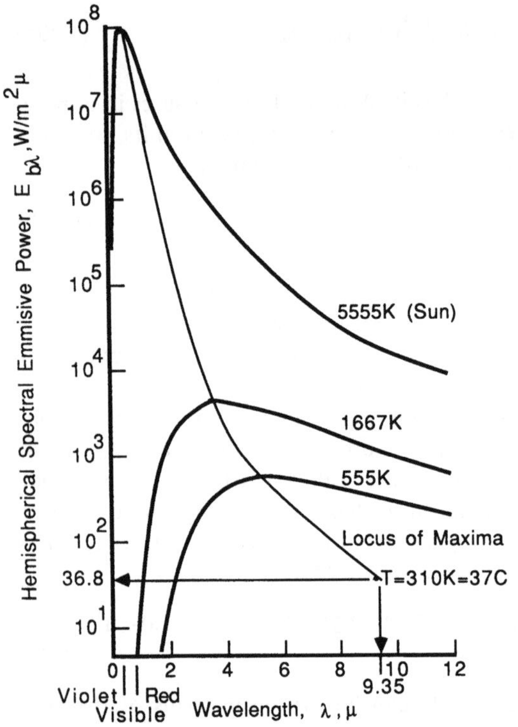

Fig. 1.8. Blackbody emissive power as a function of wavelength. Area under each curve = σT^4

1.3.4 Radiation

Every body emits electromagnetic radiation in proportion to the fourth power of its absolute surface temperature. The maximum amount of radiation that can be emitted from an *ideal black body* is

$$q_r = \sigma A T^4 = 5.676 \times 10^{-8} A T^4 = 5.676\, A (T/100)^4 \, W \tag{1.73}$$

where σ is the Stefan-Boltzmann constant in W/m^2-K^4 and T is in absolute units, K. The total black body radiation, E_b, is an integral of all spectral (or monochromatic) black body emissive powers $E_{b\lambda}$ taken over all wavelengths, i.e.,

$$E_b = \int_0^\infty E_{b\lambda} d\lambda = \sigma T^4 \tag{1.74}$$

$E_{b\lambda}$ in W/m^2-μ is a function of the wavelength, λ, according to Planck's law

$$E_{b\lambda} = 3.742 \times 10^8 / [\lambda^5 (e^{1.439 \times 10^4/\lambda T} - 1)] \tag{1.75}$$

where λ is in microns, μ. This function is plotted for various temperatures in Fig. 1.8. The value and location of the maximum for each curve is a function of temperature according to Wien's displacement law

$$\lambda_{max} T = 2897.6\, \mu K \ . \tag{1.76}$$

The highest curve in Fig. 1.8 corresponds to the sun's output, with the maximum occurring in the visible range. The implication toward the evolution of the eye is obvious. The dry, normal human skin acts very nearly as an ideal black surface. At 37 °C = 310 K the wavelength of maximum radiation is about 9.3 μ, which falls into the infrared region. The corresponding energy flux is $\sigma T^4 = 524.2\, W/m^2$. Thus our sample person with a surface area of 2 m^2 radiates about 1 kW energy. This is a rather large amount of energy, but, fortunately, the body also receives radiation from the environment. Consequently, the net energy lost by the body is not only substantially less but can even become an energy gain.

Very few surfaces are truly black bodies. In order to characterize real surfaces the concepts of *emittance*, or *emissivity*, and *absorptance* or *absorptivity* are used. The monochromatic hemispherical emittance, ε_λ is the fraction of the black body radiation, $E_{b\lambda}$, that is actually emitted at a given temperature and wavelength, i.e.,

$$\varepsilon_\lambda \equiv E_\lambda / E_{b\lambda} \ . \tag{1.77}$$

The monochromatic hemispherical absorptance α_λ is defined as the fraction of the total radiation incident on the surface which is absorbed. Kirchoff's radiation law states that at thermal equilibrium $\alpha_\lambda = \varepsilon_\lambda$. The total hemispherical emittance, ε_r, can be obtained by integration of all the emitted energies over all wavelengths

$$\varepsilon_r = \frac{\int_0^\infty \varepsilon_\lambda E_{b\lambda} d\lambda}{E_b} \ . \tag{1.78}$$

A similar expression can be written for the total hemispherical absorptance, α, with ε's replaced by α's and E's replaced by the incident radiation. Since the characteristics of the incident and emitted radiation can be different, ε and α are equal only if:

1. No net heat transfer occurs.
2. ε_λ and α_λ are uniform for all wavelengths. Such surfaces are called *gray bodies.*

Figure 1.9 shows the comparison of the emissive characteristics of a black, a gray, and a "real" body. For most practical applications the gray body concept is quite acceptable with a single emittance for the surface. For example, in thermographic applications the dry skin is usually assumed to be a gray body with $\varepsilon_r = 0.98-0.99$. If the body is covered with water, such as with profuse sweating, then the radiation properties of water will dominate the energy transfer and it will be quite different from the case of dry skin. Another problem arises from the possibility that the surface may emit radiation at different rates in different directions. Figure 1.10 shows a typical emitted radiations pattern. If ε_r is independent of the direction, then the intensity of emitted radiation depends only on the projected area in the directions of radiation, i.e., it varies as the cosine of the angle between the direction of radiation and the normal to the surface. This pattern is called Lambert's cosine law. This relation is usually assumed to hold for the dry skin, but it may not be true for other "animal" teguments.

Figure 1.10 also illustrates other radiative properties of a surface, related to the incident radiation. If the surface does not absorb all incident radiation, then some of it will be reflected and/or transmitted. The fraction of the total incident energy which is absorbed is the total absorptivity, α_r, the fraction which is reflected is the total reflectance, ϱ_r, and the fraction which transmitted is the total transmittance, τ_r. The first law of thermodynamics, or conservation of energy, requires that

$$\alpha_r + \varrho_r + \tau_r = 1 . \qquad (1.79)$$

Most materials are opaque with $\tau_r = 0$, However, many studies on the blood vessels near the skin or in various body membranes depend on the transmittance of light to at least some depth.

With these basic concepts in mind, we can now consider the net heat exchanged between two surfaces at different temperatures. The net radiant heat transferred from a body at temperature T_1 to another at temperature T_2 is

$$q_{1-2} = A_1 F_{1-2} \sigma (T_1^4 - T_2^4) . \qquad (1.80)$$

F_{1-2} is a factor involving the emittances of both surfaces and the geometry, i.e., how much of each other can the two surfaces "see." A_1 is generally the smaller of the two surfaces. For example, for two concentric cylinders or spheres:

$$F_{1-2} = \left[\frac{1}{\varepsilon_{r1}} + \frac{r_1(1-\varepsilon_{r2})}{r_2 \varepsilon_{r2}}\right]^{-1} . \qquad (1.81)$$

For two infinitely large parallel plates:

$$F_{1-2} = \left[\frac{1}{\varepsilon_{r1}} + \frac{1}{\varepsilon_{r2}} - 1\right]^{-1} . \qquad (1.82)$$

For a small gray or black body with radiating area A_1 inside a large enclosure, such as the human body in a room:

$$F_{1-2} = \varepsilon_{r1} . \qquad (1.83)$$

For this last case the energy loss from the body becomes

$$q_{1-2} = A_1 \varepsilon_1 \sigma (T_1^4 - T_2^4) . \qquad (1.84)$$

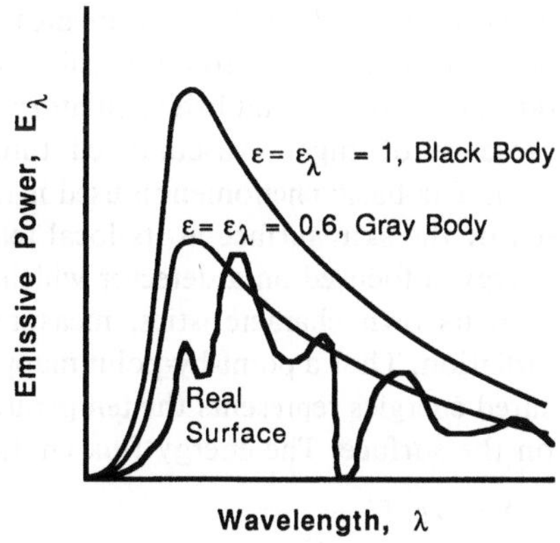

Fig. 1.9. Emissive powers of various surfaces

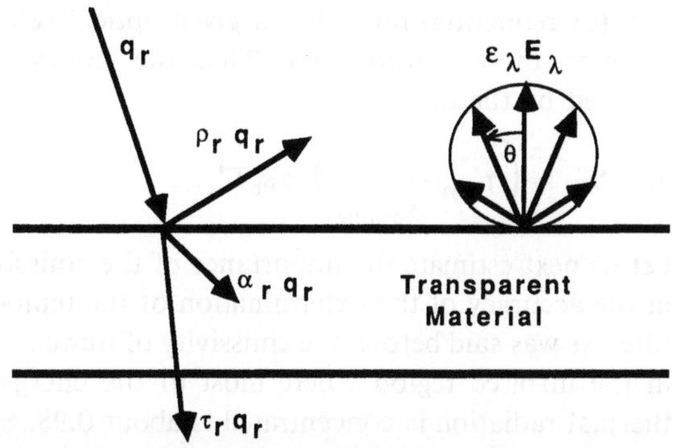

Fig. 1.10. Incident and emitted radiation patterns

This nonlinear expression can be converted into a linear one with a radiation heat transfer coefficient, h_r, if T_1 and T_2 are not too different

$$q_{12} = A_1 \varepsilon_1 \sigma (T_1^3 + T_1^2 T_2 + T_1 T_2^2 + T_2^3)(T_1 - T_2)$$
$$= 4 \varepsilon_1 \sigma T_m^3 A_1 (T_1 - T_2) = h_r A_1 (T_1 - T_2) \qquad (1.85)$$

where $h_r = 4 \varepsilon_1 \sigma T_m^3$.

In this last form the radiation heat transfer can be treated exactly as the convective heat transfer. However, care must be exercised in the combination of the two types of heat transfer because although the relevant body temperature, T_1, is the same for both, the environmental temperature, T_2, could quite likely be different: for convection it is the air temperature near the body; whereas for radiation it is the mean radiant temperature of the environment consisting of walls and windows, etc. For a radiating surface the following general expression can be written for the net energy leaving

$$q/A = \sigma \varepsilon_r T^4 - \alpha_r q_r$$

where q_r is the incident radiation energy flux.

Thermography is used to establish temperature patterns on the body surface for medical-biological purposes. Besides basic physiological studies, this method can be used to establish circulatory disorders or the presence of highly vascularized tumors under the skin. The basic phenomenon used is the energy emitted by the skin surface at its local temperature. This energy is focused on a detector which, in accordance with its own characteristics, measures this incident radiation. Thus a point-by-point mapping of the measured energies represents the temperature distribution on the surface. The energy flux emitted is

$$q/A = \sigma \varepsilon_r T^4 \ . \qquad (1.86)$$

The actual energy flux reaching the detector is modified by the transmittance, $\tau_{r,sys}$, of the elements of the optical systems as well as the area magnification (or reduction) ratio. For a given optical setting, however, these are constant. Thus the energy flux received by the detector is

$$q_{rec}/A_{det} = \left(\tau_{r,sys} \frac{A}{A_{picture}} \right) \sigma \varepsilon_r T^4 \ . \qquad (1.87)$$

Let us next estimate the importance of the emissivity in the accuracy of the determination of the temperature. As was said before, the emissivity of human skin in the infrared region where most of the energy of thermal radiation is concentrated is about 0.98. Suppose the instrument calibrated for this value reads a skin temperature of 306 K (33 °C); then the variable part of the above equation is

$$\varepsilon_r T^4 = 0.98\,(306)^4 = 85.923 \times 10^8\ K^4 \ . \qquad (1.88)$$

Now let us suppose that the emissivity of the surface is actually 0.97. Since the energy measured by the thermograph is, of course, the same, the actual temperature can be estimated from

$$0.97\ T^4 = 85.923 \times 10^8\ K^4 \qquad (1.89)$$

which yields a temperature of T = 306.786 K. That means that at the typical operating region of the thermograph there is a 0.79 K (or °C) error per 1% deviation from the assumed emissivity. Fortunately past experience indicates that the emissivity of the skin surface in the infrared region is quite constant for each individual; even birthmarks and blemishes do not seem to affect it. However, if thermograms are to be used for accurate determination of temperature differences of less than about 0.1 °C, a more rigorous examination of the skin emissivity will be required. If only temperature differences are to be measured then the above error will be approximately constant for all points and the differential readings will be quite accurate.

For more detailed discussion of thermography the reader should consult the appropriate literature (e.g., [46]).

1.3.5 Two-Phase (Solid/Liquid) Boundaries

1.3.5.1 Introduction

The inclusion of a phase change boundary into a biological heat transfer problem, such as the prediction of the growth of an ice ball around a cryosurgical probe, creates considerable difficulties. We are only going to introduce the basic concepts with some very simple examples. For more detailed discussion of the subject the reader should consult the literature (e.g., [29, 51, 56, 66]).

A pure substance freezes at a constant temperature while giving off the latent heat of freezing, h_{if}. For water this is a rather substantial amount of energy, 333.4 kJ/kg at 0 °C. Biological substances are, of course, not pure thermodynamically and their freezing occurs over a temperature range. Whether or not a single, constant freezing temperature can be used in a particular model depends on the properties of the tissue and the character of the problem itself. For example, a single temperature assumption is probably quite accurate to predict the macroscopic growth of the ice front around a cryosurgical probe. On the other hand, the study of the freezing of cells and their substructures requires a more detailed analysis of the process. We are going to deal only with the constant temperature case where freezing occurs within the solid tissue and, consequently, there are no convective effects in the unfrozen phase.

1.3.5.2 Steady State Problems

Examples 1.7: Steady State Conduction in One Direction, x or r, with a Two-Phase Boundary Inside the Body

A large, cold surface is applied to the skin, lowering its temperature to T_s, below the freezing level. Find the depth of the steady state frozen phase.

The problem is similar to the three geometries of Examples 1.1, 1.2, and 1.3, but with two layers. The simplest approach to the solution is to use the concept of two thermal resistances in series, one for each phase or domain. Then, the working equations for the Cartesian case become (see Eq. 1.19)

$$\left(\frac{q}{A}\right)_x = \frac{T_c - T_s}{L_1/k_1 + L_2/k_2} \qquad (1.90a)$$

$$= \frac{T_c - T_0}{L_1/k_1} \tag{1.90b}$$

$$= \frac{T_0 - T_s}{L_2/k_2} \tag{1.90c}$$

$$L = L_1 + L_2 \tag{1.91}$$

where the subscript 0 refers to the interface between the two domains. For a given L there are only three unknowns, L_1, L_2, and $(q/A)_x$; therefore, only two of the first three equations can be used. The solution is

$$L_1 = \frac{L k_1 (T_c - T_0)}{k_1 (T_c - T_0) + k_2 (T_0 - T_s)} \tag{1.92a}$$

$$L_2 = \frac{L k_2 (T_0 - T_s)}{k_1 (T_c - T_0) + k_2 (T_0 - T_s)} \tag{1.92b}$$

$$\left(\frac{q}{A}\right)_x = \frac{k_1 (T_c - T_0) + k_2 (T_0 - T_s)}{L} . \tag{1.93}$$

For typical values of $k_1 = 0.4$ W/m-C, $k_2 = 1.2$ W/m-C, $L = 0.04$ m, $T_c = 37\,°C$, $T_0 = 0\,°C$, and $T_s = -10\,°C$ the frozen depth and heat transfer rates are:

$L_2 = 0.018 =$ m (18 mm) and $(q/A)_x = 670$ W/m^2.

The same type of analysis applied to a one-dimensional cylindrical problem yields the following working equations (see Eq. 1.25).

$$q = \frac{2\pi H (T_c - T_s)}{[\ln (r_0/r_c)/k_1] + [\ln (r_s/r_0)/k_2]} \tag{1.94a}$$

$$= \frac{2\pi H (T_c - T_0)}{[\ln (r_0/r_c)/k_1]} \tag{1.94b}$$

$$= \frac{2\pi H (T_0 - T_s)}{[\ln (r_s/r_0)/k_2]} \tag{1.94c}$$

$$\frac{r_s}{r_c} = \frac{r_s}{r_0} \cdot \frac{r_0}{r_c} \quad \text{or} \quad \ln (r_s/r_c) = \ln (r_s/r_0) + \ln (r_0/r_c) \tag{1.95}$$

The results are:

$$\ln (r_0/r_c) = \frac{\ln (r_s/r_c) k_1 (T_c - T_0)}{k_1 (T_c - T_0) + k_2 (T_0 - T_s)} \tag{1.96a}$$

$$\ln (r_s/r_0) = \frac{\ln (r_s/r_c) k_2 (T_0 - T_s)}{k_1 (T_c - T_0) + k_2 (T_0 - T_s)} \tag{1.96b}$$

$$q = 2\pi H \frac{k_1 (T_c - T_0) + k_2 (T_0 - T_s)}{\ln (r_s/r_c)} \tag{1.97}$$

With the data of example 1.2:

$r_s - r_0 = 0.019$ m (19 mm), and $q/A = 591$ W/m^2.

For the spherical case the working equations become as follows (see Eq. 1.30)

$$q = \frac{4\pi (T_c - T_s)}{[1/r_c - 1/r_0]/k_1 + [1/r_0 - 1/r_s]/k_2} \tag{1.98a}$$

$$= \frac{4\pi k_1 (T_c - T_0)}{1/r_c - 1/r_0} \tag{1.98b}$$

$$= \frac{4\pi k_2 (T_0 - T_s)}{1/r_0 - 1/r_s} \tag{1.98c}$$

$$1/r_c - 1/r_s = (1/r_c - 1/r_0) + (1/r_0 - 1/r_s) . \tag{1.99}$$

The results are:

$$1/r_c - 1/r_0 = \frac{(1/r_c - 1/r_s) k_1 (T_c - T_0)}{k_1 (T_c - T_0) + k_2 (T_0 - T_s)} \tag{1.100a}$$

$$1/r_0 - 1/r_s = \frac{(1/r_c - 1/r_s) k_2 (T_0 - T_s)}{k_1 (T_c - T_0) + k_2 (T_0 - T_s)} \tag{1.100b}$$

$$q = 4\pi \frac{k_1 (T_c - T_0) + k_2 (T_0 - T_s)}{1/r_c - 1/r_s} . \tag{1.101}$$

With the data of example 1.3:

$r_s - r_0 = 0.019$ m (19 mm) and $q/A = 603$ W/m^2.

The depths of the frozen layer are virtually the same for all three geometries but the heat fluxes are less in the curved systems than in the Cartesian one.

Now let us estimate the required surface temperature for a spherical cryoprobe with a radius of $r_w = 2$ mm to obtain a frozen region with a radius of $r_0 = 10$ mm. To simplify the problem, assume that the tissue around the cryoprobe can be considered an infinite medium because there are no boundaries close enough to have any thermal influence. Apply Eq. 1.98 to both the frozen and unfrozen regions

$$|q| = \frac{4\pi k_2 (T_0 - T_w)}{1/r_w - 1/r_0} = \frac{4\pi k_1 (T_t - T_0)}{1/r_0} . \tag{1.102}$$

Solving for T_w gives

$$T_w = T_0 - (k_1/k_2)(r_0/r_w - 1)(T_t - T_0) . \tag{1.103}$$

With the data given above $T_w = -49.3\,°C$.

1.3.5.3 Transient Problems

The transient problems where the freezing or melting interfaces move are considerably more difficult to model, particularly because the initial conditions are hard to define. If, for example, a cold cryoprobe suddenly contacts the tissue, one should not assume that the temperature of the tissue surface will instantaneously drop to the level of the cryoprobe because

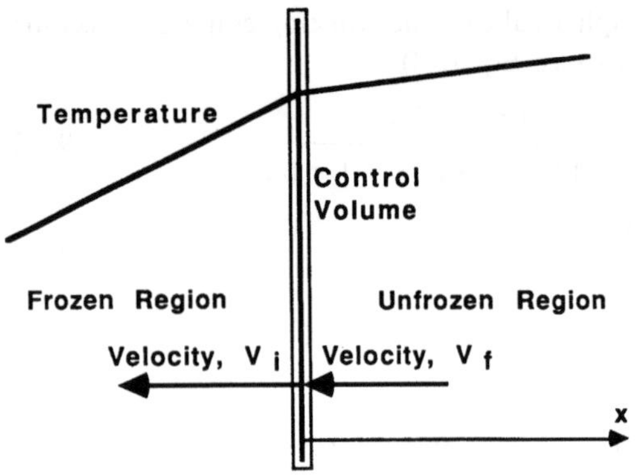

Fig. 1.11. Control volume of a freezing interface

of the phase change occurring at an intermediate temperature level. It is probably better to assume that initially the surface temperature drops to the freezing level and apply the energy balances to the problem. To understand the effect of the phase change, let us examine the energy balance of a plane ice front propagating in the positive x direction with a velocity V, as shown in Fig. 1.11. The analysis is a little easier if we consider a control volume which moves with the interface. Then the mass balance requires that

$$\varrho_i V_i = \varrho_f V_f = G \tag{1.104}$$

where both velocities are in the negative direction. Although in many cases the density difference between the two phases is neglected, we will not do so here. The energy balance of the interface becomes

$$k_1 \frac{\partial T_i}{\partial x} + \varrho_i V_i h_i = k_f \frac{\partial T_f}{\partial x} + \varrho_f V_f h_f \quad \text{or} \tag{1.105a}$$

$$k_i \frac{\partial T_i}{\partial x} = k_f \frac{\partial T_f}{\partial x} + G h_{if} \tag{1.105b}$$

where h_i and h_f are the enthalpies of the frozen and unfrozen materials, respectively, and $h_{if} = h_f - h_i$. The above expression has to be converted into a moving boundary condition in the stationary coordinate system by expressing the velocity, V_i, as the velocity of the moving boundary, dx_i/dt

$$k_i \left[\frac{\partial T_i}{\partial x}\right]_{x=x_i} = k_f \left[\frac{\partial T_f}{\partial x}\right]_{x=x_i} + \varrho_i h_{if} \frac{dx_i}{dt} \,. \tag{1.105c}$$

Unfortunately, this moving boundary condition makes the solution of the simultaneous partial differential equations, which model the frozen and unfrozen phases, very difficult, particularly in the cylindrical and spherical coordinates which correspond to the configurations of many cryoprobes. Approximate solutions, using the bioheat equation with the Pennes [58] blood perfusion term (see Sect. 1.4), that allow the estimation of the growth of the frozen region around various probe configurations, were published by Cooper and Trezek [29] and discussed by Trezek [66]. Solutions to general freezing or melting problems are given in Carslaw and Jaeger [12] and Ozisik [56].

A recent practical development has been the direct, on-line monitoring of the freezing interface, for example, during cryosurgery of liver cancer, by the use of noninvasive ultrasound [34]. This method eliminates the need for invasive temperature measurements.

1.3.6 Concluding Remarks

There exists an enormous amount of literature on heat transfer in general and even on heat transfer in biological systems. This section only introduced the basic concepts and provided some simple corrrelations which are specifically applicable to medical or biological applications. Other applications are given elsewhere in this volume. Obviously, a lot is left unsaid but we hope that the contents provide an adequate basis of understanding to the reader to be able to read the current literature with competence.

1.4 Heat Transfer to Blood Vessels

1.4.1 Introduction

The most unusual and difficult basic problem of estimating heat transfer in living biological systems is the modeling of the effect of blood circulation. The thermal interactions between a blood vessel and the surrounding tissue depend on a number of parameters, which include the geometry of the blood vessel, the blood flow rate through it, the properties of the blood and the surrounding tissue, and even the presence of another blood vessel within the thermally influenced volume around the blood vessel considered. As it will be discussed in some detail below, Chen and Homes [24] and Chato [17] have shown for individual blood vessels that the capillaries are essentially in thermal equilibrium with the surrounding tissue, the smaller arteries and veins have significant heat transfer with the surrounding tissue, but the larger blood vessels experience relatively little heat transfer. In a series of articles Weinbaum et al. [69–71], Jiji et al. [42], and Song et al. [64] developed a new, three-layer model for the heat transfer in the muscle-skin complex. This model is based on anatomical and thermal studies, which indicated that in the deep muscle tissue the "thermally significant" arteries and veins always run parallel and close to each other, such that most of the heat is transferred between these paired vessels with relatively little energy exchange with the surrounding tissue. In such a model heat exchange between parallel vessels plays the dominant role.

To lay the proper foundation for the various heat transfer models in living tissue, in the following sections we will study heat transfer between a single vessel and its surrounding tissue and between two parallel vessels.

1.4.2 Heat Transfer from Blood Flowing in a Vessel

This problem was analyzed in its simplest form by Chato [17] and the following sections are based primarily on this work. The convective heat transfer between flowing blood and the vessel wall was derived theoretically with a non-Newtonian model by Victor and Shaw [68], who assumed that the shear stress-shear rate relation of blood follows Casson's rule:

$$\sqrt{\tau_s} = \sqrt{\tau_y} + \sqrt{\mu(\partial V/\partial y)} \tag{1.106}$$

where τ_s is shear stress, τ_y is yield stress, μ is constant viscosity, V is axial velocity, and y is the direction normal to the vessel wall. Based on their literature survey, they assumed the following properties for blood:

$\mathrm{Pr} = 25$

$\mu = 3.2\times10^{-3}$ kg/m-s , or N-s/m$_2$, or g/mm-s

$\varrho_b = 1.06\times10^3$ kg/m^3 = 1.06 g/cc

$c_b = 3.9$ kJ/kg-C

$k_b = 0.5$ W/m-C .

Their steady flow solution for the variation of the mean Nusselt number, based on the diameter, $\mathrm{Nu_m}$, with Graetz number, $\mathrm{Gz} = \mathrm{Re}\cdot\mathrm{Pr}\cdot D/L = 8.333\cdot V\cdot D^2/L$ in mm-s units, at constant wall temperature can be approximated by:

$$\mathrm{Nu_m} = 4 + 0.155\exp(1.58\log\mathrm{Gz}) \quad \text{for} \quad \mathrm{Gz} < 10^3 \tag{1.107}$$

where the log is to the base 10. For $\mathrm{Gz} < 1.5$, i.e., for very long tubes with thermally fully developed flows, $\mathrm{Nu_m}$ is within 5% of its minimum value of 4, which is a little higher than the theoretical value of 3.66 for a Newtonian fluid (constant viscosity and no yield stress) with constant wall temperature. Since the Nusselt number for constant wall heat flux is much higher, we can use Eq. 1.107 as a conservative estimate

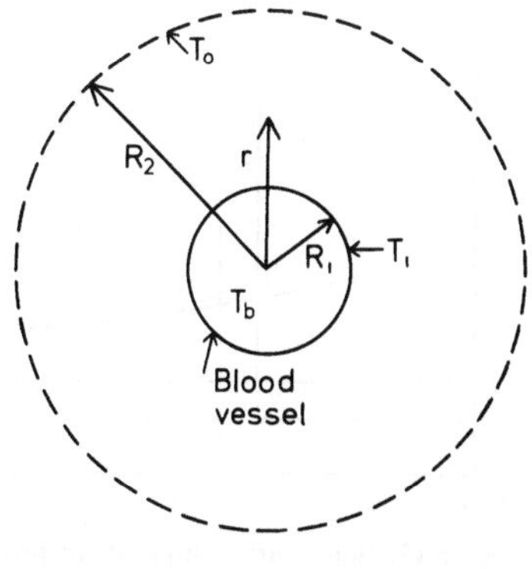

Fig. 1.12. Idealized geometry of heat transfer around a blood vessel. [17]

for convective heat transfer. To continue with the analysis, we must make two assumptions. First, we shall ignore the effects of pulsation which, generally, tend to increase heat transfer. Second, we shall assume the validity of Eq. 1.107 for all blood vessels, even though the flow patterns are quite different in the smallest vessels from those assumed in the derivation of the equation.

The two most significant questions that can be asked about heat transfer from blood flowing in a vessel are:

1. At what distance from the entrance will the blood reach tissue temperature?
2. What is the blood temperature at any given length of the blood vessel?

Let us use a very simple, but still good, model to answer these questions. Consider the heat transfer in the tissue around the blood vessel as shown in Fig. 1.12. Assume that at some radius, R_2, the tissue is held at a constant temperature, T_0, by some unspecified, physiological processes occurring in the body. Then the radial temperature distribution becomes:

$$\frac{T-T_0}{T_b-T_0} = \frac{\ln(R_2/r)}{k_t/(h_b R_1)+\ln(R_2/R_1)}$$

$$\text{for } R_1 \le r \le R_2 \,. \tag{1.108}$$

The heat transfer can be shown to be

$$q_1 = \frac{2\pi k_t(T_b-T_0)}{k_t/(h_b R_1)+\ln(R_2/R_1)} \tag{1.109a}$$

$$= h_e 2\pi R_1(T_b-T_0) \tag{1.109b}$$

where h_e is an equivalent and h_b is the local heat transfer coefficient for the blood-stream. The use of the equivalent heat transfer simplifies the solution of the differential equation, as shown below. Combining Eqs. 1.109a and 1.109b and non-dimensionalizing the

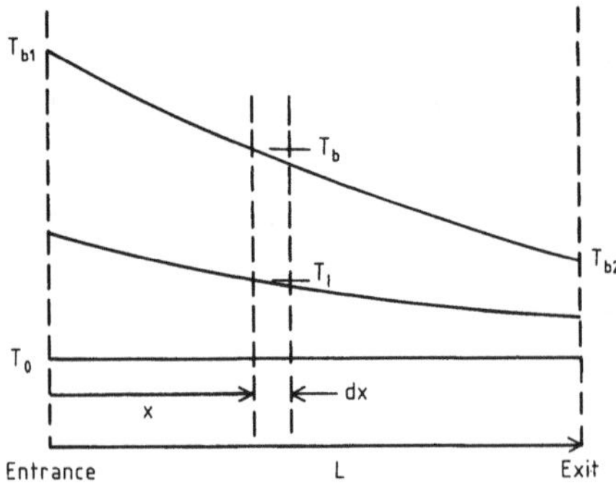

Fig. 1.13. Schematic temperature profiles along a single blood vessel corresponding to Fig. 1.12. [17]

results yields an expression for the equivalent Nusselt number, Nu_e, in terms of the local Nusselt number (based on $D = 2R_1$), Nu_D:

$$Nu_e = \frac{1}{(1/Nu_D)+(k_b/k_t)\ln\sqrt{(R_2/R_1}} \; . \qquad (1.110)$$

The results of Victor and Shah [68] for the local Nusselt number with constant wall temperature can be approximated within 3.5% by the following two correlations:

$$Nu_D = 4+0.486\ln^2(Gz_x/18) \quad \text{for } Gz_x>18 \qquad (1.111a)$$

$$Nu_D = 4 \quad \text{for } Gz_x \le 18 \qquad (1.111b)$$

where $Gz_x = Re \cdot Pr \cdot D/x$ and x is the axial distance from the entrance. It should be noted that from a practical standpoint $1<k_b/k_t<2.5$ and $R_2/R_1<10$. Therefore, the smallest value for Nu_e is about 0.32.

The governing differential equation for the axial temperature variation of the blood can be obtained by applying the energy balance to a differential length, dx, of the blood vessel as shown in Fig. 1.13. The result is

$$\frac{dT_b}{dx}+\frac{2h_e}{\varrho_b V c_b R_1}(T_b-T_0)=0 \qquad (1.112a)$$

or in dimensionless form

$$\frac{d\theta}{dX}+\lambda\theta=0 \qquad (1.112b)$$

where

$$\theta=\frac{T_b-T_0}{T_{b1}-T_0} \qquad (1.113)$$

$$X=\frac{x}{2R_1}=\frac{x}{D} \qquad (1.114)$$

$$\lambda=\frac{4Nu_e}{Re\,Pr}\ \text{(a function of X)} \; . \qquad (1.115)$$

The solution of the governing equation, Eq. 1.112b, depends on the functional dependence of λ on X. For example, in the limiting case when $R_2/R_1 = 1$, $Nu_e = Nu_D$ as given by Eqs. 1.111a, b and the result is

$$\frac{T_{b2}-T_0}{T_{b1}-T_0}=\exp\left\{-\frac{1.945}{Gz}\left[10.226+\ln^2\left(\frac{Gz}{18}\right)+2\ln\left(\frac{Gz}{18}\right)\right]\right\} \quad \text{for } Gz>18 \quad (1.116a)$$

$$\frac{T_{b2}-T_0}{T_{b1}-T_0}=0.8057\exp\left(-\frac{16}{Gz}\right) \quad \text{for } Gz\le 18 \qquad (1.116b)$$

where $Gz = Re \cdot Pr \cdot D/L$ is based on the length of the blood vessel.

For the case, $R_2/R_1 \gg 1$ and $Nu_e = 0.32$

$$\frac{T_{b2}-T_0}{T_{b1}-T_0}=\exp\left(-\frac{1.28}{Gz}\right) \; . \qquad (1.117)$$

Another way to calculate the exit temperature is to consider the average heat transfer coefficient as a constant to be evaluated using Eq. 1.107 if we assume that $Nu_e = Nu_m$, then

$$\frac{T_{b2}-T_0}{T_{b1}-T_0}=\exp\left[-\frac{16+0.62\exp(1.58\log Gz)}{Gz}\right] \qquad (1.118)$$

The heat transfer effectiveness can be defined as

$$\varepsilon=\frac{T_{b1}-T_{b2}}{T_{b1}-T_0}=1-\frac{T_{b2}-T_0}{T_{b1}-T_0} \; . \qquad (1.119)$$

Now we can answer the two questions stated before. To find the distance required for the blood to reach tissue temperature, let us assume that $\varepsilon = 0.95$ can be considered as sufficiently close to equilibrium. (We cannot choose $\varepsilon = 1$ because that requires infinite length.) The corresponding dimensionless length is 1/Gz.

From Eq. 1.116b: $1/Gz = 0.1737$ (1.120)

From Eq. 1.117: $1/Gz = 2.34$ (1.121)

From Eq. 1.118: $1/Gz = 0.1653$ (1.122)

Figure 1.14 shows ε as a function of Gz from Eqs. 1.116–1.118. Since the results of Eqs. 1.116 and 1.117 are virtually identical, the latter correlation is preferred because of its relative simplicity.

Table 1.1 was compiled by Chato [17] based on the remarkably painstaking work of Mall [49]. Even though this latter reference was published about 100 years ago, it has been used directly or indirectly by virtually everyone dealing with quantitative information on blood flow. Unfortunately, this led to some questionable values being quoted today. Probably the most significant data provided by Mall [48] was the

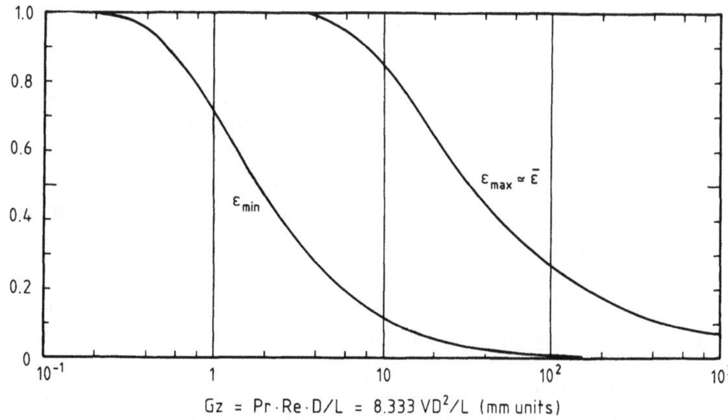

Fig. 1.14. Heat transfer effectiveness of a single blood vessel: ε_{min} from Eq. 1.117, ε_{max} from Eq. 1.116a, and $\bar{\varepsilon}$ from Eq. 1.118 [17]

length, diameter, and number of the various blood vessels in the mesentery. Others contributed additional data on blood velocities, based either on experimental work or only on theoretical calculations [49, 59]. For example, the most commonly quoted population numbers for each type of blood vessel in the human body are based on a publication by Green [35] in which he "calculated" these numbers based on the data of Mall [48]. On studying these reports, Müller-Schauenburg working with Chato [22] in 1986 discovered that these calculations simply involved the combination of similar-size blood vessels, particularly the capillaries, into fewer categories and then multiplying all the numbers resulting from Mall's data by 40. This procedure implies two very questionable assumptions:

1. The blood vessel distribution of the entire human body is essentially the same as that of the mesentery of the dog, and
2. the human body is about 40 times the size of the mesentery of a 13-kg dog.

Müller-Schauenburg and Chato estimated that the resulting population numbers must be low by at least an order of magnitude. The data given in Table 1.1, however, have the right orders of magnitude for our purposes.

When the heat transfer effectivenesses of the blood vessels are estimated from Fig. 1.14, they fall into three categories.

1. The largest vessels, the aorta and vena cava, with $Gz > 1000$ have very little heat exchange with the tissue ($\varepsilon \approx 0$). Since the human body contains much larger main blood vessels than the dog in Table 1.1, there are also more blood vessels that fall into this category.
2. The smallest blood vessels, the arterioles, capillaries, and venules, with $Gz < 0.4$, are essentially ideal heat exchangers with the blood leaving at tissue temperature. The maximum L/D for thermal equilibrium, based on Eq. 1.121, is only 1.2 in the arterioles.

Table 1.1. Estimated characteristics of blood vessels in a 13-kg dog based on Mall's [48] data. (After [17])

Blood vessel	Diameter (mm)	Length (mm)	Blood velocity (mm/s)	Reynolds number[a]	Graetz number[a]	Heat transfer effectivenesses		
						$\bar{\varepsilon}$	ε_{max}	ε_{min}
Aorta	10	400	500	1667	1042	0.08	0.06	0
Large arteries	3	200	130	130	48.7	0.40	0.41	0.026
Main arterial branches	1	100	80	27	6.75	0.93	0.92	0.17
Terminal branches	0.6	10	60	12	18	0.68	0.67	0.07
Arterioles	2×10^{-2}	2	3	2×10^{-2}	5×10^{-3}	1.0	1.0	1.0
Capillaries	8×10^{-3}	1	0.7	1.9×10^{-3}	3.8×10^{-4}	1.0	1.0	1.0
Venules	3×10^{-2}	2	0.7	7×10^{-3}	2.6×10^{-3}	1.0	1.0	1.0
Terminal veins	1.5	10	13	6.5	24.4	0.59	0.58	0.051
Main venous branches	2.4	100	15	12	7.2	0.92	0.91	0.16
Large veins	6	200	36	72	54	0.38	0.39	0.024
Vena cava	12.5	400	330	1375	1074	0.08	0.06	0

[a] Assuming the kinematic viscosity of blood $(\mu/\rho)_b = 3\ mm^2/s$ and Prandtl number $Pr = 25$

3. The intermediate blood vessels fall in a relatively narrow band of $6 < Gz < 54$ with maximum effectivenesses, based on Eqs. 1.116 or 1.119, between 0.39 and 0.92. Because of the metabolic heat generation in the tissue the actual effectivenesses are probably much closer to these values than the ones ($\varepsilon < 0.1$) based on Eq. 1.117. Thus, this group remains separate. The blood leaving these vessels can be at distinctly different temperature levels than the tissue itself, requiring some form of accounting in the energy balances.

Chen and Holmes [24] analyzed the heat transfer in the vasculature and also came to the conclusion that the primary heat transfer would occur in the small arteries and veins, not in the capillaries.

1.4.3 Heat Transfer Between Parallel Blood Vessels

The cross section of the configuration is shown in Fig. 1.15 with the y axis passing through the centers of

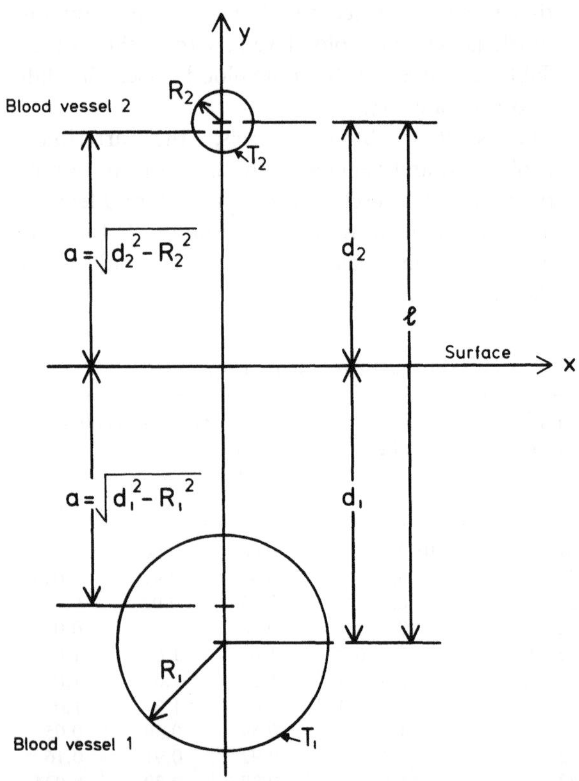

Fig. 1.15. Configuration for heat transfer between two blood vessels, or between blood vessel 1 and the skin surface at $y = 0$. a is distance of line source from $y = 0$. [17]

both circular blood vessels and the x axis ($y = 0$) located between them according to the relations

$$a = \sqrt{d_1^2 - R_1^2} = \sqrt{d_2^2 - R_2^2} \tag{1.123}$$

$$l = d_1 + d_2 \ . \tag{1.124}$$

A relatively simple solution can be obtained if we assume that the circles, i.e., the walls of the blood vessels, are at constant temperatures T_1 and T_2. The solution is based on the concept of a line source and a line sink of equal strength located at $x = 0$, $y = -a$, and $x = 0$, $y = a$, respectively. Among the several references available on this subject, the work of Awbery [2] is the most useful because it includes convective effects which will be used later for blood vessels near the skin surface.

The temperature at a point x, y in the tissue due to the source-sink pair is

$$T - T_0 = \frac{q_1}{4\pi k_t} \ln\left[\frac{x^2 + (y-a)^2}{x^2 + (y+a)^2}\right] \tag{1.125}$$

where T_0 is the uniform temperature of the reference surface $y = 0$, and q_1 is the source strength per unit length. The temperature difference between the two isothermal circles can be found by evaluating Eq. 1.125 at two convenient points, such as $x_1 = 0$, $y_1 = -d_1 + R_1$ and $x_2 = 0$, $y_2 = d_2 - R_2$. The final result is

$$T_1 - T_2 = \frac{q_1}{2\pi k_t} \ln\left[(b_1 + \sqrt{b_1^2 - 1})(b_2 + \sqrt{b_2^2 - 1})\right] \tag{1.126}$$

where $b = d/R$ or, in terms of the centerline distance, l:

$$b_i = \frac{(l/R_i)^2 - (R_k/R_i)^2 + 1}{2(l/R_i)} \tag{1.127}$$

where i, k are 1,2 or 2,1. Many references use $\cosh^{-1} b = \ln[b \pm (b^2 - 1)^{1/2}]$ which, however, is a multivalued function.

If the two blood vessels are the same size, $b = l/D$ and then

$$T_1 - T_2 = \frac{q_1}{\pi k_t} \ln[b + \sqrt{b^2 - 1}] \ . \tag{1.128}$$

Figure 1.16 shows this temperature difference in dimensionless form, i.e., the logarithmic term against b. It can be seen that for $b > 1.9$ the logarithmic term can be approximated by $\ln[2b]$ within 5%. This condition for b is satisfied in virtually all practical cases. Therefore, Eq. 1.126 can be replaced by

$$T_1 - T_2 \cong \frac{q_1}{2\pi k_t} \ln(4b_1 b_2) \quad \text{for} \quad b_1, b_2 > 1.9 \ . \tag{1.129}$$

Wissler [76] examined the effect of the film

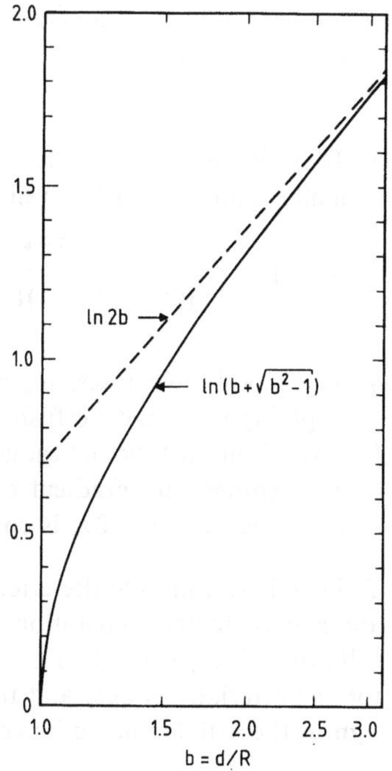

Fig. 1.16. The geometrical factor for heat transfer between two blood vessels as a function of depth-to-radius ratio. [17]

resistances in the two blood vessels and proposed the following working equations.

$$Nu_m = q_l \,|T_m - T_w| / \pi k = 4.364 \tag{1.130}$$

$$T_{a,m} - T_{v,m} = \frac{q_l}{2\pi k_t} \ln\left(2.5 \frac{l^2}{R_a R_v}\right) . \tag{1.131}$$

Here the temperatures represent cup-mixed values of the blood, whereas in Eq. 1.129 the temperatures are values at the vessel walls. The Nusselt number is based on an assumed parabolic, fully developed profile, with constant viscosity and linear temperature change in the axial direction; hence the slight discrepancy between Eqs. 1.130 and 1.107.

Next we shall develop relations for establishing the heat transfer between given lengths of two parallel blood vessels. Since parallel arteries or veins with blood flowing in the same direction would have almost identical temperatures, the important configuration consists of an artery and a parallel vein with the blood running in counterflow. This constitutes a counterflow heat exchanger and the solution can be given most conveniently in terms of the dimensionless effectiveness, ε, the number of transfer units, N, and the heat capacity rate ratio, C

$$\varepsilon = \frac{m_a(T_{a1} - T_{a2})}{m_{min}(T_{a1} - T_{v1})} = \frac{m_v(T_{v2} - T_{v1})}{m_{min}(T_{a1} - T_{v1})} \tag{1.132}$$

$$N = UA/(m_{min} c_b) \tag{1.133}$$

$$C = m_{min}/m_{max} . \tag{1.134}$$

Since the specific heat is the same for both fluids, it cancels out in the definitions for ε and C. The overall heat transfer capacity rate, UA, can be found from

$$\frac{1}{UA} = \frac{1}{h_a 2\pi R_a} + \frac{\ln B}{2\pi k_t} + \frac{1}{h_v 2\pi R_v}$$

$$= \frac{1}{2\pi k_b}\left(\frac{2}{Nu_a} + \frac{k_b}{k_t}\ln B + \frac{2}{Nu_v}\right) \tag{1.135}$$

where ln B is the logarithmic term in Eqs. 1.126, 1.128, or 1.129. Substituting into Eq. 1.133 yields

$$N = \frac{2\pi k_b L}{m_{min} c_b \,[(2/Nu_{m,a}) + (2/Nu_{m,v}) + (k_b/k_t)\ln B]} . \tag{1.136a}$$

If the blood vessels are long, $Gz < 1.5$, we may assume that both Nusselt numbers are equal to 4 and the equation can be approximated by

$$N \cong \frac{2\pi k_b L}{m_{min} c_b \,[1 + (k_b/k_t)\ln B]} . \tag{1.136b}$$

For a counterflow heat exchanger

$$\varepsilon = \frac{1 - \exp[-N(1-C)]}{1 - C\exp[-N(1-C)]} \tag{1.137}$$

when $C = 1$, this reduces to

$$\varepsilon = N/(1+N) . \tag{1.138}$$

The amount of heat transferred is

$$q = m_{min} c_b \varepsilon (T_{a1} - T_{v1}) . \tag{1.139}$$

The temperature changes for the two streams are

$$\text{for } m_{min}: \quad \Delta T = \varepsilon (T_{a1} - T_{v1}) \tag{1.140}$$

$$\text{for } m_{max}: \quad \Delta T = C\varepsilon (T_{a1} - T_{v1}) . \tag{1.141}$$

As was discussed earlier, these relations are applicable to the situation when the blood vessels are close enough such that they exchange heat only with each other through the surrounding tissue. If the blood vessels are close to the skin surface and there is heat loss to the environment, the blood temperatures will be reduced. Strong metabolic heat generation, on the other hand, will increase the temperatures.

Change in blood flow along the length of the blood vessels may have to be considered if the length is significant because the blood leaving the artery tends to enter the parallel vein at the same axial location, x. If enough anatomical and physiological data are available for the tissue under consideration, the length of the blood vessels can be divided into sections with constant mass flow rates. Then the relations developed before can be applied to each section with the additional boundary conditions arising from the equality of temperatures between the exit of an upstream section and the entrance of the next, downstream section.

Chato [17] examined the model in which the blood flow was assumed to change continuously and linearly along both parallel vessels

$$m_a = m_v = m_0(1-FZ) \tag{1.142}$$

where $Z = x/L \leq 1$, and $0 \leq F \leq 1$. The results showed that the mass transfer fraction, F, and the number of conductive heat transfer units, $N_0 = UA/(m_0 c_b)$, contribute identically to the heat transfer, which is

$$q = m_0 c_b (T_{a1} - T_{v1}) \frac{N_0 + F}{1 + N_0} . \tag{1.143}$$

The results also showed that whereas the exit temperature of the artery depended only on N_0, the exit temperature of the vein increased linearly with F and reached the entrance temperature of the artery in the limit when $F = 1$.

Most recently, articles by Baish et al. [3, 4], Wissler [75], and Weinbaum and Jiji [69, 70] presented more sophisticated but related analyses of the counterflow heat exchange between pairs of parallel arteries and veins. Wissler [75] developed the following set of equations to define the temperature field in the tissue around an arterial-venous pair of blood vessels

$$\nabla^2 T_t = 0 \tag{1.144}$$

$$m_a c_b (dT_a/dz) = -q_a \tag{1.145}$$

$$m_v c_b (dT_v/dz) = -q_v \tag{1.146}$$

$$q_a = -kR \int_0^{2\pi} (\partial T_t/\partial r)_{r=R} d\theta \tag{1.147}$$

and

$$q_v = -kR \int_0^{2\pi} (\partial T_t/\partial r)_{r=R} d\theta . \tag{1.148}$$

Now Wissler claims that the solutions to these equations are those developed by Weinbaum and Jiji [69] only if the following conditions are satisfied:

1. The mean tissue temperature in the neighborhood of an artery-vein pair is the arithmetic mean of the arterial and venous blood temperatures at the point of entry to the control volume, i.e.,

$$T_t = (T_a + T_v)/2 . \tag{1.149}$$

2. The temperature of blood draining into "thermally significant" veins from capillaries, T_c, is equal to the "cup-mixed" temperature of venous blood at the point of entry to the control volume, T_v, i.e.,

$$T_c = T_v . \tag{1.150}$$

3. There is very little net heat transfer between thermally significant artery-vein pairs and tissue, i.e.,

$$q_a \cong q_v \cong \frac{2\pi k_t}{\ln[(b_a + \sqrt{b_a^2 - 1})(b_v + \sqrt{b_v^2 - 1})]} (T_a - T_v). \tag{1.151}$$

4. The blood flow rates, m_a and m_v, are constant, implying no blood perfusion.
5. There is no metabolic heat generation in the tissue.
6. The temperature gradient of the tissue along the blood vessels, $\partial T_t/\partial z$, is constant.

To be able to estimate the effects of blood perfusion and metabolic heat generation, Wissler developed the following three, simplified energy balance equations for the arterial, venous, and tissue temperatures. (A sign in the article had to be corrected.)

$$m_b (dT_a/dz) = h_{av}(T_v - T_a) + h_t(T_t - T_a) \tag{1.152}$$

$$m_b (dT_v/dz) = h_{av}(T_v - T_a) - h_t(T_t - T_v) - m_{av}(T_t - T_v) \tag{1.153}$$

$$Ak_t (d^2T_t/dz^2) = h_t(2T_t - T_v - T_a) + m_{av}(T_t - T_a) - Aq_m . \tag{1.154}$$

Here the blood flow rates, m_b, are assumed to be the same at the same location, z; the rates of heat transfer per unit length are: $h_{av}(T_v - T_a)$ from vein to artery, $h_t(T_t - T_a)$ from tissue to artery, $h_t(T_t - T_v)$ from tissue to vein; m_{av} is the rate at which blood flows from artery to vein through intervening capillary beds per unit length of vessel. The temperatures are mean values at a given location, z. In addition, Wissler defined another parameter, the thermal coupling coefficient between artery and vein, $0 < \gamma < 1$, such that

$$h_{av} = \gamma C_{av} k_t \tag{1.155}$$

$$h_t = 2(1-\gamma) C_{av} k_t \tag{1.156}$$

where $C_{av} k_t$ is the coefficient of $(T_a - T_v)$ in Eq. 1.151. Solving these equations for various conditions, Wissler came to the conclusion that in many important cases the tissue temperature was not the average of those of the artery and vein, and, consequently, the Weinbaum and Jiji model had restricted use. An extreme case of his results, when the entering arterial temperature is lower than that of the tissue at the same point, is shown in Fig. 1.17. The tissue temperature is never even between the two blood temperatures.

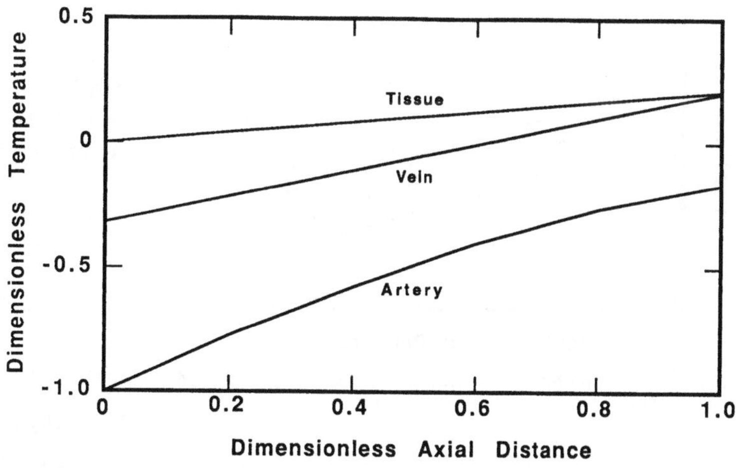

Fig. 1.17. Temperature profiles along an artery-vein pair when the entering arterial temperature is lower than the left-end tissue temperature. [75]

In a rebuttal, Weinbaum and Jiji [70] used the following relations for the heat transfer between arteries and veins, which were developed by them and by Baish et al. [3, 4]. These equations are claimed to be the correct ones to replace Eqs. 1.152 and 1.153 in Wissler's analysis. These equations are based on the heat transfer model depicted in Fig. 1.18

$$\pi \varrho_b c_b V R^2 \frac{dT_a}{dx} = -C_{av} k_t (T_a - T_v) - \frac{C_t k_t}{2} (T_m - T_t) \quad (1.157)$$

$$\pi \varrho_b c_b V R^2 \frac{dT_v}{dx} = -C_{av} k_t (T_a - T_v) + \frac{C_t k_t}{2} (T_m - T_t) \quad (1.158)$$

where $C_t = 2\pi/[\ln (r_t/r_{a \text{ or } v}) + 2k_t/(k_b Nu_b) - 1/2] \cong 2\pi/\ln (r_t/r_{a \text{ or } v})$. These two equations can be added or subtracted and the resulting equations differentiated once. After some manipulation the following set of equations results.

$$\delta^2 \frac{d^2 T_m}{dZ^2} = \frac{C_t}{C_{av}} (T_m - T_t) \quad (1.159)$$

$$\delta^2 \frac{d^2 (T_a - T_v)}{dZ^2} = \frac{C_t}{C_{av}} \left[(T_a - T_v) + \delta \frac{dT_t}{dZ} \right] \quad (1.160)$$

where $Z = x/L$ and L is a characteristic length of the temperature gradient.

$$\delta = \frac{\pi \varrho_b c_b V R^2}{k_t C_{av} L} = \frac{\pi R Pe}{2 C_{av} L} \ll 1 \ . \quad (1.161)$$

Because δ is small, of the order of 0.003 for a 0.1-mm blood vessel and 0.112 for a 0.3-mm one, Eqs. 1.159 and 1.160 are of the boundary layer type and the solutions are shown schematically in Fig. 1.19. Near the two ends, $X = 0$ and $X = 1$, there is rapid variation of T_m and $T_a - T_v$ in a narrow region of the approximate thickness δ. In the center region, however, the second-order derivative terms become insignificant and the corresponding solutions are

$$T_m = T_t \quad (1.162)$$

$$T_a - T_v = -\delta (dT_t/dZ) \ . \quad (1.163)$$

The first of these two equations indicates that the mean arterial-venous temperature must follow the average tissue temperature along most of the blood vessel pairs except near arterial or venous entrance points. The second equation relates the arterial-venous temperature difference to the local axial gradient of the average tissue temperature. Thus, this analysis substantiates the Weinbaum and Jiji [69] thermal model for tissues with the appropriate vasculature consisting of closely paired arteries and veins in the range where δ is small. However, Wissler's

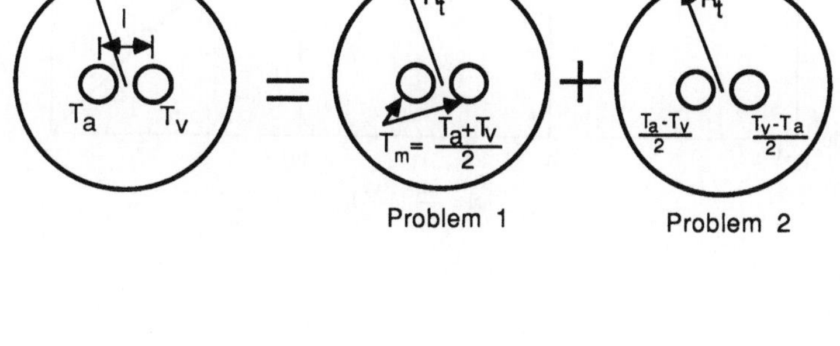

Fig. 1.18. Superposition of two heat conduction problems in the plane perpendicular to the blood vessels to obtain the thermal model. Problem 1 describes heat loss to tissue from a countercurrent pair with no heat exchange between vessels. Problem 2 describes heat exchange between vessels with no net heat loss to the far field of tissue. [70]

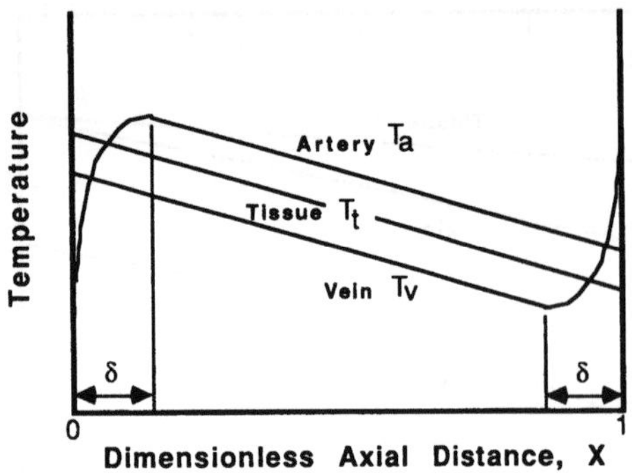

Fig. 1.19. Representative solutions to Eqs. 1.159 and 1.160. (After [70])

contention is that this parameter may not be small for some blood vessels for which L becomes very short. Thus, some care must be taken in using this formulation.

1.4.4 Heat Transfer from a Blood Vessel near the Skin Surface

If a blood vessel runs parallel to the skin surface, a significant amount of energy may be transferred from it to the environment. The resulting distortion of the temperature pattern on the skin surface can be of importance in some applications, such as thermography. Chato and Shitzer [23] developed an analytical solution to the problem when the skin above the blood vessel is cooled directly by a symmetrically placed strip. Here we shall analyze the more common situation of heat transfer form the skin to the environment, which is at a constant temperature, T_0. The configuration can be represented by the lower half ($y \leq 0$) of Fig. 1.15 with $R_1 = R_2 = R$.
A simple solution was given by Awbery [2] as

$$T - T_0 = \frac{q_1}{\pi k_t}\left\{0.25 \ln\left[\frac{x^2+(y-a)^2}{x^2+(y+a)^2}\right] + e^H \int_{-H}^{-\infty} \frac{e^u(\cos \gamma x)\,du}{u}\right\} \tag{1.164}$$

where

$$H = (a h_c/k_t)(1 - y/a) \tag{1.165}$$

$$u = (a\gamma + a h_c/k_t)(1 - y/a)\ . \tag{1.166}$$

Note that γ is the basic variable of integration. The maximum temperatures occur at $x = 0$ where the temperature difference in dimensionless form becomes

$$\theta_0 = \frac{\pi k_t (T - T_0)}{q_1} = 0.25 \ln\left[\frac{y-a}{y+a}\right]^2 + e^H \int_{-H}^{-\infty} \frac{e^u du}{u}\ . \tag{1.167}$$

Figure 1.20 shows the last integral term, designated as f(H), as a function of H. For $H < 0.5$, this term can be approximated to within 1% by

$$f(H) \approx e^H (H - H^2/4 - \ln H - 0.57716) \quad \text{for} \quad H < 0.5\ . \tag{1.168}$$

At the skin surface, $x = 0$, $y = 0$,

$$\theta_{0s} = f(H_s) \tag{1.169}$$

where

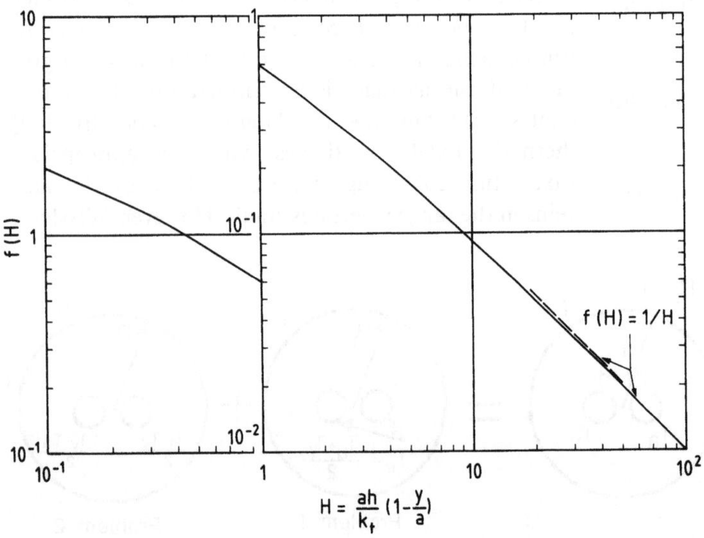

Fig. 1.20. The integral, f(H), as function of $H = (ah_c/k_t)\ (1 - y/a)$. [17]

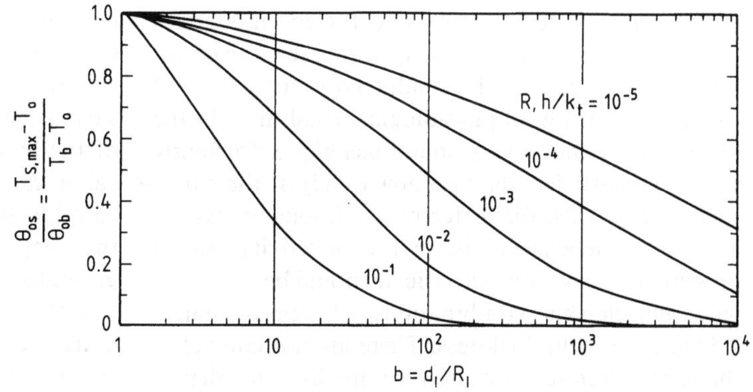

Fig. 1.21. Maximum skin to blood temperature ratio as function of depth-to-radius ratio, b, and Biot number, R_1h_b/k_t

$$H_s = \frac{a\,h_c}{k_t} = \frac{R\,h_c}{k_t}\sqrt{b^2-1} \tag{1.170}$$

at the surface of the blood vessel, $x = 0$, $y = -d+R$,

$$\theta_{0b} = 0.5\ln\left(b+\sqrt{b^2-1}\right)+f(H_b) \tag{1.171}$$

where $b = d/R$ and

$$H_b = \frac{R\,h_c}{k_t}\left(b-1+\sqrt{b^2-1}\right) . \tag{1.172}$$

These temperatures, therefore, can be expressed in terms of two dimensionless parameters: a Biot number, Rh_c/k_t, and the depth to radius ratio, d/R. The expected range of this Biot number in living tissue is between 10^{-5} and 10^{-1}. Figure 1.21 (where the subscript 1 has been retained) shows the ratio of the maximum skin temperature to the blood vessel temperature, θ_{0s}/θ_{0b}, as a function of these two parameters. In general, increasing either parameter, i.e., higher heat transfer to the environment or greater depth of the same blood vessel, forces the skin temperature toward the environmental temperature. It has been shown by Chato [17] that the maximum temperature increase (or decrease if $T_0 > T_b$) on the skin surface due to a subcutaneous blood vessel is independent of other heat fluxes and can be found from the above relations. q_1 can be expressed in terms of the blood flow and the temperature gradient in the axial, z, direction in the vessel

$$q_1 = (\pi R^2 \varrho_b c_b V_b)(\partial T_b/\partial z) \tag{1.173}$$

Since in this solution the minimum skin temperature approaches T_0 at large values of x, i.e., far from the blood vessel, the maximum temperature difference on the skin surface above a blood vessel becomes

$$T_{s,max}-T_{s,min} = \frac{q_1}{\pi k_t} f(H_s)$$

$$= \frac{\varrho_b c_b V_b R^2}{k_t}\left(\frac{\partial T_b}{\partial z}\right) f(H_s) . \tag{1.174}$$

To estimate the orders of magnitude, let us calculate this temperature difference for two different size blood vessels. First consider a capillary with $R = 4\times10^{-3}$ mm, $V_b = 0.7$ mm/s, $\partial T_b/\partial z = 0.1$ C/mm, and $d = 8\times10^{-2}$ mm. Assume $k_t = 3\times10^{-4}$ W/mm-C and $h_c = 6\times10^{-6}$ W/mm^2-C. Then

$$T_{s,max}-T_{s,min} = 1.07\times10^{-4}\,C .$$

This is indeed a very small value. Even decreasing d by one-half to 4×10^{-2} mm will increase this temperature difference only by 10%.

Next consider a terminal vein with $R = 0.75$ mm, $V_b = 13$ mm/s, $\partial T_b/\partial z = 10^{-3}$ C/mm, $d = 1.5$ mm, and k_t and h_c the same as before. Then,

$$T_{s,max}-T_{s,min} = 0.33\,°C .$$

The obvious conclusion is that the larger the blood vessel and the closer it is located to the skin surface the stronger is its effect on the temperature of the skin surface.

1.4.5 Concluding Remarks

Among the three models discussed, Pennes' [58] bioheat equation has served both the research and application-oriented communities quite well even though its physical and physiological interpretation is somewhat questionable. The equation is relatively easy to evaluate and it allows the manipulation of two blood-related parameters, the volumetric perfusion rate and the local arterial temperature, to modify the results. It is to be noted that the blood flow can serve either as a sink or a source of energy (cooling or heating of tissue), depending on whether the tissue temperature is above or below the arterial temperature.

The temperature-dependent thermal conductivity model yields faster diffusion of thermal energy with increasing local temperature and thereby moderates the high (but not the low) temperature leves reached. However, using a single conductivity curve for all tissues or even for all physiological conditions in the same tissue is not a very sound technique. Currently we have insufficient data on how to adjust the curve, such as Fig. 1.24, for different conditions or tissues. The depth-dependent thermal conductivity model presented is very tissue specific. It should be used only with muscle-skin combinations of approximately 2.5 cm (≅ 1 inch) thickness. There are no data yet in the open literature on how to modify the depth-dependent functions for other thicknesses. For example, the presence of a significant fat layer would not only create a low conductivity region under the skin surface, but would also displace the conductivity curves in some presently unspecified, manner.

It is obvious that the proper modeling of the thermal effects of blood perfusion is not a simple matter but it depends very strongly on the structure and behavior of the tissue considered, particularly on its vasculature. Some progress has already been made. However, it seems that one fruitful area of future research will be the development of appropriate thermal models for the different organs of the body and also for the different tumors which are candidates for hyperthermia treatment. Such work will require the acquisition of considerable, reliable anatomical and morphological data before the application of bioengineering analysis can begin.

1.5 System Modeling

1.5.1 Introduction

System modeling here means the description of the overall thermal behavior of some macroscopic entity in a biological system, such as an organ or the whole human body. We are going to consider only some relatively simple thermal models, including those of mammalian, particularly human live tissue. The very complex models of the whole body are of very limited use in clinical medicine and, therefore, will not be discussed. The reader is directed to use the specific literature, such as Wissler [74]. However, a few general remarks are in order.

The human thermal behavior and its models consist of passive and active elements. In the previous sections we dealt only with passive elements where the active nature of the behavior is only implied by given variations of such parameters as metabolic heat generation, blood perfusion, or sweat evaporation rates. A complete model of the thermal system includes active control elements which regulate the various body functions. For example, the temperature of the hypothalamus in the brain relative to a "set" value can be considered the control function for vasodilatation or vasoconstriction near the skin or for the magnitude of the additional metabolic heat generated due to shivering.

The three models we will be discussing here are still quite incomplete in that no active elements will be considered. This is due, in part, to the fact that this is an introductory heat transfer treatise and dealing with active feedback elements requires knowledge or development of control principles and theory which are beyond the scope of this work. The first model uses the simple but very powerful lumped element concept to predict the transient behavior of the whole human body. This concept can be (and, indeed, has been) applied to individual parts of the body, with appropriate interrelations among them in terms of heat and blood exchange, to develop a more accurate overall model for the body. The second example illustrates how a very simple model can provide solutions to important, practical thermal problems. The third section deals with the all important question of how to describe the thermal influence of blood perfusion and illustrates several models.

1.5.2 Lumped Element Models

If a system is small enough, or its conductivity is very high, then we can assume that all of its parts are essentially at the same temperature which characterizes the state of the entire system. Such a model is called a lumped element. The only relevant problem that arises from such a model is the time dependence of the temperature. Although our first impulse may be to consider such a model as too crude or simplistic, it is a very useful one which is employed in many sophisticated models of the entire body, where the total system is divided into many segments, each of which is characterized by only one temperature and interacts thermally with the others.

Let us consider a simple model of the body, as shown in Fig. 1.22, consisting of a core at a constant temperature, T_c, an outer layer of mass M at a mean temperature T_m, and the skin surface with negligible mass at temperature T_s. The thermal resistance between the core and the outer layer is R_c; the thermal resistance between the outer layer and the skin is R_s. Since the convective heat transfer can also be de-

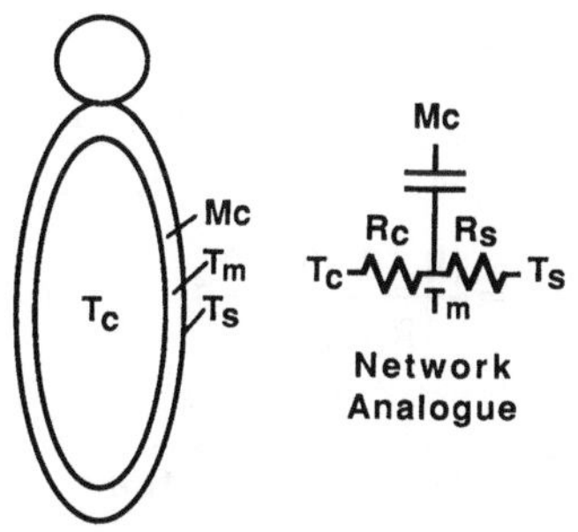

Fig. 1.22. Lumped element model of the human body

scribed by a resistance, $(1/h_c A)$, we can see that the problem remains the same if, instead of the skin temperature, we specify the air temperature and add the convective resistance to R_s. This also implies that the thermal capacitance of the air boundary layer is negligible compared with Mc, a reasonable assumption. The problem is to find the variation of T_m from an initial equilibrium value if T_s is changed in some manner.

Example 1.8: T_s Is Changed Suddenly from T_1 to T_2 (Step Function Change)

Apply the first law to the outer layer, which is the only system of interest since T_c is constant and T_s is a known function of time, using the thermal resistances

$$\frac{T_c - T_m}{R_c} + \frac{T_s - T_m}{R_s} = Mc\frac{dT_m}{dt} \ . \tag{1.175a}$$

Rearranging yields a first-order ordinary differential equation

$$\frac{dT_m}{dt} + \left(\frac{1}{R_c Mc} + \frac{1}{R_s Mc}\right) T_m = \frac{T_c}{R_c Mc} + \frac{T_s}{R_s Mc} \ . \tag{1.175b}$$

The specific solution corresponding to the steady state is

$$T_{ms} = \left(\frac{T_c}{R_c Mc} + \frac{T_s}{R_s Mc}\right) \Big/ \left(\frac{1}{R_c Mc} + \frac{1}{R_s Mc}\right) = \frac{(R_s/R_c)T_c + T_s}{R_s/R_c + 1} \ . \tag{1.176}$$

The general solution is

$$T_{mg} = C_1 e^{-\gamma t} \tag{1.177}$$

where $\gamma \equiv \left(\frac{1}{R_c Mc} + \frac{1}{R_s Mc}\right)$.

The boundary conditions are:

$$\text{Initially} \quad T_{mi} = \frac{(R_s/R_c)T_c + T_1}{R_s/R_c + 1} \ . \tag{1.178}$$

At $t > 0$: $T_s = T_2$. Thus

$$T_{ms} = \frac{(R_s/R_c)T_c + T_2}{R_s/R_c + 1} \tag{1.179}$$

and at $t = 0$: $T_m = T_{mg} + T_{ms} = T_{mi}$. Therefore,

$$C_1 = \frac{T_1 - T_2}{R_s/R_c + 1} \ . \tag{1.180}$$

The total solution then becomes

$$T_m = \frac{(T_1 - T_2)e^{-\gamma t} + (R_s/R_c)T_c + T_2}{R_s/R_c + 1} \ . \tag{1.181}$$

The temperature of the outer layer varies as a decaying exponential with a so-called time constant $(1/\gamma)$. In one time constant the decaying part is reduced to 37% of its initial value. It takes 2.3 time constants to reach 10% and 4.6 to reach 1%. Although the final steady state is reached only in infinite time we can arbitrarily define a practical transient period by the final value of the approach, e.g., 1%.

Taking $R_s = R_c = 1/40$ C/W $= 0.025$ C/W, $M = 30$ kg, $c = 4 \times 10^3$ J/kg-C. Then $\gamma = 2/(0.025 \times 30 \times 4 \times 10^3) = 0.667 \times 10^{-3}\ s^{-1}$ or the time constant is 1500 s = 25 min (which is very close to the time constant of 27 min in Example 1.6). If we further let $T_c = 37\,°C$, $T_1 = 33\,°C$, and $T_2 = 29\,°C$ then the solution is

$$T_m = 2e^{-t/1500} + 33 \ .$$

Thus the layer temperature changes 2 °C from 35 °C to 33 °C in about 2 h ($\simeq$ 4.6 time constants).

If we include an air resistance R_a and let T_s be air temperature, the following numerical results will be obtained with $h_c = 12.5\ W/m^2$-C.

$$R_a = 1/h_c A_D = 1/12.5 \times 2 = 1/25 = 0.04\ C/W \ .$$

$$R_c = 0.025\ C/W$$

$$R_s = 0.025 + 0.040 = 0.065\ C/W \ .$$

Let us find the initial, T_1, and final, T_2, air temperatures which will result in the same initial and final outer layer temperatures as above.

$$T_s = (R_s/R_c + 1)T_m - (R_s/R_c)T_c$$

$$T_1 = (0.065/0.025 + 1)35 - (0.065/0.025)37 = 29.8\,°C$$

$$T_2 = 3.6 \times 33 - 2.6 \times 37 = 22.6\,°C \ .$$

The time constant is evaluated from $\gamma = (1/0.025 \times 1.2 \times 10^5 + 1/0.065 \times 1.2 \times 10^5) = 0.4615 \times 10^{-3}\ s^{-1}$ or the time constant is 2167 s = 36 min. Thus the additional resistance slows down the transient process.

Example 1.9: T_s Is Changing Linearly with Time, $T_s = T_1 + at$ (Ramp Function Change)

Equation 1.175b becomes

$$\frac{dT_m}{dt} + \gamma T_m = \frac{T_c}{R_c Mc} + \frac{T_1}{R_s Mc} + \frac{a}{R_s Mc} t \ . \quad (1.182)$$

The general solution is the same as before, Eq. 1.177, but the specific solution is

$$T_{ms} = A_2 + B_3 t \ . \quad (1.183)$$

Substituting into Eq. 1.182 allows us to solve for A_2 and B_3

$$B_3 + \gamma(A_2 + B_3 t) = \frac{T_c}{R_c Mc} + \frac{T_i}{R_s Mc} + \frac{a}{R_s Mc} t \quad (1.184)$$

$$A_2 = \frac{(R_s/R_c) T_c + T_1 - a/\gamma}{R_s/R_c + 1} \quad (1.185)$$

$$B_3 = \frac{a}{R_s/R_c + 1} \ . \quad (1.186)$$

The total solution is

$$T_m = C_1 e^{-\gamma t} + A_2 + B_3 t \ . \quad (1.187)$$

The initial condition is

$$\frac{(R_s/R_c T_c + T_1}{R_s/R_c + 1} = C_1 + \frac{(R_s/R_c) T_c + T_1}{R_s/R_c + 1} - \frac{a/\gamma}{R_s/R_c + 1} \ . \quad (1.188)$$

Therefore,

$$C_1 = \frac{a/\gamma}{R_s/R_c + 1} \quad (1.189)$$

and

$$T_m = \frac{(A/\gamma) e^{-\gamma t} + (R_s/R_c) T_c + T_1 - a/\gamma + at}{R_s/R_c + 1} \ . \quad (1.190)$$

The transient part has the same character with the same time constant as before; however, the "steady state" part is not a constant but is a time-varying function of the same type as the boundary condition.

Example 1.10: T_s Is Changing Exponentially from T_1 to T_2, $T_s = T_2 + (T_1 - T_2) e^{-\eta t}$

The specific solution is of the form

$$T_{ms} = A_2 + B_3 e^{-\eta t} \ . \quad (1.191)$$

Following the previous procedure, we substitute into the governing Eq. 1.175b to obtain

$$-B_3 \eta e^{-\eta t} + \gamma(A_2 + B_3 e^{-\eta t}) = \frac{T_c}{R_c Mc} + \frac{T_2}{R_s Mc} + \frac{(T_1 - T_2)}{R_s Mc} e^{-\eta t} \quad (1.192)$$

$$A_2 = \frac{(R_s/R_c) T_c + T_2}{R_s/R_c + 1} \quad (1.193)$$

$$B_3 = \frac{T_1 - T_2}{R_s/R_c + 1 - R_s Mc\eta} \ . \quad (1.194)$$

The total solution is

$$T_m = C_1 e^{-\gamma t} + A_2 + B_3 e^{-\eta t} \ . \quad (1.195)$$

The initial condition is

$$\frac{(R_s/R_c) T_c + T_1}{R_s/R_c + 1} = C_1 + \frac{(R_s/R_c) T_c + T_2}{R_s/R_c + 1} + \frac{T_1 - T_2}{R_s/R_c + 1 - R_s Mc\eta} \ . \quad (1.196)$$

Therefore

$$C_1 = \frac{T_1 - T_2}{R_s/R_c + 1} \left[\frac{1}{1 - [(1/R_c + 1/R_s)/Mc\eta]} \right] \quad (1.197)$$

and

$$T_m = \frac{(R_s/R_c) T_c + T_2}{R_s/R_c + 1} + \frac{T_1 - T_2}{R_s/R_c + 1} \times \left[\frac{1}{1 - [(1/R_c + 1/R_s)/Mc\eta)]} e^{-\gamma t} + \frac{1}{1 - [Mc\eta/(1/R_c + 1/R_s)]} e^{-\eta t} \right] \ . \quad (1.198)$$

This is probably the most realistic of the three examples since the outside temperature, whether on the skin or in the air, is most likely to change in a gradual manner between some fixed limits. The next solution is applicable to various periodic variations, such as the circadian rhythms.

Example 1.11: T_s Is Changing from T_1 in a Sinusoidal Manner, $T_s = T_1 + a \sin \omega t$

The specific solution can be expressed either in terms of $\sin \omega t$ and $\cos \omega t$, or more conveniently in terms of a phase shift, $\sin(\omega t - \phi)$

$$T_s = C_2 + C_3 \sin(\omega t - \phi) \ . \quad (1.199)$$

Substitute into Eq. 1.175b

$$C_3 \omega \cos(\omega t - \phi) + \gamma [C_2 + C_3 \sin(\omega t - \phi)] = \frac{T_c}{R_c Mc} + \frac{T_1}{R_s Mc} + \frac{a}{R_s Mc} \sin \omega t \quad (1.200)$$

$$C_2 = \frac{(R_s/R_c)T_c + T_1}{R_s/R_c + 1} \tag{1.201}$$

$$C_3[\omega \cos(\omega t - \phi) + \gamma \sin(\omega t - \phi)] = \frac{a}{R_s Mc} \sin \omega t \ . \tag{1.202}$$

Expanding the trigonometric functions and letting the coefficient of $\cos \omega t$ be zero yields

$$C_3[(\omega \cos \phi - \gamma \sin \phi) \cos \omega t + (\omega \sin \phi + \gamma \cos \phi) \sin \omega t] = \frac{a}{R_s Mc} \sin \omega t \ . \tag{1.203}$$

Therefore

$$\omega \cos \phi - \gamma \sin \phi = 0 \tag{1.204a}$$

or

$$\tan \phi = \frac{\omega}{\gamma} \tag{1.204b}$$

$$\omega \sin \phi + \gamma \cos \phi = \gamma(\tan \phi \sin \phi + \cos \phi) = \frac{\gamma}{\cos \phi}(\sin^2 \phi + \cos^2 \phi) = \frac{\gamma}{\cos \phi} \tag{1.205}$$

$$C_3 = \frac{a \cos \phi}{\gamma R_s Mc} = \frac{a \cos \phi}{R_s/R_c + 1} \ . \tag{1.206}$$

The complete solution is

$$T_m = C_1 e^{-\gamma t} + \frac{(R_s/R_c)T_c + T_1}{R_s/R_c + 1} + \frac{a \cos \phi}{R_s/R_c + 1} \sin(\omega t - \phi) \ . \tag{1.207}$$

The initial condition is

$$\frac{(R_s/R_c)T_c + T_1}{R_s/R_c + 1} = C_1 + \frac{(R_s/R_c)T_c + T_1}{R_s/R_c + 1} - \frac{a \cos \phi \sin \phi}{R_s/R_c + 1} \tag{1.208}$$

$$C_1 = \frac{a \cos \phi \sin \phi}{R_s/R_c + 1} \tag{1.209}$$

where $\cos \phi \sin \phi = 1/(\omega/\gamma + \gamma/\omega)$. Thus the final solution becomes

$$T_m = \frac{a \cos \phi \sin \phi e^{-\gamma t} + (R_s/R_c)T_c}{R_s/R_c + 1} + \frac{T_1 + a \cos \phi \sin(\omega t - \phi)}{R_s/R_c + 1} \ . \tag{1.210}$$

The time constant is the same as before. The steady state response of T_m to the sinusoidal variation of T_s is a sinusoidal oscillation with an amplitude $a \cos \phi/(R_s/R_c + 1)$ and a phase shift of ϕ.

This lumped element model can be made more sophisticated for smaller sections of the body by including internal metabolic heat generation and blood supply and drainage, and by making some of these parameters, including the thermal resistance, variable functions of time and/or temperature. This model is actually the basis of most of the system models used today as described, for example, by Wissler [74].

1.5.3 Estimation of the Maximum Surface Temperature of a Material for Thermal Safety

If the skin comes in contact with a hot surface, burn or permanent damage will occur depending on the properties and temperatures of the material contacted and of the skin, and on the length of exposure. Since tissue damage occurs at most at a depth of 80 μm, the thickness of the epidermal layer, the estimation of the temperatures can be based on the assumptions that

1. the skin and the material can be considered as semi-infinite bodies near the contact,
2. the initial temperatures are constant, and
3. the heat flow is one-dimensional, perpendicular to the contacting surface.

This problem has been treated by Wu [78]. Burn thresholds have been given as temperature-time relations at the skin surface by Wu [78] and by Henriques and Moritz [38], Moritz and Henriques [52], and Henriques [37] as shown in Fig. 1.23; and as temperatures at 80 μm depth by Wu [78] and Stoll [65] or at 1500 μm depth by Dussan and Weiner [32]. To estimate the time required to reach a given temperature at some location, x, from the skin surface, the one-

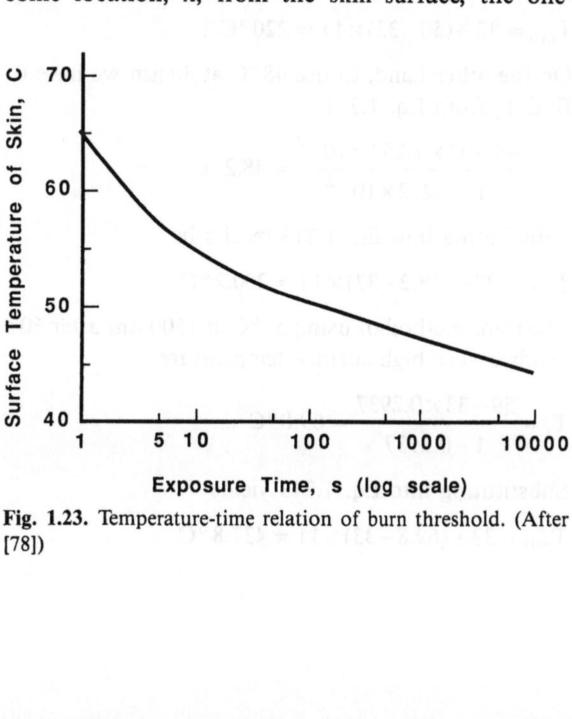

Fig. 1.23. Temperature-time relation of burn threshold. (After [78])

dimensional heat conduction equation can be applied to both the tissue and the material (e.g., [12, pp. 59–60]).

$$\frac{T_s-T}{T_s-T_0} = \operatorname{erf}\frac{x}{2\sqrt{\alpha t}} \tag{1.211}$$

$$\frac{q}{A} = \frac{(T_s-T_0)k_t}{\sqrt{\pi\alpha t}}\, e^{-x^2/4\alpha t} \; . \tag{1.212}$$

Since at the interface both the temperature and heat flux must be the same for the two bodies in contact, this interface temperature can be shown to be constant for all times $t>0$

$$T_s-T_0 = \frac{T_{m0}-T_0}{1+\sqrt{(k\varrho c)_t/(k\varrho c)_m}} \tag{1.213}$$

where the subscript m refers to the material in contact with the skin and 0 to initial values.

Example 1.12

Let us find the maximum allowable temperature for a plastic whose thermal inertia, $k\varrho c$, is one hundredth that of tissue, for glass with the same thermal inertia as tissue, and for a brass with hundred times the thermal inertia of tissue. From a safety consideration we must accept the possibility of a very moist skin with high thermal conductivity. Thus we should take a high thermal diffusivity as well: $\alpha = 1.3\times10^{-7}\ \mathrm{m^2/s}$. Let us also assume that the normal skin temperature is $T_0 = 33\ °C$ and the maximum exposure time is 100 s. Then from Fig. 1.23 the maximum skin temperature is about 50 °C; from Stoll [65] we could choose 48 °C as a reasonable limit at 80 µm; whereas Dussan and Weiner [32] suggest 59 °C at 1500 µm depth after 60 s. For the plastic, with $T_s = 50\ °C$, Eq. 1.213 yields

$$T_{m0} = 33+(50-33)\times11 = 220\ °C \; .$$

On the other hand, to use 48 °C at 80 µm we have to find T_s from Eq. 1.211

$$T_s = \frac{48-33\times1.252\times10^{-2}}{1-1.252\times10^{-2}} = 48.2\ °C \; .$$

Substituting into Eq. 1.213 results in

$$T_{m0} = 33+(48.2-33)\times11 = 200.2\ °C \; .$$

The third method of using 59 °C at 1500 µm after 60 s yields a very high surface temperature

$$T_s = \frac{59-33\times0.2937}{1-0.2937} = 69.8\ °C \; .$$

Substituting into Eq. 1.213 yields

$$T_{m0} = 33+(69.8-33)\times11 = 437.8\ °C \; .$$

This third method gives much higher temperatures, with definite burns near the skin, than the other two methods and is, therefore, not recommended for use. The same calculations for the other two materials yield the following values.

For the glass:
$T_s = 50\ °C$, $T_{m0} = 67\ °C$
$T_s = 48.2\ °C$, $T_{m0} = 63.4\ °C$
$T_s = 69.9\ °C$, $T_{m0} = 106.8\ °C$.

For the brass:
$T_s = 50\ °C$, $T_{m0} = 50.2\ °C$
$T_s = 48.2\ °C$, $T_{m0} = 48.4\ °C$
$T_s = 69.9\ °C$, $T_{m0} = 70.3\ °C$.

1.5.4 Thermal Models of the Tissue Perfused by Blood

This topic has been treated partially in the section on heat transfer to blood vessels. We will emphasize the system-oriented aspects here. The most complete model of a perfused tissue was developed by Chen and Holmes [24]

$$\varrho c\frac{\partial T}{\partial t} = \nabla\cdot(k+k_b)\nabla T + m_b^* c_b(T_a^*-T) - \varrho_b c_b V_b\cdot\nabla T + q_i \tag{1.214a}$$

where k_b is an apparent increase of the thermal conductivity due to blood perfusion in the small blood vessels; the starred quantities refer to the blood perfusion and arterial temperature at a specific size level; and V_b is an overall vectorial perfusion velocity. Various aspects of this equation have been proposed previously by workers in the field of bioheat transfer. For example, Pennes [58] developed what has become known as the bioheat equation. This is still being used successfully

$$\varrho c\frac{\partial T}{\partial t} = \nabla\cdot k\nabla T + m_b c_b(T_a-T) + q_i \; . \tag{1.214b}$$

Here T_a is an appropriate arterial temperature which has been frequently assumed to be the temperature of the body's core (≈ 37 °C).
Gautherie [33] proposed a temperature-dependent conductivity function for $(k+k_b)$ shown in Fig. 1.24. Hurlburt and Chato [41] accurately approximated this function as

$$k+k_b = 4.82-4.44833\,[1.00075^{-1.575^{(T-25)}}]\ \mathrm{W/m\text{-}C} \; . \tag{1.215}$$

For this model only the conduction term and internal heat generation is used

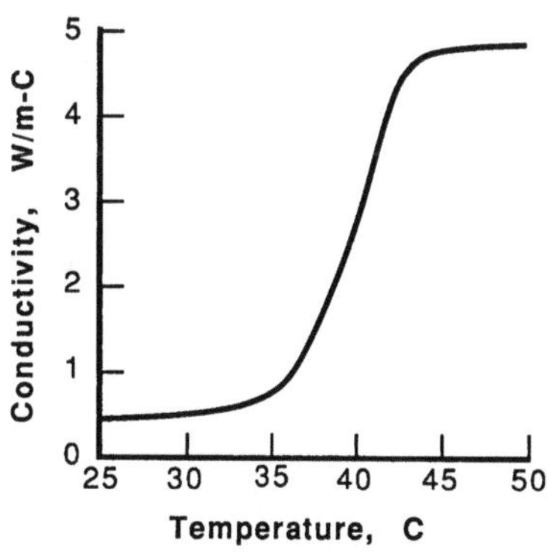

Fig. 1.24. Temperature-dependent thermal conductivity of live tissue as suggested by Gautherie [33]

$$\varrho c \frac{\partial T}{\partial t} = \nabla\cdot(k+k_b)\nabla T + q_i \ . \qquad (1.214c)$$

In an extensive study of the details of the effects of the circulatory system in the peripheral tissue Keller and Seiler [44] proposed overall effective thermal conductivities across the peripheral layer. For a resting muscle-skin combination they derived

$$\frac{k_{eff}}{k} = \frac{k+k_b}{k} = \frac{\sqrt{m_b c_b L^2/k}}{\tanh\sqrt{m_b c_b L^2/k}} \qquad (1.216a)$$

where L is the depth of the peripheral tissue. This expression, however, can only be used as an overall conductivity. The corresponding overall, thermal conductance, k_{eff}/L, between the skin surface and the body core is

$$\frac{k_{eff}}{L} = \frac{\sqrt{m_b c_b k}}{\tanh\sqrt{m_b c_b L^2/k}} \ . \qquad (1.216b)$$

Wulff [79] claimed that the only proper term for the effects of blood perfusion was the vectorial one containing V_b. Unfortunately we have, as yet, no way of determining its magnitude and, therefore, it has not been used in practice.

A quite realistic steady-state model of the muscle-skin complex has been developed by Weinbaum, Jiji, Lemons, and coworkers (see [42, 69–71]). In particular, Song et al. [64] developed a relatively simple, four-layer model based on their observations of the structure of the microcirculation and on their temperature measurements taken in the hind leg of anesthetized rabbits. These data showed only very minor temperature excursions of the blood vessels from the temperature of the surrounding tissue. Some of the details have been presented in Sect. 4 on heat transfer to blood vessels. The following set of equations is their relatively simple, one-dimensional model of a 25-mm-thick muscle-skin combination.

For the deepest 20-mm muscle layer the following dimensionless equation is used. This is based on the assumption of nearly (but not completely) perfect heat exchange between the parallel running and almost touching smaller arteries and veins.

$$\frac{d}{dZ}\,[1+A(Z)Pe_0^2]\,\frac{d\theta}{dZ} - B(Z)Pe_0^2\,\frac{d\theta}{dZ} + q_0 = 0 \qquad (1.217)$$

where

$$\theta = \frac{T-T_s}{T_a-T_s}\ ,$$

$Z = \dfrac{z}{L_1}$ where $L_1 = 20\,\text{mm}$, the depth of the layer,

$Pe_0 = \left(\dfrac{\varrho c D V}{k}\right)_b$ an arterial inflow Peclet number in the deep tissue with a normal range of about 60–240, and

$$q_0 = \frac{q_i L_1^2}{k(T_c-T_s)}$$

with a normal range of about 0 to 1.

The functions A(Z) and B(Z) are shown in their original graphical form in Fig. 1.25. They were approximated by Hurlburt and Chato [41] in dimensional form as

$$A(z) = 1.946\times10^{-7}(18-z)^2 \quad \text{for} \quad 0\le z<18 \qquad (1.218a)$$
$$A(z) = 0 \quad \text{for} \quad 18\le z\le 20 \qquad (1.218b)$$

and

$$B(z) = 2.32\times10^{-7}(14-z)^2 \quad \text{for} \quad 0\le z<14 \qquad (1.219a)$$
$$B(z) = 0 \quad \text{for} \quad 14\le z\le 20 \qquad (1.219b)$$

where z is in millimeters measured from the boundary at the core. Both of these functions decrease monotonically from the core outward. Therefore, they have

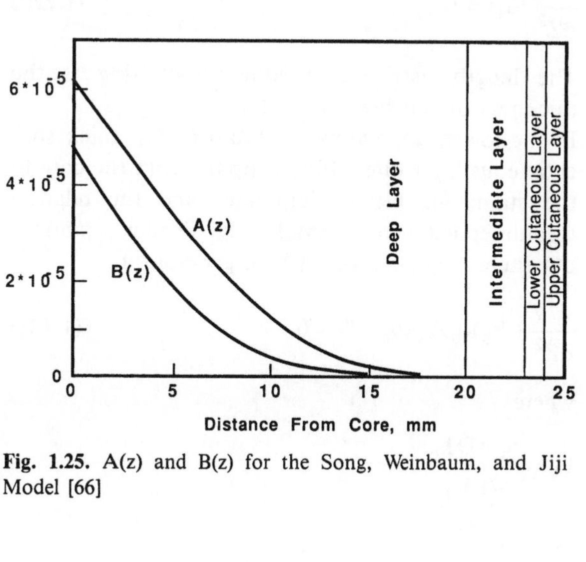

Fig. 1.25. A(z) and B(z) for the Song, Weinbaum, and Jiji Model [66]

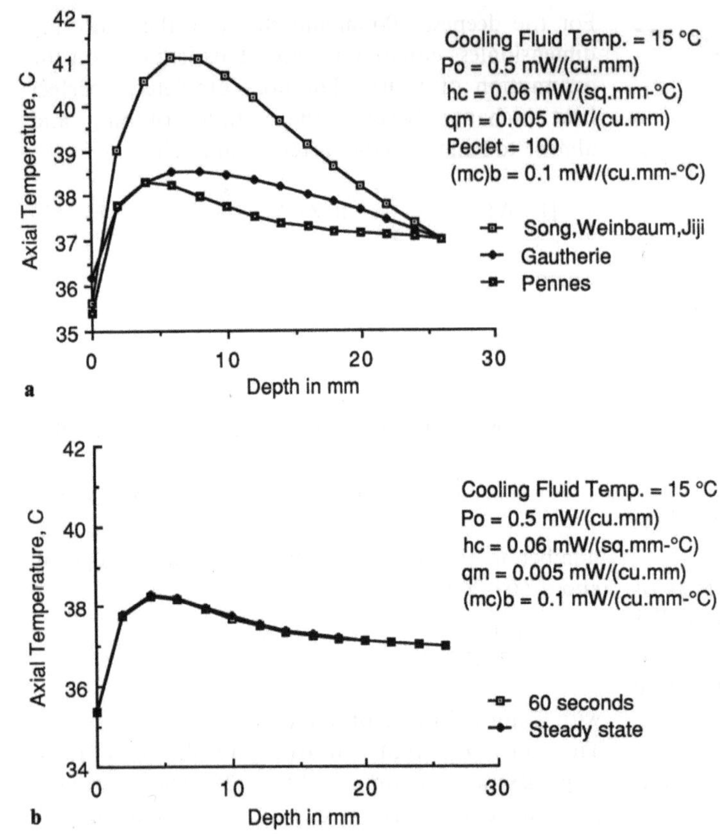

Fig. 1.26. a Steady-state comparison of three models. (After [41]. **b** Transient Pennes model. (After [41])

no influence near the next, intermediate layer and the heat transfer becomes a simple conduction process with internal heat generation and constant thermal conductivity, just like in the next layer.

In the next, 3-mm-thick intermediate layer the arterial-venous heat exchange does not exist in this model and the governing equation consists of only conduction and heat generation terms

$$\frac{d^2\theta}{dZ^2}+q_0=0\ . \qquad (1.220)$$

The length used for nondimensionalizing is the thickness of this layer, $L_2 = 3$ mm.

In the lower, approximately 1 mm ($= L_3$) thick subcutaneous layer direct blood supply from the core to the cutaneous plexus dominates and the relation recommended here resembles the Pennes equation, but there is no significant heat generation

$$\frac{d^2\theta}{dZ^2}+F_b R_b Pe_0(\theta_a-\theta)=0 \qquad (1.221)$$

where

$$F_b=\frac{n_0 \pi D k_b}{4 k L_3}\ ,$$

R_b is the blood supply ratio between this cutaneous layer and all the lower layers, and θ_a is the dimensionless, local arterial temperature.

Finally, in the last, 1-mm ($= L_4$)-thick surface layer only conduction is assumed to exist

$$\frac{d^2\theta}{dZ^2}=0\ . \qquad (1.222)$$

Hurlburt and Chato [41] made a comparison of the temperatures obtained from three different models for the problem of axially and radially decaying, axisymmetric heating of the tissue from the skin inward. Such a pattern may be generated by a microwave applicator. The power deposition in the tissue was assumed to follow the following form

$$P_t = P_0 \exp(-C_1 r^2 - C_2 z) \qquad (1.223)$$

where z is inward from the skin surface.

The skin was assumed to be cooled by a liquid-filled pad with an assumed convective film coefficient. Typical temperature distributions are shown in Fig. 1.26. The Pennes and Gautherie models produced similar temperature patterns with relatively short, 1- to 2-min, transient times. The Song, Weinbaum, and Jiji model generated significantly higher temperature

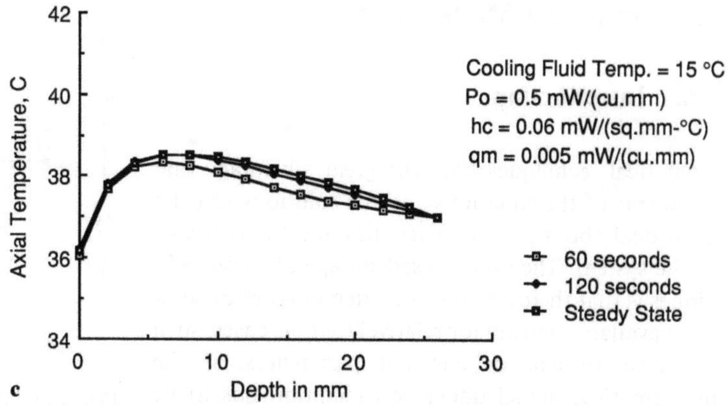

c

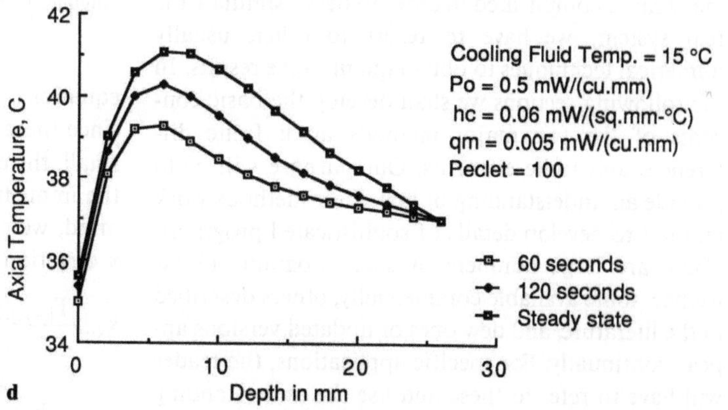

d

Fig. 1.26. **c** Transient Gautherie model. (After [41]). **d** Transient Song, Weinbaum, and Jiji model. (After [41])

levels and longer transient periods. Although these latter results are due, in part, to our assumption of negligible blood supply to the cutaneous plexus ($R_b \cong 0$), the general behavior of this model is to enhance heat transfer only as the core is approached because of the character of the conductivity function A(z) as shown in Fig. 1.25. Since the energy is deposited most strongly near the skin surface, where the thermal conductivity is the lowest in this model, higher temperatures should be expected to be generated near the skin surface than in both of the other two models where either the conductivity (Gautherie) or cooling due to blood perfusion (Pennes) increases with temperature. It is also to be noted that if a tumor is to be heated, the Song, Weinbaum, and Jiji model would probably not apply because the tumor usually lacks the close parallel arterial-venous vasculature which forms the basis of this model.

1.5.5 Whole Body Models

As it has been briefly mentioned before the complete thermal model of the human body contains a number of active control functions. Some of these are triggered by local temperatures, others by a central temperature such as that of the hypothalamus in the brain. The controls regulate such functions as the metabolic heat generation or blood perfusion which appear as input parameters in the passive models. The passive elements, such as the various tissues, can be modeled as distributed systems with internal temperature distribution or as lumped element systems characterized by a single temperature for each element. The chief difference between these two approaches is that the whole system requires fewer distributed elements with more complicated mathematical equations than lumped elements with simpler relations. For example, an arm or a leg may be modeled as a distributed cylindrical core surrounded by a distributed cylindrical model of the muscle and the skin, which may have as many as four layers (e.g., the Song, Weinbaum, and Jiji 1987 model described above [64]). Temperature conditions and energy balances at the boundaries have to be satisfied. With lumped element modeling a larger number of concentric cylinders, each characterized by a single temperature, are needed with appropriate interconnections in terms of energy transport via thermal conductances and blood exchange.

Comprehensive reviews of this subject have been written by Shitzer [61] and Wissler [74].

1.6 Numerical Methods

1.6.1 Introduction

Analytical techniques have the great advantage that the forms of the equations and the solutions reveal a great deal about the characteristics and the behavior of the system. The major disadvantage of these techniques is that there are only a limited number of solutions available, mostly for relatively simple cases, such as linear systems or constant parameters. If the mathematical model under consideration has to be made more complicated in order to better simulate the real system, we have to resort to other, usually numerical techniques to obtain quantitative results. In the following sections we shall develop the basic concepts of the two major methods used: finite differences and finite elements. Our purpose will be to provide an understanding of how these methods work and not to develop details of sophisticated programs. There are large numbers of such programs in existence, some available commercially, others described in the literature, and new ones or updated versions appear continually. For specific applications, the reader will have to refer to these and use the understanding gained from this treatise to comprehend, evaluate, and use them. There are also several textbooks on both finite difference (e.g. [1]) and finite element techniques (e.g. [40]). Perhaps the most concise of these, dealing only with heat conduction, is the one by Myers [54].

1.6.2 Finite Difference Method

The analytical methods described earlier start out by applying the appropriate physical relations, such as the conservation of energy, to differential elements, e.g., $dx \cdot dy \cdot dz$. If we treat these differentials as small but finite differences, $\Delta x \cdot \Delta y \cdot \Delta z$, and apply the physical relations the same way as before in the analytical methods, we have the essential basic procedure for the development of the finite difference equations. One might describe the analytical equation as the limit of the corresponding finite difference equation as the differences approach zero.

Consider the three-dimensional field in Cartesian coordinates as shown in Fig. 1.27 and develop the energy balance for a typical element located at i, j, k, in the x, y, z directions, respectively, of size $\Delta x \cdot \Delta y \cdot \Delta z$, which is identified by a single node at its center (i, j, k). We need to make several assumptions here which will determine the complexity of the final

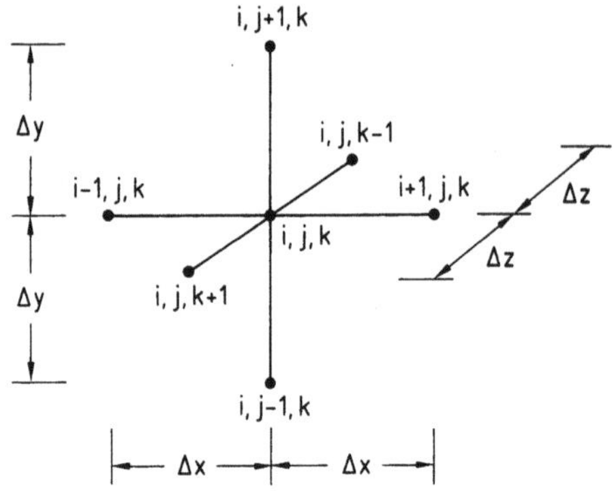

Fig. 1.27. Three-dimensional, finite difference field in rectangular, Cartesian coordinates

equations. The most practical assumption is that, since these finite differences can be made arbitrarily small, the energy relations can be considered linear in the immediate vicinity of each element. With this in mind, we can write the heat conduction terms in the x direction as follows:

$$k_{x-} \frac{T_{i-1,j,k} - T_{i,j,k}}{\Delta x} \Delta y \Delta z - k_{x+} \frac{T_{i,j,k} - T_{i+1,j,k}}{\Delta x} \Delta y \Delta z \ .$$

The two thermal conductivities can be expressed in different ways. If the conductivity is changing relatively strongly, then perhaps the best approximations are:

$$k_{x-} = (k_{i-1,j,k} + k_{i,j,k})/2 \tag{1.224}$$

$$k_{x+} = (k_{i,j,k} + k_{i+1,j,k})/2 \ . \tag{1.225}$$

Energy will be generated or dissipated in the control volume at a rate of

$$q_i \Delta x \Delta y \Delta z$$

where q_i is positive for heat generation and negative for dissipation. As discussed earlier, in biological systems the two major parameters of this type are metabolic heat, q_m, and blood perfusion, q_b. For example, Pennes' blood perfusion term in finite difference from becomes

$$m_b c_b (T_a - T)_{i,j,k} \Delta x \Delta y \Delta z \ .$$

The next thermal quantity to be considered is the internal energy storage in the control volume. With the assumptions described earlier, during the development of the analytical expressions, this term becomes

$$\varrho c \Delta x \Delta y \Delta z \frac{T^{n+1}_{i,j,k} - T^{n}_{i,j,k}}{\Delta t}$$

where the superscripts n and n+1 represent successive time steps. Combining these terms and dividing by the volume, $\Delta x \Delta y \Delta z$, yields the basic, finite difference energy equation for a general node at i, j, k, with conduction occurring only in the x direction

$$\frac{\varrho c}{\Delta t}(T^{n+1}_{i,j,k} - T^{n}_{i,j,k}) = \frac{k_{x-}}{\Delta x^2}(T_{i-1,j,k} - T_{i,j,k}) - \frac{k_{x+}}{\Delta x^2}(T_{i,j,k} - T_{i+1,j,k}) + q_i \quad (1.226)$$

or

$$T^{n+1}_{i,j,k} = \frac{k_{x-}\Delta t}{\varrho c \Delta x^2} T_{i-1,j,k} + T^{n}_{i,j,k} - \frac{(k_{x-} + k_{x+})\Delta t}{\varrho c \Delta x^2} T_{i,j,k} + \frac{k_{x+}\Delta t}{\varrho c \Delta x^2} T_{i+1,j,k} + \frac{q_i \Delta t}{\varrho c} . \quad (1.226a)$$

For the conduction terms in the other directions, expressions similar to the two terms given in Eq. 1.226 have to be added. Thus, conduction in the y direction can be represented by

$$\frac{k_{y-}}{\Delta y^2}(T_{i,j-1,k} - T_{i,j,k}) - \frac{k_{y+}}{\Delta y^2}(T_{i,j,k} - T_{i,j+1,k})$$

whereas in the z direction we need

$$\frac{k_{z-}}{\Delta z^2}(T_{i,j,k-1} - T_{i,j,k}) - \frac{k_{z+}}{\Delta z^2}(T_{i,j,k} - T_{i,j,k+1}) .$$

Where no superscript time indices are given on the right-hand side for the temperatures, those values are arbitrary and they determine the character of the calculations needed to solve the problem. The simplest computational scheme results if all the temperatures on the right-hand side are taken as the current, known values (superscript n). In this case, each node equation becomes explicit for $T^{n+1}_{i,j,k}$ and can be solved directly using the current, known values for all temperatures. This explicit or Euler method, however, has two disadvantages. The first is illustrated in Fig. 1.28 on a simple, one-dimensional case. The explicit method finds the next value of the variable, f^{n+1}, by using the current slope to extrapolate from the current value of the variable, f^n. Thus, it tends to overshoot the "real" value in the direction of the convex side of the variable versus time curve. The second disadvantage of this method is that it becomes unstable if the time increments are too big, such that the coefficient of $T^{n}_{i,j,k}$ becomes negative. For the one-dimensional case, for example, the coefficient is (see Eq. 1.226 where q_i is assumed not to contribute)

$$1 - \frac{(k_{x-} + k_{x+})\Delta t}{\varrho c \Delta x^2} .$$

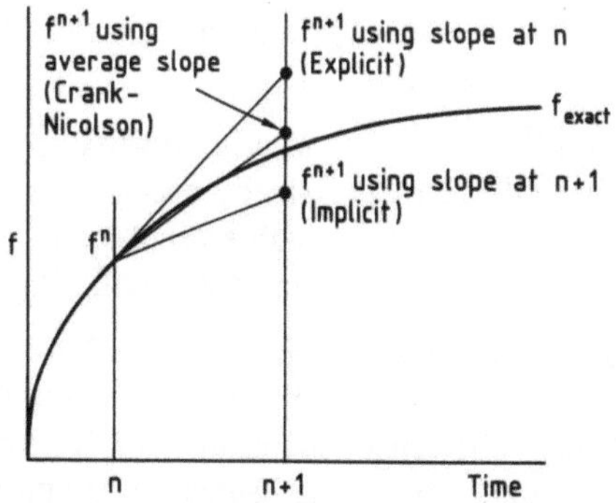

Fig. 1.28. One-dimensional illustration of the explicit and implicit time extrapolation

Therefore, the maximum time increment becomes

$$\Delta t_{max} = \frac{\varrho c \Delta x^2}{k_{x-} + k_{x+}} . \quad (1.227)$$

This may be very small, requiring many steps to explore the required time range.

One way to overcome this problem is to make the temperatures on the right-hand side equal to their next, future value, T^{n+1}, or a combination of the present and future values, i.e.,

$$T = \eta T^{n+1} + (1-\eta) T^n \quad (1.228)$$

where $0 \le \eta \le 1$ is the implicitness of the method. For any nonzero value of η the resulting equations require simultaneous solution, such as a matrix inversion technique. The fully implicit method, $\eta = 1$, is unconditionally stable for all values of Δt. However, it tends to undershoot the "real" value in the direction of the concave side of the variable versus time curve because it uses the future slope to find the next, n+1, value of the variable as shown in Fig. 1.28. If Δt is too big, the error can be considerable. If $\eta = 0.5$, we have the Crank-Nicolson method.

To illustrate the stability of the solution in terms of the coefficient of the $T^{n}_{i,j,k}$ term, let us examine the simple heat conduction equation with constant thermal conductivity, k, constant diffusivity, $\alpha = k/\varrho c$, and no internal heat generation. Equation 1.226 can be written for the temperature at time (n+1) as

$$T^{n+1}_{i,j,k} = \frac{Fo}{1 + C \cdot Fo \cdot \eta} \sum [\eta T^{n+1}_{(,,)} + (1-\eta) T^{n}_{(,,)}] + \frac{1 - C \cdot Fo \cdot (1-\eta)}{1 + C \cdot Fo \cdot \eta} T^{n}_{i,j,k} \quad (1.229)$$

where $Fo = \alpha \Delta t / \Delta x^2$ is the Fourier number and C = 2, 4, or 6 for the one-, two-, or three-dimensional equation, respectively, and the summation term contains $T^{n+1}_{i,j,k}$ but not $T^{n}_{i,j,k}$. Designating the coefficient of $T^n_{1,j,k}$ as COEF, the following stability conditions can be identified.

COEF > 1	steady growth
0 < COEF < 1	steady decay
−1 < COEF < 0	stable oscillation
COEF < −1	unstable oscillation

Thus, the second range, from 0 to 1, is the stable one. Now let us examine briefly the development of the finite difference equations for various, common boundary conditions. Since the boundary temperatures are of great importance, it is preferable to assume that the boundary nodes are right on the surface, i.e., the dimension of the element around the boundary node perpendicular to the surface is only 1/2 of the distance between the nodes in the same direction as illustrated by $\Delta x/2$ in Fig. 1.29. As a consequence, the heat transfer areas perpendicular to the boundary and the element volume are only half that of a regular node away from the surface. Then typical boundary conditions can be formulated as follows.

1.6.2.1 Temperature Specified at the Boundary

This is the simplest case because the boundary nodes need not be calculated and they contribute only a constant term to the equation of the next node. For example, if $T_{1,j,k} = T_0$, a constant, then all $T_{2,j,k}$ node equations will contain that constant in the $T_{i-1,j,k} = T_{1,j,k} = T_0$ term.

1.6.2.2 Nonzero Heat Flux

If the heat flux, $(q/A)_w$, is given, the energy balance for the boundary node for the case when k_x, k_y, and k_z are constants becomes

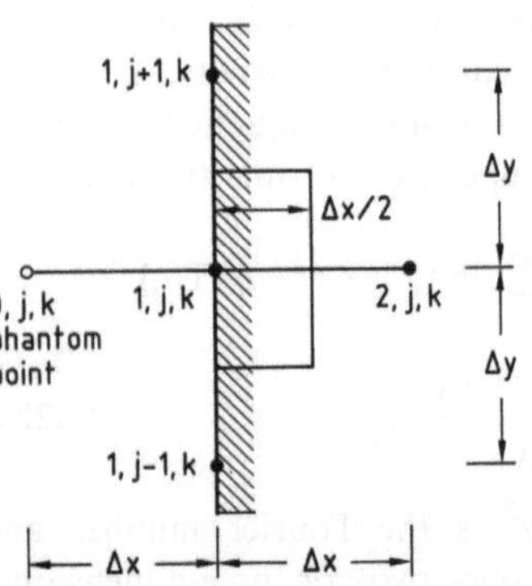

Fig. 1.29. Typical configuration of a boundary node in Cartesian coordinates

$$\varrho c \frac{\Delta x}{2} \Delta y \Delta z \frac{T^{n+1}_{1,j,k} - T^n_{1,j,k}}{\Delta t} = k_x \Delta y \Delta z \frac{T_{2,j,k} - T_{1,j,k}}{\Delta x} + k_y \frac{\Delta x}{2} \Delta z \frac{T_{1,j-1,k} - 2T_{1,j,k} + T_{1,j+1,k}}{\Delta y} + k_z \frac{\Delta x}{2} \Delta y \frac{T_{1,j,k-1} - 2T_{1,j,k} + T_{1,j,k+1}}{\Delta z} + (q/A)_w \Delta y \Delta z + q_i \frac{\Delta x}{2} \Delta y \Delta z \,. \quad (1.230)$$

No time indicator superscripts are given to the temperatures on the right-hand side to indicate a choice for the user. The equation would be most likely divided by the coefficient of the $T^{n+1}_{1,j,k}$ term to develop the working equation in terms of temperatures. If $\Delta x = \Delta y = \Delta z$, this equation is

$$T^{n+1}_{1,j,k} = \frac{2k_x \Delta t}{\varrho c \Delta x^2} T_{2,j,k} + \frac{k_y \Delta t}{\varrho c \Delta x^2} (T_{1,j-1,k} + T_{1,j+1,k}) + \frac{k_z \Delta t}{\varrho c \Delta x^2} (T_{1,j,k-1} + T_{1,j,k+1}) + T^n_{1,j,k} - \frac{2(k_x + k_y + k_z)\Delta t}{\varrho c \Delta x^2} T_{1,j,k} + \frac{2(q/A)_w \Delta t}{\varrho c \Delta x} + \frac{q_i \Delta t}{\varrho c} \,. \quad (1.230\text{a})$$

Here, again, the temperatures without superscripts will have to be defined according to Eq. 1.228.

1.6.2.3 Zero Heat Flux

The simplest and most accurate means of modeling this boundary condition is to assume the presence of a phantom node outside the boundary, as shown in Fig. 1.29, with a temperature, $T_{0,j,k}$, which is set equal to that of the node just inside the boundary, $T_{2,j,k}$. Then the equation for $T_{1,j,k}$ will have a $2T_{2,j,k}$ term in it. For example, in the two-dimensional case with constant thermal conductivities the governing equation becomes

$$\frac{\varrho c \Delta x^2}{k_x \Delta t} (T^{n+1}_{1,j} - T^n_{1,j}) = 2T_{2,j} + \frac{k_y \Delta x^2}{k_x \Delta y^2} (T_{1,j-1} + T_{1,j+1}) - \left(2 + 2\frac{k_y \Delta x^2}{k_x \Delta y^2}\right) T_{1,j} + \frac{q_i \Delta x^2}{k_x} \,. \quad (1.231)$$

It is to be noted that this relation can also be obtained without the phantom node by considering the energy balance for the half element at the boundary.

1.6.2.4 Convection

If there is convective heat transfer at the boundary, its magnitude is $h_c \Delta y \Delta z(T_\infty - T_{1,j})$ and the corresponding equation for the two-dimensional case with constant conductivities becomes

$$\frac{\varrho c \Delta x^2}{k_x \Delta t}(T_{1,j}^{n+1} - T_{1,j}^{n}) = 2T_{2,j} + \frac{k_y \Delta x^2}{k_x \Delta y^2}(T_{1,j-1} + T_{1,j+1}) - 2\left(1 + \frac{h_c \Delta x}{k_x} + \frac{k_y \Delta x^2}{k_x \Delta y^2}\right) T_{1,j} + \frac{2h_c \Delta x}{k_x} T_\infty + \frac{q_i \Delta x^2}{k_x} . \quad (1.232)$$

In curvilinear, orthogonal coordinate systems the conduction terms become more complicated because the conduction areas vary with position, such as the radius. Figure 1.30 illustrates the case for the cylindrical coordinate system. Here the radius, r_i, was assumed to be halfway between the $i-1, j, k$ and the i, j, k nodes which are separated by Δr. Then the heat conduction terms in the radial direction can be written as

$$k_{r-} \frac{T_{i-1,j,k} - T_{i,j,k}}{\Delta r} r_i \Delta \theta \Delta z + k_{r+} \frac{T_{i+1,j,k} - T_{i,j,k}}{\Delta r}(r_i + \Delta r) \Delta \theta \Delta z .$$

The radius, r_i, could also have been assumed to be at the i, j, k node, in which case the first term above would have an $(r_i - \Delta r/2)$ in it and the second term an $(r_i + \Delta r/2)$. The expression given, however, corresponds to a solution presented later in the section on thermal modeling.

In a spherical coordinate system the area varies as r^2 in the radial direction. The conduction terms have to be adjusted accordingly.

As indicated before, the solutions of these numerical equations have two major approaches, the explicit and the implicit. The explicit transient system can be solved directly, node by node, since each equation has only one unknown and, consequently, each is independent of the others. Thus, the computer program is quite simple although, because of the limitation on the time increment discussed above, it may require a very large number of time steps. It is useful to note that in many cases it is simple to obtain the steady-state solution by letting the transient program run long enough, starting from any initial temperature distribution until the changes in all temperatures become less than some arbitrarily small value relative to some characteristic temperature difference of the thermal system. This approach may be preferable to solving the matrix equation associated with the steady-state equations.

The implicit systems of equations have to be treated with matrix solution techniques usually involving matrix inversions. For details on such techniques the reader should examine a specialty book on the subject, such as Anderson et al. [1].

As an example, let us consider the square, two-dimensional body with sides L shown in Fig. 1.31. Two sides, $x = 0$ and $y = 0$, are insulated and the other two, $x = L$ and $y = L$, are at $T = T_0$. There is uniform internal heat generation, q_i. This is a typical example to be found in many texts (e.g., [54]). In the simple geometry assumed there are only for unknown temperatures, T_1, T_2, T_4, and T_5. However, there are three different size volumes associated with them. Applying the energy balances to the four volumes yields the following set of four simultaneous equations expressed in matrix notation.

$$\begin{bmatrix} 2 & -1 & -1 & 0 \\ -1 & 4 & 0 & -2 \\ -1 & 0 & 4 & -2 \\ 0 & -1 & -1 & 4 \end{bmatrix} \begin{bmatrix} T_1 \\ T_2 \\ T_4 \\ T_5 \end{bmatrix} = \begin{bmatrix} q_i L^2/8k \\ q_i L^2/4k + T_0 \\ q_i L^2/4k + T_0 \\ q_i L^2/4k + 2T_0 \end{bmatrix} \quad (1.233)$$

These equations can be solved by various methods such as the gaussian elimination or the Gauss-Seidel iteration. In the gaussian technique the square coefficient matrix is converted to an upper triangular matrix by using the first equation to convert all terms in the first column, below the diagonal, to zero; then using the second equation to convert all terms in the second column, below the diagonal, to zero, and so on. In the above equation, for example, the first equation should be divided by two and added to the second and third equations to change the two -1 values to zero in the first column. Then proceed with the second and third equations to convert the lower halves of

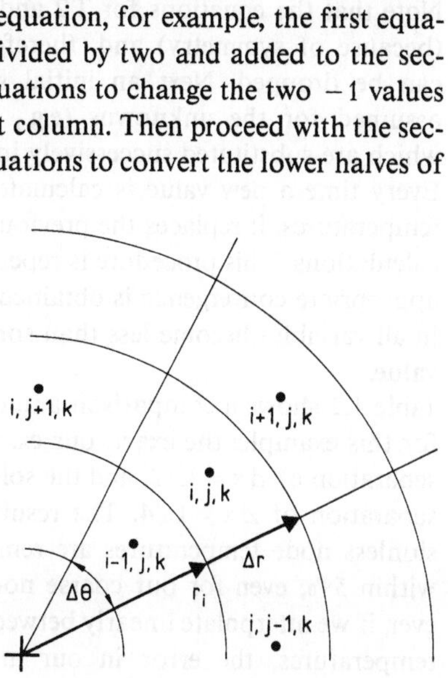

Fig. 1.30. Typical node in the cylindrical coordinate system

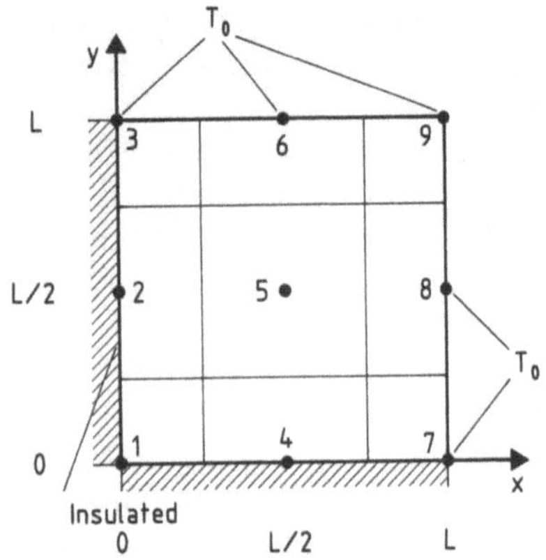

Fig. 1.31. Two-dimensional, finite difference example with internal heat generation

the second and third columns to zeros. In the end the last equation will contain only one unknown which can be found directly. This value can be substituted into the equation before the last to make it directly solvable for the next unknown. This back substitution continues until all unknowns are found.

In the Gauss-Seidel iteration method the equations are rearranged to have the diagonal terms appear by themselves on the left-hand side with all the other terms on the right-hand side. In the above example the equations become

$$T_1 = T_2/2+T_4/2+q_i L^2/16\,k \tag{1.234a}$$

$$T_2 = T_1/4+T_5/2+q_i L^2/16\,k+T_0/4 \tag{1.234b}$$

$$T_4 = T_1/4+T_5/2+q_i L^2/16\,k+T_0/4 \tag{1.234c}$$

$$T_5 = T_2/4+T_4/4+q_i L^2/16 +T_0/2\ . \tag{1.234d}$$

Note that the equations for T2 and T4 are identical (because of symmetry) and, therefore, one of them can be dropped. Next an initial set of values are assumed for the unknowns (e.g., all equal to T_0) which are substituted successively into the equations. Every time a new value is calculated for one of the temperatures, it replaces the previous value in further calculations. This procedure is repeated in order until appropriate convergence is obtained, i.e., the changes in all variables become less than some predetermined value.

Table 1.2 shows a comparison among three solutions for this example: the exact, our example with a node separation of $\Delta x = L/2$, and the solution with a node separation of $\Delta x = L/4$. The results for the dimensionless node temperatures are remarkably accurate, within 5%, even for our coarse node spacing. However, if we interpolate linearly between nodes for other temperatures, the error in our arrangement could reach above 20%, whereas it remains much smaller

Table 1.2. Comparison of three solutions for the example. The values are given for $Tk/q_i L^2$

Node No.	Exact	$\Delta x = L/2$	% Error	$\Delta x = L/4$[a]	% Error
1	0.2947	0.2813	−4.55	0.2911	−1.22
2 and 4	0.2293	0.2188	−4.58	0.2266	−1.18
5	0.1811	0.1719	−5.08	0.1787	−1.33

[a] From [54]

with $\Delta x = L/4$. This is to be expected because finer divisions generally produce more accurate results. Another approach, the use of a "spreadsheet" program, will also be discussed here because it is rather easy to set up for two-dimensional problems if the equations are simple, such as when the material properties are constant [31]. Spreadsheets are programmed internally to calculate the value at a position based on the values of any combination of other positions which can be specified relative to the position itself. These relative expressions can be quickly and automatically copied to all positions with the same type of governing equation by identifying the field of positions and specifying that the copying be done in a relative mode. As an example let us consider the internal nodes in a two-dimensional, rectangular body in the solution of a steady-state heat conduction problem with constant properties and constant internal heat generation. The equation for a typical node internal to the body is

$$T_{i,j} = (T_{i-1,j}+T_{i+1,j}+T_{i,j-1}-T_{i,j+1})/4 + q_i \Delta x^2/4k\ . \tag{1.235}$$

In a spreadsheet program the positions may be identified by lettered columns and numbered rows. Thus, the first internal position may be **B2**. Defining the entire heat generation term as Q, the following expression has to be typed in the proper space for position B2

$$\text{T at B2 (not typed)} = (\text{B1}+\text{B3}+\text{A2}+\text{C2})/4 + \text{Q (a number)}\ . \tag{1.236}$$

Now the field with identical type equations has to be identified, the copying instruction in the relative mode given, and the programming for these positions is finished. The boundary positions can be handled in a similar fashion with the appropriate equations. For example, if the boundary represented by the first row is at a constant temperature, T_0, one can start at position A1 by typing the value T_0. Next the first row up to the column representing the right boundary has to be identified and the copying instruction given. Since the expression is a constant it does not matter if the copying is done in the relative or absolute mode.

1.6.3 Finite Element Method

1.6.3.1 Derivation of the Governing Equations

In contrast to the finite difference technique, the finite element method is based on the calculus of variations. The relevant aspects can be summarized as follows using a one-dimensional example.
Let us find the function u(x) which minimizes the integral

$$I = \int_{x=0}^{L} F(x, u, u')\,dx \tag{1.237}$$

where $u' = du/dx$. Now let $u(0) = u_0$ and $u(L) = u_L$ and define a complete set of functions

$$\hat{u}(x, \varepsilon) = u(x) + \varepsilon\eta(x) \tag{1.238}$$

where we define $\eta(0) = 0$ and $\eta(L) = 0$ and, thus, satisfy the boundary conditions. From Eq. 1.238 we can see that $\hat{u}(x, 0) = u(x)$. Now let

$$I(\varepsilon) = \int_{0}^{L} F(x, \hat{u}, \hat{u}')\,dx\ , \tag{1.239}$$

To minimize the integral we simply take the derivative and set it equal to zero.

$$\frac{dI(\varepsilon)}{d\varepsilon} = \int_0^L \frac{\partial}{\partial\varepsilon} F(x, \hat{u}, \hat{u}')\,dx = \int_0^L \left[\frac{\partial F}{\partial \hat{u}}\frac{\partial \hat{u}}{\partial \varepsilon} + \frac{\partial F}{\partial \hat{u}'}\frac{\partial \hat{u}'}{\partial \varepsilon}\right] dx$$

$$= \int_0^L \left[\frac{\partial F}{\partial \hat{u}}\eta + \frac{\partial F}{\partial \hat{u}'}\frac{d\eta}{dx}\right] dx = 0\ . \tag{1.240}$$

The second term in the brackets can be integrated by parts to yield

$$\frac{dI(\varepsilon)}{d\varepsilon} = \int_0^L \eta \left[\frac{\partial F}{\partial \hat{u}} - \frac{d}{dx}\left(\frac{\partial F}{\partial \hat{u}'}\right)\right] dx = 0\ . \tag{1.241}$$

Therefore minimization requires that the expression in the brackets be zero. Now if we let ε go to zero, $\hat{u} = u$, and we obtain the differential equation which corresponds to the minimization of the integral

$$\frac{\partial F}{\partial u} - \frac{d}{dx}\left(\frac{\partial F}{\partial u'}\right) = 0\ . \tag{1.242}$$

This expression is called the Euler-Lagrange equation. Let us examine the one-dimensional heat conduction equation for a fin-type structure as shown in Fig. 1.32. Heat is transferred between the fin and the surrounding fluid across a perimeter, P, and internal heat generation in the material is also included

$$h_c P T - q_i A - \frac{d}{dx}\left(kA\frac{dT}{dx}\right) = h_c P T$$

$$-q_i A - \frac{d}{dx}(kAT') = 0\ . \tag{1.243}$$

The temperature, T, here is relative to the temperature of the surrounding fluid, T_∞, i.e., $T = T_{actual} - T_\infty$. Comparing Eqs. 1.242 and 1.243 reveals that in the heat conduction equation $u = T$ and $u' = T'$. Therefore,

$$\frac{\partial F}{\partial T} = h_c P T - q_i A \tag{1.244a}$$

$$\frac{\partial F}{\partial T'} = kAT'\ . \tag{1.244b}$$

Integrating both equations yields

$$F = 0.5 h_c P T^2 - q_i A T + f(T') \tag{1.245a}$$

$$F = 0.5 k A T'^2 + g(T)\ . \tag{1.245b}$$

Comparing these two equations leads us to the conclusion that

$$F(x, T, T') = 0.5(kAT'^2 + h_c P T^2) - q_i A T\ . \tag{1.246}$$

Thus the solution of the differential equation is equivalent to minimizing the integral of Eq. 1.237 with F given by Eq. 1.246. Although we are using a fin example to illustrate the method in a one-dimensional model, it should be noted that if the convective coefficient $h_c P$ is replaced by the blood perfusion term $m_b c_b$ and the reference temperature is taken as the arterial temperature, then we have the bioheat equation.

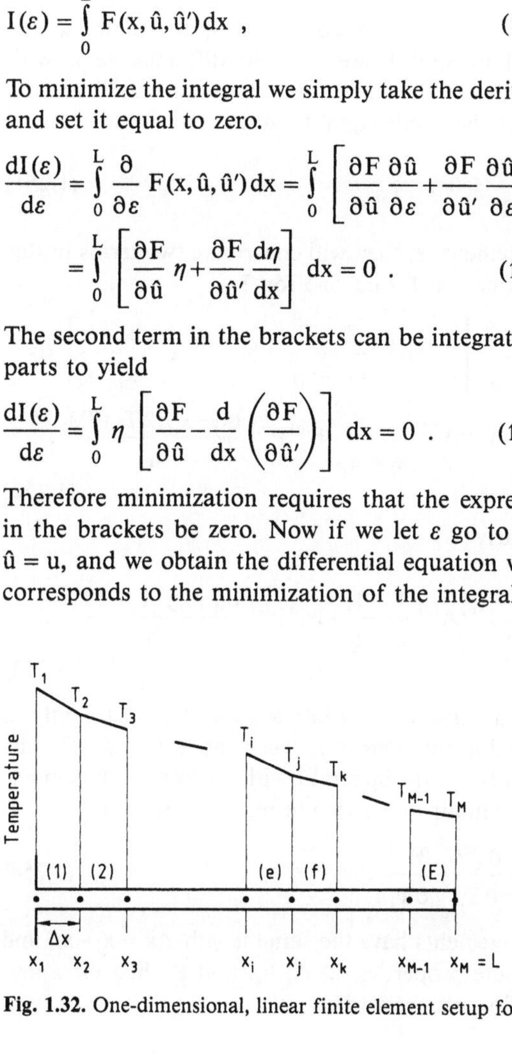

Fig. 1.32. One-dimensional, linear finite element setup for a fin

1.6.3.2 Boundary Conditions

Specified temperatures on any boundary can be handled directly by the above equations by simply substituting the known values into the appropriate equations. Based on the variational principles, expressions can be derived for the heat transferred at boundaries with specified heat flux, with convection, or with radiation. Actually, we already have the basic concept expressed in Eqs. 1.244a and 1.246. The former represents heat quantities (other than conduction) leaving the differential element and the latter results, in part, from the integration of these heat quantities with respect to the temperature difference, T. Thus we can directly modify Eq. 1.237 by adding the temperature integrals obtained from the boundary conditions for convection on S_c, specified conduction on S_{cd}, and radiation on S_r

$$\frac{1}{2}\int_{S_c} h_c T^2 dS - \int_{S_{cd}} (q/A)_{in} T\, dS + \int_{S_r} \left[\frac{1}{5}\sigma\varepsilon_r (T+T_0)^5 - \alpha_r q_r T\right] dS \; .$$

It is to be emphasized again that T represents a temperature difference with respect to T_0, which must be in absolute temperature units (Kelvin). q_r is the radiation energy flux incident on the surface S_r.

1.6.3.3 Transient Model

The transient term in the heat conduction equation can be handled similarly to the boundary conditions. Thus the additional integral in Eq. 1.237 becomes

$$+\frac{1}{2}\int_0^L \varrho c \frac{\partial (T^2)}{\partial t} dx \; .$$

Now the one-dimensional heat conduction equation 1.237 can be written in its complete form as

$$\begin{aligned} I = & \int_0^L \left[\frac{1}{2}(kAT'^2 + h_c P T^2) - q_i A T\right] dx \\ & + \frac{1}{2}\int_{S_c} h_c T^2 dS - \int_{S_{cd}} (q/A)_{in} T\, dS \\ & + \int_{S_r} \left[\frac{1}{5}\sigma\varepsilon_r (T+T_0)^5 - \alpha_r q_r T\right] dS \\ & + \frac{1}{2}\int_0^L \varrho c \frac{\partial (T^2)}{\partial t} dx \; . \end{aligned} \tag{1.237a}$$

1.6.3.4 Linear Approximation

Figure 1.32 shows the setup for a one-dimensional fin problem without internal heat generation. It was assumed that the temperature distribution within each element is linear and, therefore, can be characterized by the two end temperatures. Thus, for the element (e) the temperature at any point can be expressed as

$$T^{(e)} = \frac{T_i(x_j - x) + T_j(x - x_i)}{x_j - x_i} \tag{1.247}$$

and

$$\frac{dT^{(e)}}{dx} = \frac{T_j - T_i}{x_j - x_i} \; . \tag{1.248}$$

The integral to be minimized was derived earlier

$$I = \frac{1}{2}\int_0^L \left[kA\left(\frac{dT}{dx}\right)^2 + h_c P T^2\right] dx$$

also

$$I = \sum_{e=1}^{E} I^{(e)} \; . \tag{1.249}$$

Therefore, we can deal with the individual integrals pertaining to each element, such as (e)

$$I^{(e)} = \frac{1}{2}\int_{x_i}^{x_j} \left[k^{(e)}A^{(e)}\left(\frac{T_j - T_i}{x_j - x_i}\right)^2 + h_c^{(e)} P^{(e)} (T^{(e)})^2\right] dx \tag{1.250}$$

where $T^{(e)}$ is given above. Now, to minimize the overall integral I, we need to differentiate it with respect to all the end temperatures, such as T_i and T_j, and set the result equal to zero

$$\sum_{i=1}^{M} \frac{\partial I}{\partial T_i} = 0 \; . \tag{1.251}$$

The element (e) then will contribute two terms to this sum: one for T_i and one for T_j

$$\begin{aligned} \frac{\partial I^{(e)}}{\partial T_i} & = \int_{x_i}^{x_j} \left[k^{(e)}A^{(e)} \frac{T_i - T_j}{(x_j - x_i)^2} + h_c^{(e)} P^{(e)} T^{(e)} \frac{x_j - x}{x_j - x_i}\right] dx \\ & = k^{(e)}A^{(e)} \frac{T_i - T_j}{x_j - x_i} + h_c^{(e)} P^{(e)} \frac{(x_j - x_i)(2T_i + T_j)}{6} \; . \end{aligned} \tag{1.252}$$

Similarly

$$\frac{\partial I^{(e)}}{\partial T_j} = k^{(e)}A^{(e)} \frac{T_j - T_i}{x_j - x_i} + h_c^{(e)} P^{(e)} \frac{(x_j - x_i)(T_i + 2T_j)}{6} \; . \tag{1.253}$$

Since an end temperature, such as T_j, occurs only in two adjacent elements, such as (e) and (f), the derivative of the integral I with respect to any temperature contains only two terms. For example,

$$\frac{\partial I}{\partial T_j} = \frac{\partial I^{(e)}}{\partial T_j} + \frac{\partial I^{(f)}}{\partial T_j} \; . \tag{1.254}$$

If all elements have the same length $\Delta x = x_j - x_i$, and the same properties, k, A, h_c, and P, then the above equation can be written as

$$\frac{\partial I}{\partial T_j} = kA\,\frac{-T_i+2T_j-T_k}{\Delta x} + h_c P\,\frac{\Delta x(T_i+4T_j+T_k)}{6} = 0\ . \qquad (1.255)$$

If we rearrange the equation and define

$$D = \frac{12+4h_cP\Delta x^2/kA}{6-h_cP\Delta x^2/kA} \qquad (1.256)$$

then the governing equation for each derivative, $\partial I/\partial T_j$, becomes simply

$$-T_i+DT_j-T_k = 0\ . \qquad (1.257)$$

This expression can be easily modified for various boundary conditions. For example, if $T_1 = T_0$, a constant, then the equation for T_2 is

$$DT_2-T_3 = T_0\ . \qquad (1.258)$$

If at the outer edge at T_M the fin is insulated, i.e., there is no heat flow, then, as was discussed earlier, we can assume a phantom temperature point $T_{M+1} = T_{M-1}$ (see Fig. 1.29). Thus the equation for T_M becomes

$$-2T_{M-1}+DT_M = 0\ . \qquad (1.259)$$

If there is convective heat transfer at the outer edge, then the derivative of the convective boundary integral in Eq. 1.237a with respect to T_M yields an additional term, $h_cA_MT_M$, in the equation for T_M, which becomes

$$-T_{M-1}+\frac{6+2h_cP\Delta x^2/kA+6h_cA_M\Delta x/kA}{6-h_cP\Delta x^2/kA}T_M = 0\ . \qquad (1.260)$$

Thus we have a set of M simultaneous equations, each containing only three terms; except for the first equation, which is only a constant ($T_1 = T_0$), and the second and last equations with only two terms. Such a set of equations can be expressed in terms of a tri-diagonal matrix and can be solved by simple methods, such as the Thomas algorithm.
If the properties vary along the length of the fin, then Eq. 1.254 will become

$$\frac{\partial I}{\partial T_j} = \frac{k^{(e)}A^{(e)}}{\Delta x}(T_j-T_i)+\frac{k^{(e)}A^{(f)}}{\Delta x}(T_j-T_k) + \frac{h_c^{(e)}P^{(e)}\Delta x}{6}(T_i+2T_j) + \frac{h_c^{(f)}P^{(f)}\Delta x}{6}(2T_j+T_k) = 0\ . \qquad (1.261)$$

Collecting the coefficients of the temperatures yields the general expression

$$-\left[\frac{k^{(e)}A^{(e)}}{\Delta x}-\frac{h_c^{(e)}P^{(e)}\Delta x}{6}\right]T_i + \left[\frac{k^{(e)}A^{(e)}}{\Delta x}+\frac{k^{(f)}A^{(f)}}{\Delta x}+\frac{h_c^{(e)}P^{(e)}\Delta x}{3}+\frac{h_c^{(f)}P^{(f)}\Delta x}{3}\right]T_j - \left[\frac{k^{(f)}A^{(f)}}{\Delta x}-\frac{h_c^{(f)}P^{(f)}\Delta x}{6}\right]T_k = 0\ . \qquad (1.262)$$

The resulting set of equations can still be represented by a tri-diagonal matrix, as before.
The total heat transferred at the base, $x = 0$, can be estimated in two ways: by integrating the convective heat transfer along the length or by calculating the heat conducted through the base.

$$q_0 = \int_0^L h_cPT\,dx = \sum_1^E \int_{x_i}^{x_j} h_c^{(e)}P^{(e)}\frac{T_i(x_j-x)+T_j(x-x_i)}{\Delta x}dx + h_cA_MT_M = \sum_{e=1}^{E} h_c^{(e)}P^{(e)}\Delta x\frac{T_i+T_j}{2}+h_cA_MT_M \qquad (1.263\,a)$$

or approximately

$$q_0 \cong k^{(1)}A^{(1)}\frac{T_1-T_2}{\Delta x}\ . \qquad (1.263\,b)$$

1.6.3.5 Quadratic Approximation

In the derivations above we assumed a linear approximation of the temperature function within each element. If the boundaries of the temperature field have strong curvatures then a higher order approximation can give better results with fewer nodes because these curvilinear approximations can follow the curved contours of the boundaries more accurately. In most cases, however, a quadratic approximation is quite satisfactory and going to higher orders is not only more complicated but could also produce less accurate results.
The quadratic finite element setup for the previous one-dimensional problem is shown in Fig. 1.33. The element (e) now contains three temperatures, T_i, T_j, T_k, instead of two. The temperature in the element is given by the following equation

$$T^{(e)} = C_0^{(e)}+C_1^{(e)}x+C_2^{(e)}x^2\ . \qquad (1.264)$$

The coefficients can be evaluated in terms of the three temperatures

$$T_i = C_0+C_1x_i+C_2x_i^2 \qquad (1.265\,a)$$

$$T_j = C_0+C_1x_j+C_2x_j^2 \qquad (1.265\,b)$$

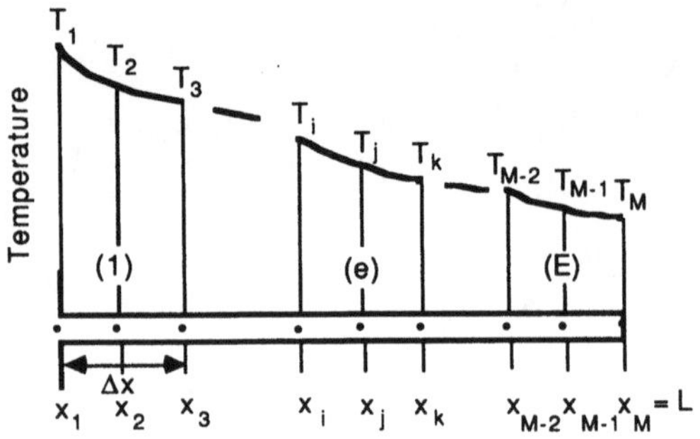

Fig. 1.33. One-dimensional, quadratic finite element setup for a fin

$$T_k = C_0 + C_1 x_k + C_2 x_k^2 \ . \tag{1.265 c}$$

In determinant form define

$$|D| = \begin{vmatrix} 1 & x_i & x_i^2 \\ 1 & x_j & x_j^2 \\ 1 & x_k & x_k^2 \end{vmatrix} \tag{1.266}$$

Then, again in determinant from, the coefficients become

$$C_0 = \begin{vmatrix} T_i & x_i & x_i^2 \\ T_j & x_j & x_j^2 \\ T_k & x_k & x_k^2 \end{vmatrix} / |D| \tag{1.267 a}$$

$$C_1 = \begin{vmatrix} 1 & T_i & x_i^2 \\ 1 & T_j & x_j^2 \\ 1 & T_k & x_k^2 \end{vmatrix} / |D| \tag{1.267 b}$$

$$C_2 = \begin{vmatrix} 1 & x_i & T_i \\ 1 & x_j & T_j \\ 1 & x_k & T_k \end{vmatrix} / |D| \ . \tag{1.267 c}$$

As an example let us consider the first element with the boundary condition that the heat flux $(q/A)_1$ is specified at the left end, i.e., at point $1\,(x = 0)$. To make the example more general, let us also include the volumetric heat generation term, q_i. Designate the length of the element (from 1 to 3) as Δx. The temperature in the element is

$$T = T_1 + C_1 x + C_2 x^2 \tag{1.268}$$

then

$$T_2 = T_1 + C_1 \Delta x/2 + C_2 \Delta x^2/4 \tag{1.269}$$

$$T_3 = T_1 + C_1 \Delta x + C_2 \Delta x^2 \ . \tag{1.270}$$

Solving these two equations for the coefficients yields

$$\begin{aligned} T &= T_1 - \frac{x}{\Delta x}(3T_1 - 4T_2 + T_3) + \frac{2x^2}{\Delta x^2}(T_1 - 2T_2 + T_3) \\ &= \left(1 - \frac{3x}{\Delta x} + \frac{2x^2}{\Delta x^2}\right) T_1 + \left(\frac{4x}{\Delta x} - \frac{4x^2}{\Delta x^2}\right) T_2 \\ &\quad - \left(\frac{x}{\Delta x} - \frac{2x^2}{\Delta x^2}\right) T_3 \ . \end{aligned} \tag{1.271}$$

Consequently,

$$\begin{aligned} \frac{dT}{dx} &= -\frac{3T_1 - 4T_2 + T_3}{\Delta x} + \frac{4x}{\Delta x^2}(T_1 - 2T_2 + T_3) \\ &= -\left(\frac{3}{\Delta x} - \frac{4x}{\Delta x^4}\right) T_1 + \left(\frac{4x}{\Delta x} - \frac{8x}{\Delta x^2}\right) T_2 \\ &\quad - \left(\frac{1}{\Delta x} - \frac{4x}{\Delta x^2}\right) T_3 \ . \end{aligned} \tag{1.272}$$

Although Eq. 1.271 can be solved as one of a set of simultaneous equations, it is instructive to solve for the temperature distribution in this first element by applying the energy balance to it. The various energy terms are as follows.

Conduction at $x = 0$:

$$-kA(dT/dx)|_{x=0} = (q/A)_1 A \quad \text{entering}$$

This condition can be satisfied by setting the coefficient of x in Eq. 1.271 which is also the constant term in Eq. 1.272, $(3T_1 - 4T_2 + T_3)/\Delta x$ equal to $(q/A)_1/k$. Then,

Conduction at $x = \Delta x$:

$$-k\frac{dT}{dx}A = (q/A)_1 A - \frac{4kA(T_1 - 2T_2 + T_3)}{\Delta x} \quad \text{leaving}$$

Convection:

$$\int_0^{\Delta x} h_c P \left[T_1 - \frac{(q/A)_1}{k} x + \frac{2(T_1 - 2T_2 + T_3)}{\Delta x^2} x^2\right] dx$$

$$= h_c P \left[T_1 \Delta x - \frac{(q/A)_1}{2k} \Delta x^2 + \frac{2(T_1 - 2T_2 + T_3)}{3} \Delta x\right] \quad \text{leaving}$$

Internal heat generated: $q_i A \Delta x$ entering.

For steady state the entering heat quantities have to be set equal to the leaving ones and the resulting equation can be solved for the coefficient of the quadratic term, x^2, in Eq. 1.271 for the temperature. Thus,

$$T = T_1 - \frac{(q/A)_1}{k} x - \frac{q_i A - h_c P \left(T_1 - \dfrac{(q/A)_1 \Delta x}{2k}\right)}{2kA - h_c P \Delta x^2/3} x^2 \ . \tag{1.273}$$

Note that in the linear model only the first two terms exist and, consequently, if we tried to apply this method, the temperature at the end of the first element, $x = \Delta x$, could be in error, unless the heat flux boundary condition, $(q/A)_1$, is modified with convective and heat generation terms, or Δx is made sufficiently small to minimize the error.

1.6.3.6 Two-Dimensional Steady-State Model

Equation 1.243 can be easily modified to include conduction in the y direction and convection on one (P = 1) or both (P = 2) $\Delta x-\Delta y$ surfaces.

$$h_c P T - q_i - \frac{\partial}{\partial x}\left(k_x \frac{\partial T}{\partial x}\right) - \frac{\partial}{\partial y}\left(k_y \frac{\partial T}{\partial y}\right) = 0 \; . \tag{1.274}$$

The integral to be minimized now becomes

$$I = \int_0^{L_1}\int_0^{L_2} F(T, T_x, T_y, x, y)\,dx\,dy \tag{1.275}$$

where the x and y subscripts indicate differentiation with respect to the variable in the subscript. The new Euler's equation can be derived similarly as before to yield

$$\frac{\partial F}{\partial T} - \frac{\partial}{\partial x}\left(\frac{\partial F}{\partial T_x}\right) - \frac{\partial}{\partial y}\left(\frac{\partial F}{\partial T_y}\right) = 0 \; . \tag{1.276}$$

Again proceeding as before we can obtain the working form of the minimization integral

$$I = \int_0^{L_1}\int_0^{L_2} \left[\frac{1}{2}(k_x T_x^2 + k_y T_y^2 + h_c P T^2) - q_i A T\right] dx\,dy$$

+boundary and heat capacitance integrals from Eq. 1.237a . (1.277)

This integral can be applied to each element. Then, the integral for the entire temperature field becomes the sum of all the integrals for the elements

$$I = \sum I^{(e)} \; . \tag{1.278}$$

To minimize this integral, its derivatives with respect to all node temperatures have to be set equal to zero

$$\sum_e \sum_j \frac{\partial I^{(e)}}{\partial T_j} = 0 \; . \tag{1.279}$$

The summation with respect to the elements (e) will involve two or more elements, depending on the geometry. The temperature T_j occurs in six of the

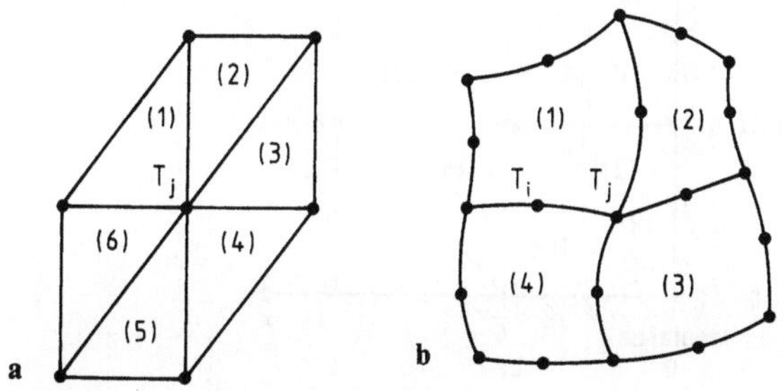

Fig. 1.34a, b. Typical geometries for nodes and elements. **a** Linear elements; **b** quadratic elements

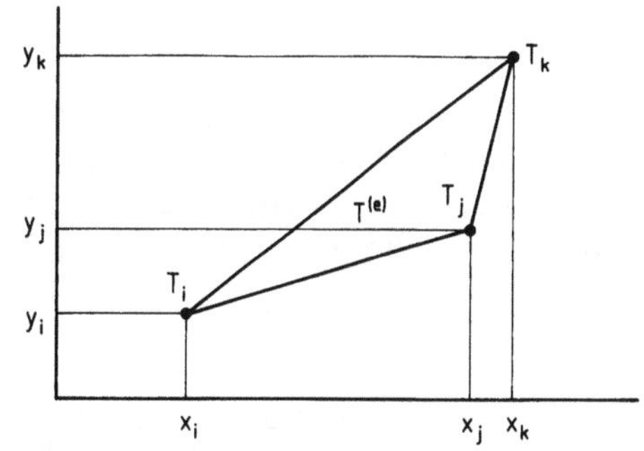

Fig. 1.35. Finite element arrangement for sample problem

linear, triangular elements of Fig. 1.34a and it occurs in four of the quadratic, four-sided elements of Fig. 1.34b. On the other hand, T_i occurs only in two of these elements.

1.6.3.7 Linear Triangular Elements

These are the simplest and most often used elements. A typical configuration is shown in Fig. 1.35. The temperature inside the triangle can be expressed as

$$T^{(e)} = C_0^{(e)} + C_1^{(e)} x + C_2^{(e)} y \; . \tag{1.280}$$

The three coefficients can be evaluated in terms of the three nodal temperatures and the nodal coordinates. The resulting expression in matrix form is

$$T^{(e)} = \frac{[1\,x\,y]}{x_{ij}y_{jk} - x_{jk}y_{ij}} \tag{1.281}$$

$$\times \begin{bmatrix} x_j y_k - x_k y_j & x_k y_i - x_i y_k & x_i y_j - x_j y_i \\ -y_{jk} & y_{ik} & -y_{ij} \\ x_{jk} & -x_{ik} & x_{ij} \end{bmatrix} \begin{bmatrix} T_i \\ T_j \\ T_k \end{bmatrix}$$

where the double subscript indicates the distance between the corresponding coordinates. For example, $x_{ij} = x_j - x_i$.

Let us examine the development of the set of simultaneous, linear equations by outlining the major steps for a two-dimensional conduction problem with internal heat generation. Details of such derivations can be found in texts dealing with finite element methods, such as Myers [54] or Huebner and Thornton [40]. Dividing Eq. 1.277 into two separate integrals, one for the conduction term and one for the internal heat generation, and applying these to the element (e), we obtain

$$I_{cd}^{(e)} = \frac{k^{(e)}}{2} \iint_{A^{(e)}} (T_x^{(e)2} + T_y^{(e)2})\,dx\,dy \tag{1.282}$$

and

$$I_q^{(e)} = q_i^{(e)} \iint_{A^{(e)}} T^{(e)} dx\,dy \qquad (1.283)$$

where $q_i^{(e)}$ is assumed to be constant over the area of the element. The derivative of the conduction integral with respect to the temperatures can be written in matrix form as (for details see e.g. [54]).

$$\frac{dI_{cd}}{dT} = \sum_e \frac{dI_{cd}^{(e)}}{dT^{(e)}} = \mathbf{KT}$$

$$= \sum_e \frac{k^{(e)}}{4A^{(e)}} \begin{bmatrix} x_{jk}^2+y_{jk}^2 & -(x_{ik}x_{jk}+y_{ik}y_{jk}) & x_{ij}x_{jk}+y_{ij}y_{jk} \\ \text{sym} & x_{ik}^2+y_{ik}^2 & -(x_{ij}x_{ik}+y_{ij}y_{ik}) \\ \text{sym} & \text{sym} & x_{ij}^2+y_{ij}^2 \end{bmatrix} \begin{bmatrix} T_i \\ T_j \\ T_k \end{bmatrix} \qquad (1.284)$$

where "sym" means symmetrical term. The bold letter **T** represents the column matrix for the temperatures. The area, $A^{(e)}$, can be shown to be the positive value

$$A^{(e)} = |x_{ij}y_{jk} - x_{jk}y_{ij}|/2 \ . \qquad (1.285)$$

The square matrix **K** is built up of the terms of the typical matrix shown in Eq. 1.284. For example the term in the i-th row and i-th column is

$$\frac{k^{(e)}(x_{jk}^2+y_{jk}^2)}{4A^{(e)}}$$

whereas the term in the k-th row and j-th column is

$$-\frac{k^{(e)}(x_{ij}x_{ik}+y_{ij}y_{ik})}{4A^{(e)}} \ .$$

The derivative of the integral for internal heat generation can be derived in matrix form also

$$\frac{dI_q}{dT} = \sum_e \frac{dI_q^{(e)}}{dT^{(e)}} = Q = \sum_e \frac{q_i^{(e)}A^{(e)}}{3} \begin{bmatrix} 1 \\ 1 \\ 1 \end{bmatrix} \ . \qquad (1.286)$$

Similar expressions can be derived for other energy terms such as Pennes' blood perfusion or convective heat transfer at the surface of the elements.
We can now combine these derivatives into a single expression which then has to be set equal to zero to obtain the final set of governing equations.

$$\frac{dI}{dT} = \mathbf{KT} - \mathbf{Q} = 0 \quad \text{or} \quad \mathbf{KT} = \mathbf{Q} \ . \qquad (1.287)$$

Let us consider again the square, two-dimensional body with sides L shown in Fig. 1.36. As in the finite difference example, two sides, $x = 0$ and $y = 0$, are insulated and the other two, $x = L$ and $y = L$, are at $T = T_0$; and there is uniform internal heat generation, q_i. The element and node numbering is shown on the figure. The coordinates can be read directly from the sketch. Let us look at the first element to develop the equations. The geometric characteristics are:

i = node 1	j = node 4	k = node 5
$x_{ij} = L/2$	$x_{ik} = L/2$	$x_{jk} = 0$
$y_{ij} = 0$	$y_{ik} = L/2$	$y_{jk} = L/2$
$A^{(1)} = L^2/8$	$k(1)/4A^{(1)} = 2k/L^2$	

Then the $\mathbf{K}^{(1)}$ matrix, representing the 1st, 4th, and 5th rows and columns in the global matrix **K**, becomes

Column no. 1 4 5 Row no.

$$\mathbf{K}^{(1)} = \frac{k}{2} \begin{bmatrix} 1 & -1 & 0 \\ \text{sym} & 2 & -1 \\ \text{sym} & \text{sym} & 1 \end{bmatrix} \begin{matrix} 1 \\ 4 \\ 5 \end{matrix} \ . \qquad (1.288)$$

The symmetry is indicated to show that the computer does not have to store these values separately. Similarly, the $\mathbf{K}^{(2)}$ matrix, representing the 1st, 2nd, and 5th rows and columns in the global matrix, looks identical to $\mathbf{K}^{(1)}$ above except that the values have to be added at different places in the global matrix. Designating places in the matrices as (row, column), we can see that, because elements (1) and (2) share nodes 1 and 5, the values in $\mathbf{K}^{(1)}$ and $\mathbf{K}^{(2)}$ at points (1,1), (1,5) = (5,1), and (5,5) should be added, whereas the values at the other points remain as they were in the individual matrices. Thus, the combined matrix becomes

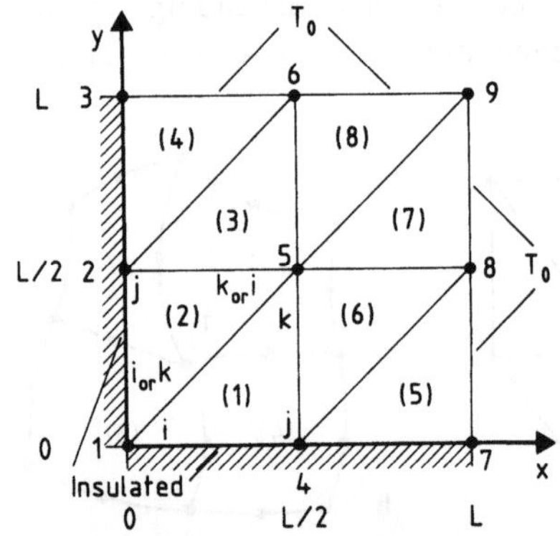

Fig. 1.36. Two-dimensional finite element example with internal heat generation

$$\begin{array}{l} \text{Column no.} \quad 1 \quad 2 \quad 4 \quad 5 \qquad \text{Row no.} \\ \mathbf{K}^{(1)}+\mathbf{K}^{(2)}=\frac{k}{2}\begin{bmatrix} 1+1=2 & -1 & -1 & 0+0=0 \\ \text{sym} & 2 & \text{blank} & -1 \\ \text{sym} & \text{sym} & 2 & -1 \\ \text{sym} & \text{sym} & \text{sym} & 1+1=2 \end{bmatrix} \begin{array}{c} 1 \\ 2 \\ 4 \\ 5 \end{array} . \end{array} \tag{1.289}$$

This process is repeated for all elements to fill up the global **K** matrix which becomes

$$\mathbf{K}=\frac{k}{2}\begin{bmatrix} 2 & -1 & 0 & -1 & & & & & \\ -1 & 4 & -1 & 0 & -2 & & & & \\ 0 & -1 & 2 & 0 & 0 & -1 & & & \\ -1 & 0 & 0 & 4 & -2 & 0 & -1 & & \\ & -2 & 0 & -2 & 8 & -2 & 0 & -2 & \\ & & -1 & 0 & -2 & 4 & 0 & 0 & -1 \\ & & & -1 & 0 & 0 & 2 & -1 & 0 \\ & & & & -2 & 0 & -1 & 4 & -1 \\ & & & & & -1 & 0 & -1 & 2 \end{bmatrix} . \tag{1.290}$$

The **Q** matrix can be quite easily constructed from Eq. 1.286, even if the $q_i^{(e)}$s are different for each element. However, if they are all equal, then in the column matrix 1 is added in each line for each element which contains the particular node. Thus

$$\mathbf{Q}=\frac{q_i L^2}{24}\begin{bmatrix} 2 \\ 3 \\ 1 \\ 3 \\ 6 \\ 3 \\ 1 \\ 3 \\ 2 \end{bmatrix} . \tag{1.291}$$

We still have to satisfy the boundary conditions where T_0 is specified. The insulated boundaries have been taken care of already by not having any heat fluxes specified. One way to take care of the given temperatures, in this case $T_3 = T_6 = T_7 = T_8 = T_9 = T_0$, is to substitute them into the equations, i.e., matrix rows, for the rest of the temperatures and transfer the resulting constant terms to the right-hand side. Then simply delete all rows and columns with the same numbers as the known temperatures. The resulting matrix equation is

$$\begin{bmatrix} 2 & -1 & -1 & 0 \\ -1 & 4 & 0 & -2 \\ -1 & 0 & 4 & -2 \\ 0 & -2 & -2 & 8 \end{bmatrix}\begin{bmatrix} T_1 \\ T_2 \\ T_4 \\ T_5 \end{bmatrix} = \begin{bmatrix} q_i L^2/6k \\ q_i L^2/4k+T_0 \\ q_i L^2/4k+T_0 \\ q_i L^2/2k+4T_0 \end{bmatrix} \tag{1.292}$$

In most cases an additional simplification can be made by letting $T_0 = 0$. In some computer programs it may be easier not to delete the rows and columns pertaining to the known temperatures but to leave the equivalent of the identity $T_i = T_0$ in the matrix, i.e., the i-th row and column will have zeros everywhere except at their intersection, where a 1 is placed. Table 1.3 shows the solution of Eq. 1.292 with $T_0 = 0$, together with the exact values and those of the corresponding finite difference scheme from Table 1.2. The results of the finite element technique are slightly worse for point 1 but are better than those of the finite difference scheme for the other points. It is important to note that if the diagonal lines in Fig. 1.36 are changed by 90°, the results would be different.

Table 1.3. Comparison of three solutions for the example. The values are given for $Tk/q_i L^2$

Node No.	Exact	Finite difference		Finite element	
		$\Delta x = L/2$	% Error	$\Delta x = L/2$	% Error
1	0.2947	0.2813	−4.55	0.3125	+6.04
2 and 4	0.2293	0.2188	−4.58	0.2292	−0.04
5	0.1811	0.1719	−5.08	0.1771	−2.21

1.6.3.8 Transient Case

We can apply the linear temperature assumption of Eq. 1.247 to the transient integral term of Eq. 1.237a and take the derivative with respect to the nodal temperatures to obtain for the one-dimensional element with unit area perpendicular to the heat flow

$$\frac{dI_c^{(e)}}{d\mathbf{T}^{(e)}}=\frac{(\varrho c)^{(e)} x_{ij}}{6}\begin{bmatrix} 2 & 1 \\ 1 & 2 \end{bmatrix}\begin{bmatrix} \partial T_i/\partial t \\ \partial T_j/\partial t \end{bmatrix}=\mathbf{C}^{(e)}\frac{\partial \mathbf{T}^{(e)}}{\partial t} \tag{1.293}$$

where $\mathbf{C}^{(e)}$ is the elemental capacitance matrix. The global capacitance matrix, **C**, can be built up exactly the same way as the conduction matrix, **K**, was developed before. Then a typical global capacitance term, with identical values of $\varrho c x_{ij} = \varrho c \Delta x$ for all elements, becomes

$$\frac{dl_c}{dT} = \frac{\varrho c \Delta x}{6} \begin{bmatrix} 2 & 1 & . & & & \\ 1 & 4 & 1 & . & . & \\ . & . & . & . & . & . \\ & . & . & 1 & 4 & 1 \\ & . & . & . & 1 & 2 \end{bmatrix} \begin{bmatrix} T_n^{n+1} - T_1^n \\ T_2^{n+1} - T_2^n \\ \cdots \\ T_{M-1}^{n+1} - T_{M-1}^n \\ T_M^{n+1} - T_M^n \end{bmatrix} / \Delta t$$

$$= \mathbf{C}(\partial \mathbf{T}/\partial t) \; . \tag{1.294}$$

The two-dimensional element of thickness 1 can be handled in a similar way. The resulting capacitance matrix is

$$\mathbf{C}^{(e)} = \frac{(\varrho c A 1)^{(e)}}{12} \begin{bmatrix} 2 & 1 & 1 \\ 1 & 2 & 1 \\ 1 & 1 & 2 \end{bmatrix} \; . \tag{1.295}$$

The elemental capacitances have to be combined to form the global capacitance **C**. When this term, multiplied by the temperature derivative matrix, is added to the other derivative terms, e.g., the conduction term, **KT**, and then the sum is set equal to zero, we obtain the final set of working equations. These have to be solved by using any of the previously described methods, such as Euler's in which all temperatures, except the single set of T^{n+1} in $\partial\mathbf{T}/\partial t$, are the current values, T^n. For this finite element case, however, Euler's method is also implicit and does not have the advantage of simplicity. Consequently, a more accurate implicit scheme, such as the Crank-Nicolson, can be used just as easily.

1.6.4 Approximate Finite Element Methods

For many differential equations no exact Lagrangian integrals can be found. In these cases other, approximate integral methods can be used. The most common technique is called the weighted residual method in which, first, the differential equation is multiplied by a weighting function, w, then an approximate function is introduced into the differential equation and the entire expression is integrated over the entire domain such that this overall integral is set equal to zero. The integration yields the values for the variables of the problem, such as the nodal temperatures. The weighting function is arbitrary but the most common practice is to make it identical to the approximating function. This approach is called the Galerkin method. Considering the two-dimensional heat conduction equation, we can write

$$T^{(e)} = \sum N_i(x,y) T_i = [N][T]^{(e)} \; . \tag{1.296}$$

Then a typical equation for an element (e) with the Galerkin method is

$$\iint_{S^{(e)}} N_i \left[\frac{\partial}{\partial x}\left(k_x \frac{\partial T^{(e)}}{\partial x}\right) + \frac{\partial}{\partial y}\left(k_y \frac{\partial T^{(e)}}{\partial y}\right) + q_i \right] \times dx\,dy = 0 \; . \tag{1.297}$$

Integrate by parts to introduce the "natural" boundary conditions.

$$-\iint_{S^{(e)}} \left[k_x \frac{\partial T^{(e)}}{\partial x}\frac{\partial N_i}{\partial x} + k_y \frac{\partial T^{(e)}}{\partial y}\frac{\partial N_i}{\partial y} - N_i q_i \right] dx\,dy + \int_{L_b^{(e)}} \left[k_x \frac{\partial T^{(e)}}{\partial x} n_x + k_y \frac{\partial T^{(e)}}{\partial y} n_y \right] N_i \, dL_b^{(e)} = 0 \tag{1.298}$$

where n_x and n_y are the two components of the unit outward normal at the boundary, $L_b^{(e)}$, of the element. On each boundary the heat flux can be expressed in terms of the boundary conditions as follows:

$$k_x \frac{\partial T^{(e)}}{\partial x} n_x + k_y \frac{\partial T^{(e)}}{\partial y} n y = (q/A)_{in} - h_c(T^{(e)} - T_\infty) - \sigma \varepsilon_r T^{(e)^4} + \alpha_r q_r \; . \tag{1.299}$$

Substituting this expression into Eq. 1.298 yields the working equation for this finite element technique.

$$-\iint_{S^{(e)}} \left[k_x \frac{\partial T^{(e)}}{\partial x}\frac{\partial N_i}{\partial x} + k_y \frac{\partial T^{(e)}}{\partial y}\frac{\partial N_i}{\partial y} - N_i q_i \right] dx\,dy + \int_{L_b^{(e)}} [(q/A)_{in} - h_c(T^{(e)} - T\infty) - \sigma \varepsilon_r T^{(e)^4} + \alpha_r q_r] \times N_i \, dL_b^{(e)} = 0 \tag{1.300}$$

or in matrix notation

$$-\iint_{S^{(e)}} \left\{ k_x \left[\frac{\partial N}{\partial x}\right] [T]^{(e)} \frac{\partial N_i}{\partial x} + k_y \left[\frac{\partial N}{\partial y}\right] [T]^{(e)} \frac{\partial N_i}{\partial y} - N_i q_i \right\} dx\,dy + \int_{L_b^{(e)}} \{(q/A)_{in} - h_c [N][T]^{(e)} + h_c T_\infty - \sigma \varepsilon_r \{[N][T]^{(e)}\}^4 + \alpha_r q_r\} N_i \, dL_b^{(e)} = 0 \; . \tag{1.301}$$

All terms can be readily evaluated except the fourth-order radiation term which yields rather complicated expressions. For example, in the one-dimensional case

$$[N][T]^{(e)} = \left[\frac{x_j - x}{x_{ij}} \; \frac{x - x_i}{x_{ij}} \right] \begin{bmatrix} T_i \\ T_j \end{bmatrix} \; ; \tag{1.302}$$

therefore,

$$N_i = \frac{x_j - x}{x_{ij}} \; ; \quad \frac{\partial N_i}{\partial x} = -\frac{1}{x_{ij}} \; ; \quad \left[\frac{\partial N}{\partial x}\right] = \left[-\frac{1}{x_{ij}} \; \frac{1}{x_{ij}}\right] ;$$

and

$$k_x \left[\frac{\partial N}{\partial x}\right] [T]^{(e)} \frac{\partial N_i}{\partial x} = \frac{k_x (T_i - T_j)}{x_{ij}^2}$$

and its integral with respect to dx becomes

$$A^{(e)} \frac{k_x (T_i - T_j)}{x_{ij}^2} = \frac{k_x (T_i - T_j)}{x_{ij}} \; .$$

As it has been described in the section on radiation, it is advisable to replace the fourth-order term with a linearized, equivalent, radiative heat transfer expression, which can be quite accurate if the temperature differences are relatively small compared with the absolute temperatures. For biological systems this is almost always the case. For example, consider a body at temperature T in a large enclosure at temperature T_∞, both in absolute units (K). The radiative heat flux is, as in Eqs. 1.85,

$$q_r = \sigma \varepsilon_r (T_\infty^4 - T^4) = \sigma \varepsilon_r (T_\infty^3 + T_\infty^2 T + T_\infty T^2 + T^3) \cdot (T_\infty - T) \qquad (1.303\,a)$$

$$\cong \sigma \varepsilon_r 4 T_m^3 (T_\infty - T) \qquad (1.303\,b)$$

$$= h_r (T_\infty - T) \qquad (1.303\,c)$$

where $T_m = (T_\infty + T)/2$ is the average absolute temperature. The above expression can be treated the same way as the convective term.

Let us apply these relations to the two-dimensional example treated previously and shown in Fig. 1.36

$$T^{(e)} = \underbrace{\left[1 - \frac{x - x_i}{x_{ij}}\right]}_{N_i} T_i + \underbrace{\left[\frac{x - x_i}{x_{ij}} - \frac{y - y_i}{y_{ik}}\right]}_{N_j} T_j + \underbrace{\left[\frac{y - y_i}{y_{ik}}\right]}_{N_k} T_k \; . \qquad (1.304)$$

Therefore,

$$\frac{\partial N_i}{\partial x} = -\frac{1}{x_{ij}} \, , \quad \frac{\partial N_i}{\partial y} = 0 \, , \quad \frac{\partial N_j}{\partial x} = \frac{1}{x_{ij}} \, , \quad \frac{\partial N_j}{\partial y} = -\frac{1}{y_{ik}} \, ,$$

$$\frac{\partial N_k}{\partial x} = 0 \, , \quad \frac{\partial N_k}{\partial y} = \frac{1}{y_{ik}}$$

$$\left[\frac{\partial N}{\partial x}\right] = \left[-\frac{1}{x_{ij}} \; \frac{1}{x_{ij}} \; 0\right] \text{ and } \left[\frac{\partial N}{\partial y}\right] = \left[0 \; -\frac{1}{y_{ik}} \; \frac{1}{y_{ik}}\right] .$$

Substituting these relations into Eq. 1.301 yields the following set of equations for a typical element.

$$T_i - T_j = q_i x_{ij} y_{ik} / 3k \qquad (1.305\,a)$$

$$-T_i - 2T_j - T_k = q_i x_{ij} y_{ik} / 3k \qquad (1.305\,b)$$

$$-T_j + T_k = q_i x_{ij} y_{ik} / 3k \qquad (1.305\,c)$$

Or in matrix notation, with $x_{ij} = y_{ik} = L/2$,

$$\begin{bmatrix} 1 & -1 & 0 \\ -1 & 2 & -1 \\ 0 & -1 & 1 \end{bmatrix} \begin{bmatrix} T_i \\ T_j \\ T_k \end{bmatrix} = \frac{q_i L^2}{12k} \begin{bmatrix} 1 \\ 1 \\ 1 \end{bmatrix} \; . \qquad (1.306)$$

It is important to note that these equations depend on the unique characteristics of the geometry of the equilateral triangles used. In particular $x_{ij} = x_{ik} = y_{ik} = y_{jk} = L/2$ and the i−j line must be parallel to the x axis with j point at the 90° corner. If we compare these equations with the ones obtained by the Lagrange integral, i.e., Eqs. 1.286 and 1.288, we can see that they are identical. Consequently, the working equations are also the same as given by Eq. 1.292, and all the results and comments made previously, including Table 1.3, apply. Thus, although the computation of the coefficients in the two finite element methods is different, in this case the results are identical.

1.6.5 Concluding Remarks

The complexity of many real life problems in heat transfer mandates the use of numerical techniques with the analytical methods serving as checks on the numerical algorithms used as well as guides to the understanding of the controlling parameters and their magnitudes. We have provided an introduction to the two most important techniques, finite differences and finite elements, which will help the reader to understand the relevant literature and to develop specialized applications if needed.

The finite difference method needs the most straightforward computer program, but irregularly shaped boundaries require a great number of nodes for proper modeling. The programs for the finite element techniques are more complicated, but they can handle irregularly shaped boundaries with relatively few elements. Although the finite element Lagrangian integral method is more exact, the weighted residual methods, such as Galerkin's, are less complicated and they can be used with any partial differential equation. A newer method, the boundary element method which was not discussed here, can reduce the number of calculations required, but it seems to be ill suited for problems with complicated boundaries, such as in the case of several, distinct organs included simultaneously in a problem.

For very complicated programs or other methods the reader will need to use books and other references dealing with these techniques in detail. There are also numerous software packages available on the market, and new ones are continually introduced, which can eliminate the need for developing one's own algorithms. These, however, do require close scrutiny to ascertain that any inherent limitations will not conflict with the user's needs.

1.7 Properties and Measurements

1.7.1 Introduction

To quantify the various models described, we need to know the magnitudes of the various parameters involved and we need to have appropriate measured data from experiments both as input to the models and for comparison with the calculated results. The most prominent measurable data are temperatures at various locations. These can be used, in addition to their basic values as temperatures, to estimate other characteristics of the tissue, such as thermophysical properties or blood perfusion rates. In thermal studies of biological systems there are very few other measurements that can be made. Pressures, velocities, and overall flow rates can be determined in the blood vessels. Overall metabolic rates can be calculated from measured volume flow rates and changes in component concentration of inhaled and exhaled air. Of course, there are numerous other measurements that are made routinely in the biological sciences, such as pH, concentrations, or electrical potentials. However, in the study of bioheat transfer the most significant measurements are temperature, blood perfusion or flow, and metabolic heat generation. Even the last two are frequently derived from temperature data.

There are a few books that deal with the basic engineering aspects of measuring temperatures, pressures, and flows (e.g. [6]). There were periodic, very comprehensive symposia held on *Temperature: Its measurement and control in science and industry*, the last two volumes of which are of interest here [7, 60]. The older one [7] is significant, in spite of its age, because it contains a separate section on biology and medicine. One of the latest reviews of temperature measurements in these field was written by Cetas [13]. Overviews of the measurement of thermophysical properties as well as tabulation of their values were given by Chato [15, 16, 20–22], Bowman et al. [9], and Shitzer [61]. The state of the art of using thermal methods to determine blood perfusion rates was described by Bowman [8] and by Kress and Roemer [45]. We are not going to deal with the separate and very large topic of blood flow measurement in blood vessels.

1.7.2 Temperature

Perhaps the most important statement one can make about temperature measuring devices is that they all need careful installation and frequent calibration. For installation purposes it is to be remembered that any device measures only the temperature of its own sensor, which may not be exactly the same as the temperature of the surrounding tissue. The major reasons for this difference can be:

1. Heat conduction along the lead wires or supporting structure. To reduce this error the lead wires or supports should be as small as possible and they should be placed along the isotherms (constant temperature lines) going through the measuring point. Thermometers should be immersed into the medium as deeply as possible. The required depth is indicated on the more accurate models.
2. Energy generated by the device itself. This effect is due either to its operational requirements, e.g., the electric current passing through a resistive sensor, or to its interaction with an externally applied energy field, such as ultrasound or microwave. To reduce this error, minimization of the operating current and of the size of the sensor and its leads is helpful.
3. Insufficient thermal contact between the sensor and the surrounding medium. This problem could arise if the insertion is made with a cutter, such as a hypodermic needle, which is much larger in diameter than the size of the sensor, and it is more likely to occur in hard tissue, e.g., bone, that in a soft one.

Periodic calibration is important with all measuring devices, particularly the modern, sophisticated electronic thermometers. This can be performed fairly simply by inserting the probe into a constant temperature bath, preferably inside a vacuum-insulated flask such as a thermos bottle, which is monitored by a calibrated, precision standard thermometer. For very accurate measurements fixed-point temperature baths are needed in the physiological range, such as ice-filled water (0 °C), the melting point of gallium (29.772 °C), or the hydration points of some salt solutions recommended by Magin et al. [47].

Since any temperature-dependent property could potentially be used as the basis for measurement, there exist numerous devices, many of which were developed for specific applications. The most common thermometers are:

- Liquid in glass, using thermal expansion
- Electrical resistance or other parameter (platinum resistance, thermistors, and semiconductor devices)
- Thermocouples, using electrical potential generated at metallic junctions
- Quartz crystals, using resonant frequency
- Liquid crystals, usually embedded in a flexible sheet, using color change
- Thermography, using infrared emission of surfaces
- Bimetallic strips, using the deflection caused by differential expansion of bonded solid strips
- Fiberoptic devices, using various temperature sensor at their tips

Many of these employ electrical circuitry for transmission and processing the measuring signal. Strong electromagnetic fields tend to interfere with their operation. Some of the newer devices, particularly fiberoptic ones, are insensitive to such fields and can, therefore, be easily used with electromagnetically induced hyperthermia. Unfortunately, most of these devices are quite expensive.

1.7.3 Thermophysical Properties

The most important properties needed for thermal studies are the thermal conductivity, k, and the thermal diffusivity, $\alpha = k/\varrho c$, or its component the volumetric heat capacity, ϱc. Since most tissues can be considered as combinations of water, proteins, and fat, the magnitudes of these properties can be estimated from the proportions of these components. Cooper and Trezek [30] recommended the following relations:

$$k,\ \mathrm{W/m\text{-}C} = \varrho \times 10^{-3}(0.628\ \mathrm{mf_{water}} + 0.117\ \mathrm{mf_{protein}} + 0.231\ \mathrm{mf_{fat}}) \tag{1.307}$$

$$1/\varrho, \mathrm{m^3/kg} = \mathrm{mf_{water}}/1000 + \mathrm{mf_{protein}}/1540 + \mathrm{mf_{fat}}/815 \tag{1.308}$$

$$c,\ \mathrm{kJ/kg\text{-}C} = 4.2\ \mathrm{mf_{water}} + 1.09\ \mathrm{mf_{protein}} + 2.3\ \mathrm{mf_{fat}} \tag{1.309}$$

where mf is the mass fraction.

Table 1.4 shows selected data from the literature cited above. It can be observed or calculated that water has the highest values of thermal conductivity and diffusivity among the three components. Therefore, tissues with high water content are the best thermal conductors and they also respond the fastest to a thermal disturbance. High fat and protein content produces relatively good thermal insulation. If we consider the thermal field around a heated or cooled probe, a material with high conductivity will have a larger affected volume than a material with low conductivity.

The currently successful measuring methods for thermophysical properties of tissues, particularly in vivo, use some kind of transient technique with a relatively short measuring period of about $\frac{1}{2}-2$ min. Chato [14] described a spherical thermistor bead with a controlled step change in temperature to measure both thermal conductivity, k, and inertia, $k\varrho c$, of tissue

Table 1.4. Reported intrinsic[a] properties of biological materials. (Adapted from [21] and its references)

Material	Conductivity, k (W/m-C)	Diffusivity, α (m^2/s)	Inertia, $k\varrho c$ (W^2-s/m^4-C^2)
Skin	0.21 – 0.41	$0.82-1.2\times10^{-7}$	$1.2-2.2\times10^{6}$
Muscle	0.34 – 0.68	$1.2-2.3\times10^{-7}$	$0.94-2.0\times10^{6}$
Fat	0.094 – 0.37	$0.32-2.7\times10^{-7}$	$0.28-0.51\times10^{6}$
Bone	0.41 – 0.63		0.87×10^{6}
Dry bone and bone marrow	0.22		
Brain	0.16 – 0.57	$0.44-1.4\times10^{-7}$	
Heart	0.48 – 0.59	$1.4-1.5\times10^{-7}$	
Liver	0.42 – 0.57	$1.1-2.0\times10^{-7}$	1.0×10^{6}
Tumors, general range @ 37 °C	0.4 – 0.6		
Blood	0.48 – 0.60		
Blood plasma	0.57 – 0.60		
Frozen tissue, general range	1.0 – 1.6		
Frozen blood, – 10° to – 100 °C	1.6 – 2.7	$8.7-23.7\times10^{-7}$	
Frozen plasma, – 10° to – 100 °C	2.0 – 3.2	$9.7-26.9\times10^{-7}$	

[a] Without blood flow; from room to body temperature, except as noted

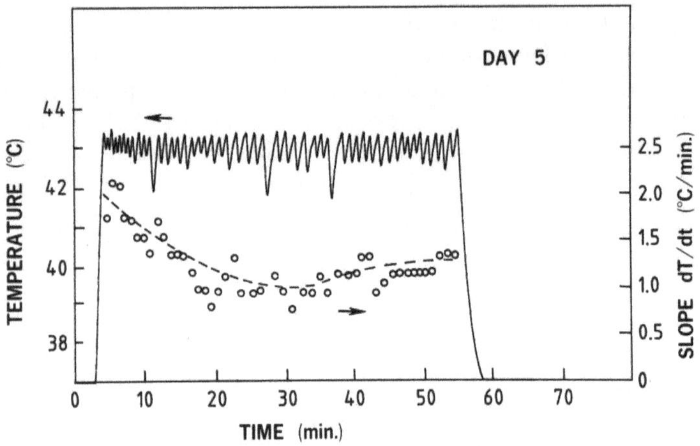

Fig. 1.37. Tumor temperature and its time derivative during hyperthermia. (Courtesy of T. Knittel 1986, personal communication. Artwork by Dept. Med. Illustration, University of NSW and Teaching Hospitals)

both in vitro and in vivo. Balasubramaniam and Bowman [5] improved this technique, primarily, by a more sophisticated and accurate way of modeling the real system. Chen et al. [26] developed a pulse-decay method using a very small thermistor. The bead delivers an initial thermal energy pulse to the tissue; afterwards the bead simply monitors the decay of the temperature. This method has the advantage that the bead can be very small because its size does not appear in the analysis of the data. Although other geometries (e.g., cylindrical probes) and protocols (e.g., constant power input) have also been reported, the above two seem to be currently the most effective, with the Chen method having a slight advantage.

1.7.4 Blood Perfusion

All methods used for the measurement of thermophysical properties can be employed, potentially, for the measurement of blood perfusion rates. The experimental procedure remains the same but the data obtained are evaluated with a mathematical model which includes blood perfusion, such as the Pennes [58] equation (Eq. 1.214b). The technique using a spherical thermistor bead with a step change in temperature was described by Chato [14] and Valvano et al. [67]. Chen and Holmes [25] adapted their pulse-decay method. Johnson et al. [43] developed a spherical probe with constant power input. A cylindrical probe configuration was studied by Patera et al. [57]. In a comparative study of the various thermistor probes, Kress and Roemer [45] found them about equally effective.

T. Knittel (1986, personal communication) Prince of Wales Hospital, Randwick, NSW, Australia estimated the change of blood perfusion in a tumor heated by RF current from the temperature data. The power was applied in short intervals and the temperature decay rate, $\partial T/\partial t$, immediately after each power cut-off was assumed to be proportional to the perfusion rate. This

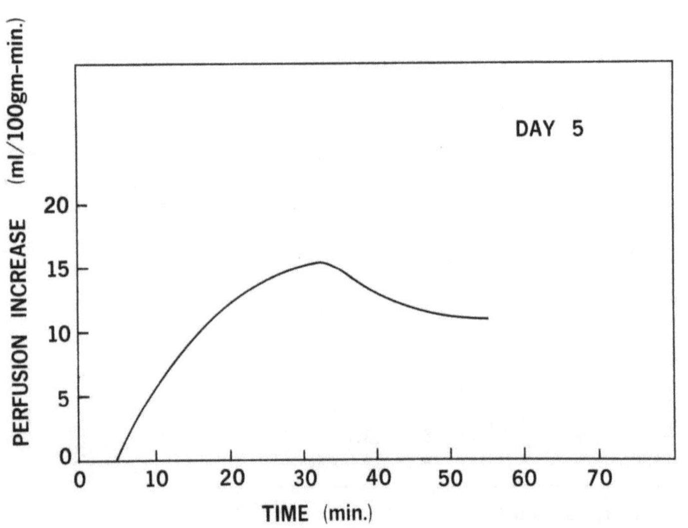

Fig. 1.38. Change of blood perfusion calculated by applying Eq. 1.310 to the data of Fig. 1.37 and to similar other data. (Courtesy of T. Knittel 1986, personal communication. Artwork by Dept. Med. Illustration, University of NSW and Teaching Hospitals)

approach is related to the heat clearance method developed by Muller-Schauenburg et al. [53]. The very simple working equation he developed was:

$$m_{b2} - m_{b1} = \frac{c_t}{\varrho_b c_b (T_a - T)} \left[\left(\frac{\partial T}{\partial t} \right)_2 - \left(\frac{\partial T}{\partial t} \right)_1 \right] \quad (1.310)$$

which for the data shown in Figs. 1.37 and 1.38 reduces to

$$m_{b2} - m_{b1} = -15.5 \left[\left(\frac{\partial T}{\partial t} \right)_2 - \left(\frac{\partial T}{\partial t} \right)_1 \right]$$

in ml/100 g-s . (1.310a)

Although this equation is based on a very simplistic analysis, it does provide a reasonable indication of the trends of blood perfusion during the hyperthermia protocol performed.

Bowman [8] summarized the various methods reported in the literature, including some based on venerable heat clearance methods. These include, for example, Hensel's [39] work, which uses the temperature difference between a heated and an unheated probe; and Cameron's [11] thermal dilution technique, which depends on the evaluation of the temperature response to an injected bolus of cold saline solution.

Nomenclature[1]

a	Length, m, or constant
A	Area, m^2
b	$= d/R$
c	Specific heat at constant pressure, J/kg-C or kJ/kg-C
C	Constant or heat capacity rate ratio $(m_1 c_1/m_2 c_2)$
d	Length, m
D	Vessel diameter, m
e	Specific energy, J/kg
E	Stored internal energy, J, or radiative power density, W/m^2
F	Fraction of blood flow leaving an artery and entering a parallel vein
F_{1-2}	Factor for radiative heat exchange, defined by Eq. 1.80
Fo	$= \alpha \Delta t/\Delta x^2$, Fourier number
g	Gravitational acceleration, 9.81 m/s^2 on earth
G	$= \varrho V$, mass flux, kg/s-m^2
Gz	$= Re \cdot Pr \cdot D/L$, Graetz number. Any subscript replaces L
h	$= u + pv$, specific enthalpy, J/kg
h_{fg}	Latent heat of vaporization, J/kg
$h_{()}$	Convective heat transfer coefficient, W/m^2-C
H	Elevation above reference level, m, height, or defined by Eq. 1.165
k	Thermal conductivity, W/m-C
ln	Natural logarithm
log	Logarithm to the base 10
l, L	Length, m
m	Mass flow rate, kg/s
m_b	Volumetric blood perfusion rate, kg/s m^3
M	Mass, kg
N	Number of transfer units, defined by Eq. 1.133
Nu	$= h_c \cdot D/k$, Nusselt number
p	Pressure, Pa (N/m^2)
P	Perimeter (wetted), m
P_t	Power deposition in the tissue per unit volume, W/m^3
Pe	$= Re \cdot Pr$, Peclet number
Pr	$= c \cdot \mu/k$, Prandtl number
q	Heat transfer rate, W
q_b	Volumetric heat generation rate due to blood perfusion, W/m^3
q_i	Volumetric heat generation rate, W/m^3
q_l	Heat transfer per unit length, W/m
q_m	Volumetric heat generation rate due to metabolism, W/m^3
q_r	Radiative heat flux incident on surface, W/m^2
q_0	Dimensionless volumetric heat generation rate
Q	Heat, J
r	Radius, m
R	Radius, m, or thermal resistance, C/W
Re	$= \varrho \cdot V \cdot D/\mu$, Reynolds number
S	Surface, m^2
t	Time, s
T	Temperature (absolute or relative as defined in text), K or C
u	Specific internal energy, J/kg, or defined by Eq. 1.166
v	Specific volume, m^3/kg
V	Velocity, m/s
$\mathcal{V}$	Volume, m^3
w	Weighting function
W	Work, J
x, y, z	Cartesian coordinates, m
X	$= x/D$, dimensionless distance
Z	$= x/L$ or z/L, dimensionless distance

[1] A consistent set of units is given here. However, in the text the units may be different for practical reasons; e.g., mm instead of m.

Greek Letters

α	Thermal diffusivity, m^2/s
α_r	Absorptivity of the surface
β	$= -(1/\varrho)(\partial\varrho/\partial T)_p = (1/v)(\partial v/\partial T)_p$, volumetric expansion coefficient, T^{-1}
γ	Defined in Eq. 1.35, Eqs. 1.155, 1.156, Eqs. 1.164, 1.166 or Eq. 1.177
δ	Defined by Eq. 1.161
Δ	Change in a variable
ε_r	Emissivity of the surface
η	Implicitness or constant
θ	Dimensionless temperature, e.g. Eq. 1.113, or angle
λ	Dimensionless parameter, e.g., Eq. 1.115, or wavelength, μ
μ	Dynamic viscosity, kg/m s, or micron (10^{-6} m)
ν	$= \mu/\varrho$, kinematic viscosity, m^2/s
ϱ	Density, kg/m^3
$\tau(t)$	Time-dependent component of temperature
τ_s	Shear stress, N/m^2
τ_y	Yield stress, N/m^2
ω	Circular frequency, s^{-1}

Superscipts

n	Index of time step
–	Time rate
′	Derivative or shifted value

Subscripts

a	Artery
abs	Absolute value, e.g., K instead of C
av	Artery to vein
b	Blood or black body
c	Convective, capillary, or body core
cd	Conductive
cv	Control volume
e	Electric, equivalent, or exhaled
env	Environment
evap	Evaporation
f	Liquid phase
g	Vapor phase
i	Internal, or solid phase (ice)
m	Magnetic, mean value, or metabolic
max	Maximum or larger value
min	Minimum or smaller value
p	Constant pressure
r	Radiative
s	Surface
t	Tissue or derivative with respect to time
v	Vein
w	Wall or water vapor
x, y, z	Direction or derivative with respect to variable
0	Reference or initial condition
1	Entrance or initial condition
2	Exit or final condition
∞	Fluid bulk quantity

References

1. Anderson DA, Tannehill JC, Pletcher RH (1984) Computational fluid mechanics and heat transfer. McGraw-Hill, New York
2. Awbery JH (1929) Heat flow when the boundary condition is Newton's law. Philos Mag 7(7):1145–1153
3. Baish JW, Ayyaswamy PS, Foster KR (1986) Small-scale temperature fluctuations in perfused tissue during local hyperthermia. Trans ASME J Biomech Eng 108:246–250
4. Baish JW, Ayyaswamy PS, Foster KR (1986) Heat transport mechanisms in vascular tissues: a model comparison. Trans ASME J Biomech Eng 108:324–331
5. Balasubramaniam TA, Bowman HF (1977) Thermal conductivity and thermal diffusivity of biomaterials: a simultaneous measurement technique. Trans ASME J Biomech Eng 99:148–154
6. Benedict RP (1984) Fundamentals of temperature, pressure, and flow measurements, 3rd edn. Wiley Interscience, New York
7. Berger RL (ed) (1972) Temperature: its measurement and control in science and industry, vol. 4. Part 3. Biology and medicine. Instrument Society of America, Pittsburgh, pp 2035–2233
8. Bowman HF (1985) Estimation of tissue blood flow. In: Shitzer A, Eberhart RC (eds) Heat transfer in medicine and biology: analysis and applications, vol 1. Plenum, New York, pp 193–230
9. Bowman HF, Cravalho EG, Woods M (1975) Theory, measurement, and application of thermal properties of biomaterials. Annu Rev Biophys Bioeng 4:43–80
10. Brebner DF, Kerslake DMcK, Waddell JL (1958) The relation between the coefficients for heat exchange by convection and by evaporation in man. J Physiol (Lond) 141:164–168
11. Cameron BD (1970) Determination of regional cerebral cortical blood flow using a heat clearance technique. Phys Med Biol 15:715–721
12. Carslaw HS, Jaeger JC (1959) Conduction of heat in solids, 2nd edn. Oxford University Press, London
13. Cetas TC (1985) Temperature measurement. In: Shitzer A, Eberhart RC (eds) Heat transfer in medicine and biology: analysis and applications, vol 2. Plenum, New York, pp 373–392
14. Chato JC (1968) A method of the measurement of the thermal properties of biological materials. In: Chato JC (ed) Thermal problems in biotechnology. ASME symposium series. American Society of Mechanical Engineers, New York, pp 16–25
15. Chato JC (1969) Heat transfer in bioengineering. In: Chao BT (ed) Advanced heat transfer. University of Illinois Press, Champaign, pp 395–414
16. Chato JC (1980) Measurement of thermal properties of growing tumors. Ann NY Acad Sci 335:67–85
17. Chato JC (1980) Heat transfer to blood vessels. Trans ASME J Biomech Eng 102:110–118

18. Chato JC (1981) Reflections on the history of bioengineering heat and mass transfer. Trans ASME J Biomech Eng 103:97–101
19. Chato JC (1983) Heat transfer in bioengineering. Heat Transfer Eng, Hemishere Publ Corp, Washington, DC 4:81 ff
20. Chato JC (1985) Measurement of thermal properties of biological materials. In: Shitzer A, Eberhart RC (eds) Heat transfer in medicine and biology: analysis and applications, vol 1. Plenum, New York, pp 167–192
21. Chato JC (1985) Selected thermophysical properties of biological materials. In: Shitzer A, Eberhart RC (eds) Heat transfer in medicine and biology: analysis and applications, vol 2. Plenum, New York, pp 413–418
22. Chato JC (1986) Thermal properties of tissues. In: Skalak R, Chien S (eds) Handbook of bioengineering. McGraw-Hill, New York, pp 9.1–9.13
23. Chato JC, Shitzer A (1975) Analytical prediction of the heat transfer from a blood vessel near the skin surface cooled by a symmetrical strip. Trans ASME J Eng Ind 97:61–65
24. Chen MM, Holmes KR (1980) Microvascular contributions in tissue heat transfer. Ann NY Acad Sci 335:137–150
25. Chen MM, Holmes KR (1980) The thermal pulse-decay method for simultaneous measurement of thermal conductivity and local blood perfusion rate of living tissues. ASME, Adv. Bioeng 113–115
26. Chen MM, Holmes KR, Rupinskas V (1981) Pulse-decay method for measuring the thermal conductivity of living tissues. Trans ASME J Biomech Eng 103:253–260
27. Clifford J, Kerslake DMcK, Waddell JL (1959) The effect of wind speed on maximum evaporative capacity in man. J Physiol (Lond) 147:253–259
28. Colin J, Houdas Y (1967) Experimental determination of coefficient of heat exchanges by convection on human body. J Appl Physiol 22:31–38
29. Cooper TE, Trezek GJ (1971) Rate of lesion growth around spherical and cylindrical cryoprobes. Cryobiology 7:183–190
30. Cooper TE, Trezek GJ (1971) Correlation of thermal properties of some human tissues with water content. Aerospace Med 42:24–27
31. Crowley JM (1985) Electrostatic fields on PC spreadsheets. IEEE-IAS annual meeting conference record, Toronto
32. Dussan BI, Weiner RI (1971) Study of burn hazard in human tissue and its implication on consumer product design. Paper no 71-WA/HT-39. American Society of Mechanical Engineers, New York
33. Gautherie M (1969) Etude par thermométrie infrarouge des properties thermiques de tissues humains "in vivo". Influence de la température et de la vascularization. Rev Fr Etud Clin Biol 14:885–901
34. Gilbert JC, Onik GM, Hoddick W, Rubinski B (1984) The use of ultrasound imaging for monitoring cryosurgery. Proceedings 6th annual conference IEEE engineering in medicine and biology, pp 107–112
35. Green HD (1944) Circulation: physical principles. In: Glasser O (ed) Medical physics, vol 1. Year Book Publishers, Chicago, pp 208–232
36. Gryzagoridis J (1971) Natural convection from a vertical flat plate in the low Grashof number range. Int J Heat Mass Transfer 14:162–164
37. Henriques FC (1947) Studies of thermal injury. V. The predictability and the significance of thermally induced rate processes leading to irreversible epidermal injury. Arch Pathol 43:489–502
38. Henriques FC, Moritz AR (1947) Studies of thermal injury. I. The conduction of heat to and through the skin and the temperatures attained therein. A theoretical and an experimental investigation. Am J Pathol 23:531–549
39. Hensel H (1953/54) Fortlaufende Wärmeleitfähigkeits- und Durchblutungsmessung im Gewebe mit einer Differential-Calorimetersonde. Ber Gesamte Physiol 162:360 ff
40. Huebner KH, Thornton EA (1982) The finite element method for engineers, 2nd edn. Wiley, New York
41. Hurlburt E, Chato JC (1987) Computer aided modeling of tissue temperatures using finite difference methods. In: BT Chao symposium volume, Department of Mechanical and Industrial Engineering, University of Illinois, Urbana
42. Jiji LM, Weinbaum S, Lemons DE (1984) Theory and experiment for the effect of vascular microstructure on surface tissue heat transfer. Part II. Model formulation and solution. Trans ASME J Biomech Eng 106:331–341
43. Johnson WR, Abdelmessih AH, Grayson J (1979) Blood perfusion measurements by the analysis of the heated thermocouple probe's temperature transients. Trans ASME J Biomech Eng 101:58–65
44. Keller KH, Seiler L (1971) An analysis of peripheral heat transfer in man. J Appl Physiol 30:779–786
45. Kress R, Roemer R (1987) A comparative analysis of thermal blood perfusion measurement techniques. Trans ASME J Biomech Eng 109:218–225
46. Love TJ (1985) Analysis and application of thermography in medical diagnosis. In: Shitzer A, Eberhart RC (eds) Heat transfer in medicine and biology: analysis and applications, vol 2. Plenum, New York, pp 333–352
47. Magin RL, Mangum BW, Statler JA, Thorton DD (1981) Transition temperatures of the hydrates of Na_2SO_4 Na_2HPO_4, and KF as fixed points in biomedical thermometry. J Res Natl Bur Stand 86:181–192
48. Mall F (1887) Die Blut- und Lymphwege im Dünndarm des Hundes. Ber Saech Gesamte Akad Wiss 14:151–200
49. Mall FP (1906) A study of the structural unit of the liver. Am J Anat 5:227–308
50. McAdams WH (1954) Heat transmission, 3d edn. McGraw-Hill, New York
51. McGrath JJ (1985) Preservation of biological materials by freezing and thawing. In: Shitzer A, Eberhart RC (eds) Heat transfer in medicine and biology: analysis and applications, vol 2. Plenum, New York, pp 185–238
52. Moritz AR, Henriques FC (1947) Studies of thermal injury. II. The relative importance of time and surface temperature in the causation of cutaneous burns. Am J Pathol 23:695–720
53. Müller-Schauenburg W, Apfel H, Benzing H, Betz E (1975) Quantitative measurement of local blood flow with heat clearance. Basic Res Cardiol 70:547–567
54. Myers GE (1987) Analytical methods in conduction heat transfer, 2nd edn. Genium, Schenectady
55. Nielsen M, Pedersen L (1953) Man's heat loss by convection and radiation. Wärme 18:1–12, 17–27
56. Ozisik MN (1980) Heat conduction. Wiley, New York
57. Patera AT, Mikic BB, Bowman HF (1978) The effect of cylindrical probe geometry on the accuracy of tissue perfusion measurements made with the thermal diffusion probe. Adv Bioeng ASME Bioeng Proc 157–159
58. Pennes HH (1948) Analysis of tissue and arterial blood temperatures in the resting human forearm. J Appl Physiol 1(2):93–122
59. Schleier J (1919) Der Energieverbrauch in der Blutbahn. Pflugers Arch Ges Physiol 173:172–204
60. Schooley JF (ed) (1982) Temperature: its measurement and

control in science and industry vol 5. American Institute of Physics, New York
61. Shitzer A (1975) Studies of bio-heat transfer in mammals. In: Gutfinger C (ed) Topics in transport phenomena. Halsted, pp 211–343
62. Shitzer A, Eberhart RC (eds) (1985) Heat transfer in medicine and biology: analysis and applications, vols 1, 2. Plenum, New York
63. Sieder EN, Tate CE (1936) Heat transfer and pressure drop of liquids in tubes. Ind Eng Chem 28:1429
64. Song WJ, Weinbaum S, Jiji LF (1987) A theoretical model for peripheral tissue heat transfer using the bioheat equation of Weinbaum and Jiji. Trans ASME J Biomech Eng 109:72–78
65. Stoll AM (1967) Heat transfer in biotechnology. In: Hartnett JP, Irvine TF (eds) Advances in heat transfer, vol 4. Academic, New York, pp 65–141
66. Trezek GJ (1985) Thermal analysis for cryosurgery. In: Shitzer A, Eberhart RC (eds) Heat transfer in medicine and biology: analysis and applications, vol 2. Plenum, New York, pp 239–259
67. Valvano JW, Allen JT, Bowman HF (1984) The simultaneous measurement of thermal conductivity, thermal diffusivity, and perfusion in small volumes of tissue. Trans ASME J Biomech Eng 106:192–197
68. Victor SA, Shaw VL (1976) Steady state heat transfer to blood flowing in the entrance region of a tube. Int J Heat Mass Transfer 19:777–783
69. Weinbaum S, Jiji LM (1985) A new simplified bioheat equation for the effect of blood flow on local average tissue temperature. Trans ASME J Biomech Eng 107:131–139
70. Weinbaum S, Jiji LM (1987) Discussion of papers by Wissler and Baish et al. concerning the Weinbaum-Jiji bioheat equation. Trans ASME J Biomech Eng 109:234–237
71. Weinbaum S, Jiji LM , Lemons DE (1984) Theory and experiment for the effect of vascular microstructure on surface tissue heat transfer. Part 1. Anatomical foundation and model conceptualization. Trans ASME J Biomech Eng 106:321–330
72. Whitaker S (1972) Forced convection heat transfer correlations for flow in pipes, past flat plates, single cylinders, single spheres, and for flow in packed beds and tube bundles. AIChE J 18:361–171
73. Winslow C-EA, Gagge AP, Herrington LP (1939) The influence of air movement upon heat losses from the clothed human body. J Physiol 127:505–518
74. Wissler EH (1985) Mathematical simulation of human thermal behavior using whole-body models. In: Shitzer A, Eberhart RC (eds) Heat transfer in medicine and biology: analysis and applications, vol 1. Plenum, New York, pp 325–373
75. Wissler EH (1987) Comments on the new bioheat equation proposed by Weinbaum and Jiji. Trans ASME J Biomech Eng 109:226–233
76. Wissler EH (1987) An analytical solution for countercurrent heat exchange between parallel vessels with a linear axial temperature gradient. In: Diller KR (ed) Network thermodynamics, heat and mass transfer in biotechnology. American Society of Mechanical Engineers, New York, pp 81–85 (ASME symp series BED-vol 5, HTD-vol 90)
77. Woodcock AH, Pratt RL, Breckenridge JR (1956) Man's thermal balance in warm environments. Technical Report EP-30, US Quartermaster Res and Dev Ctr
78. Wu YC (1972) Material properties criteria for thermal safety. J Materials 7:572–579
79. Wulff W (1974) The energy conservation equation for living tissue. IEEE Trans Biomed Eng BME-21:494–495
80. Yuge T (1960) Experiments on heat transfer from spheres including combined natural and forced convection. Trans ASME J Heat Transfer 82:214–220

Appendix

Conversion Factors

To convert the units in the first column to those in the second, multiply values of first column by factor in third.

k, W/m C = mW/mm C	W/cm-C	10^{-2}
k, W/m C	gcal/s cm C	2.39×10^{-3}
k, W/m C	Btu/h ft F	0.5778
α, m^2/s	cm^2/s	10^4
α, m^2/s	mm^2/s	10^6
α, m^2/s	ft^2/h	3.875×10^4
$k\varrho c$, W^2 s/m^4 C^2	W^2 s/cm^4 C^2	10^{-8}
$k\varrho c$, W^2 s/m^4 C^2	W^2 s/mm^4 C^2	10^{-12}
$k\varrho c$, W^2 s/m^4 C^2	$gcal^2$/s cm^4 C^2	5.712×10^{-10}
$k\varrho c$, W^2 s/m^4 C^2	Btu^2/h ft^4 F^2	8.616×10^{-6}
q, W	gcal/s	0.239
q, W	Btu/h	3.412

2 Calculation of Power Deposition Patterns in Hyperthermia

K. D. PAULSEN

2.1 Introduction

Interest in simulating hyperthermia treatments has increased dramatically over the last several years. Such modeling is now viewed as a way of reaching better understandings of many facets of the treatment process. Not only is modeling being used to illuminate the parameters which lead to successful heating, but also to aid in the understanding of the physical mechanisms of power absorption and heat transfer. The simulation of hyperthermia treatments has been identified as a two-step procedure:

1. compute the heating rate or power deposition pattern produced in the body by the heating source and
2. compute the redistribution of energy due to thermal conduction and blood flow.

To date these two steps have been regarded as decoupled such that the solution to the second step does not impact that of the first. This assumption of independence is based on the relative insensitivity of the medium properties which influence power absorption to temperature changes on the order of those found in hyperthermia therapy [102]. Further, the transient behavior of the heating sources typically decays much faster than the thermal response time, thus allowing power transients to be ignored in the thermal simulation process [6]. Note, however, that the second step cannot be undertaken until the first step has been completed (i.e., the output from the first step provides input needed for the second step). While the second step is generic to all heating systems, the first step is dependent on the specific heating device under consideration. The second step is discussed in detail elsewhere in this volume (see Chaps. 1 and 3). Thus, the first step – the calculation of power deposition patterns produced within the body for hyperthermic intent – will be the focus of the present chapter.

Although the process of hyperthermia treatment simulation has been computationally decoupled, it is important that analyses based on hyperthermia simulations remain coupled. The computational decoupling conveniently allows the two facets of treatment simulation – power absorption and heat transfer – to be discussed separately, but care must be exercised in interpreting any results based solely on one of these aspects or the other. This is especially true of power deposition calculations which, if interpreted in isolation, can result in misleading conclusions due to the profound effects of blood flow on heat transfer. Hence, the present chapter will view power deposition patterns as intermediary quantities and not as end results. This approach leaves much of the task of interpreting simulated results to other chapters, where discussions are in terms of the primary quantity of interest (i.e., temperature). Instead, the emphasis of this chapter will center on the formulation and implementation of power deposition calculations with a cognizance of their use in heat transfer simulations. While they involve secondary quantities which alone are of less interest in clinical hyperthermia, power deposition calculations are essential ingredients to all thermal simulations of hyperthermic treatment.

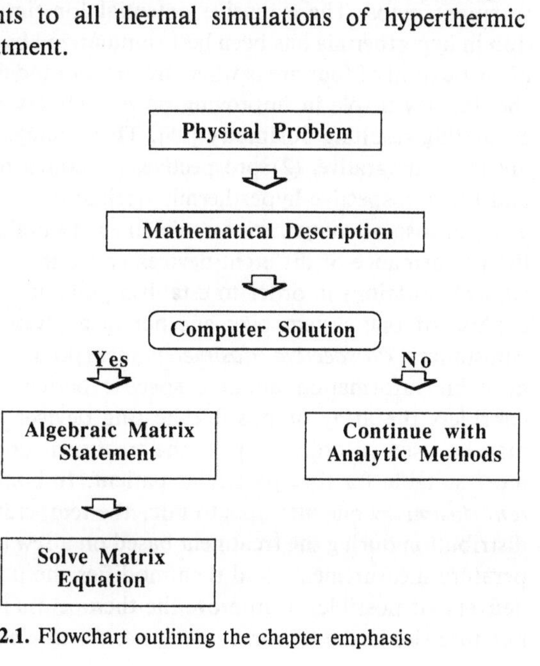

Fig. 2.1. Flowchart outlining the chapter emphasis

The concept for this chapter is illustrated by the flowchart shown in Fig. 2.1. Each of the topics in this logical progression will be discussed in varying amounts of detail with the majority of effort devoted to computer solutions and the generation of algebraic matrix statements from the functional equations which provide the mathematical descriptions of the physical problem of interest. As already indicated the physical problem of concern is the power absorption produced in the biological tissue during hyperthermia therapy and it will be introduced as the motivation for proceeding down the flowchart in Fig. 2.1. While taking this path may lead to discussions that seem to be somewhat removed from the hyperthermia context, special effort will be made to maintain a focus on the clinical hyperthermia problem. As such, discussions of numerical solutions will be favored over analytical methods since numerical schemes are more amenable to the complexities that typically occur in the clinic.

The importance of the use of treatment modeling as a tool in clinical hyperthermia arises from the present impracticality of detailed temperature or SAR (specific absorption rate) measurements throughout the treatment region, particularly for deep-seated sites, and the degree of variability/complexity among individual patients in terms of parameters (e.g., tumor size, shape, location, blood flow) which can significantly influence the treatment outcome. The impact of modeling in hyperthermia research is further magnified when one considers the time, effort, and expense needed for the carefully planned laboratory experiments that are required to extract detailed measurement maps. The extensive potential for simulation in hyperthermia has been best summarized by the identification of four areas where treatment modeling should play a role in improving power delivery and evaluating resulting dosimetry [95]. These categories are (1) comparative, (2) prospective, (3) concurrent, and (4) retrospective hyperthermic dosimetry.

The purpose of *comparative dosimetry* is to evaluate the performance of different devices under the same clinical situations in order to establish guidelines for the use of one system over another in a given circumstance. *Prospective dosimetry* incorporates all available information about a specific patient and considers the array of possible heating devices that may be used in order to plan the treatment course most suitable for that particular patient. In *concurrent dosimetry* one attempts to infer the temperature distribution during the treatment based on a few temperature measurements and then modifies the power delivery (if possible) to improve the therapeutic temperature rise in the tumor. In *retrospective dosimetry* the complete temperature profile is also inferred from measured data, but this inference occurs after the treatment in order to correlate temperature distributions with observed therapeutic benefit and to evaluate the ability of a device to elevate the entire tumor volume above some predefined therapeutic threshold.

While these four types of hyperthermic dosimetry have been conceived and developed in terms of the thermal problem, one can envision how such categories could be applied in the context of the power deposition problem as well. Comparative examination of power absorption patterns produced by various devices would result in valuable information for improving treatment quality. Prospective and concurrent studies of only power depositions, while certainly possible in theory, would not seem to be advisable since treatment decisions would result based on secondary quantities which are subject to misinterpretations. The same can be said about retrospective evaluation of power deposition patterns. Given that similar power absorptions could easily result in completely different thermal profiles due to varying blood perfusions, the correlation of power deposition patterns with successful treatment outcome would be difficult to establish. Thus, these four classes of hyperthermic dosimetry are much more appropriately discussed in Chap. 3. However, even with the brief descriptions given above, it is clear why a computational model is needed and how it can greatly facilitate the understanding of hyperthermic dosimetry which should lead to patient treatments of the highest possible quality.

A computational model can have significant impact on clinical hyperthermia or hyperthermia research in general only if it can be formulated with mathematical rigor and precision which adheres to the underlying physics of the situation to be simulated. This chapter discusses the issues involved in developing such models for calculating power deposition patterns in hyperthermia. The chapter is divided into three major sections entitled: "*General Considerations*," "*Modeling Progress*," and "*Numerical Methods*." The first two are intended for a general audience while the third is written assuming some sophistication in numerical techniques. Each part is self-contained such that those interested in the clinical relevance of this topic can read the chapter, understand the basic issues involved, but not get lost in the mathematics. However, the details of the numerical methods are intimately connected with this research, and, as such, are also discussed. Hopefully, this portion of the chapter will also be of interest to many readers as well.

Since the power deposition problem tends to be device-specific, the first section begins with some general considerations of power sources. Both the ultrasonic and electromagnetic cases are considered. Also provided here is an overview of the analytical and numerical solution techniques that have been used in the hyperthermia context. The emphasis is on general issues such as the strengths and limitations of competing methods and the impact that these techniques have had in hyperthermia research, both past and present. This section concludes with some sample calculations for three classes of electromagnetic applicators. The second section traces the progress in the development of models for making power deposition calculations. Again the emphasis is on the strengths, weaknesses, and current status of the modeling efforts in this area of research. Both two- and three-dimensional formulations are considered and their contributions to present understanding as well as their role in future research are addressed. While examples are drawn from the literature and a number of recent studies are cited, this section is not intended to be an exhaustive literature review, but rather to provide the reader with an appreciation of the progress that has been made and the current capabilities and limitations of methods employed to calculate power deposition patterns in hyperthermia. The final section discusses five major numerical techniques which are being used to simulate hyperthermia treatments:

1. domain integral equations,
2. finite element methods,
3. finite differences,
4. boundary element methods, and
5. hybrid element techniques.

The basic formulation and numerical implementation issues for each of the various techniques are addressed. Further, the strengths and weaknesses of each method are considered both in general as well as in the context of hyperthermic simulations. Analysis of simulated results is reserved for other chapters within this volume where the interpretations include the crucial influence of heat transfer mechanisms.

2.2 General Considerations

2.2.1 Heat Sources

Considerable engineering effort has gone into the design and development of hyperthermia delivery systems and in general two approaches have been implemented most often:

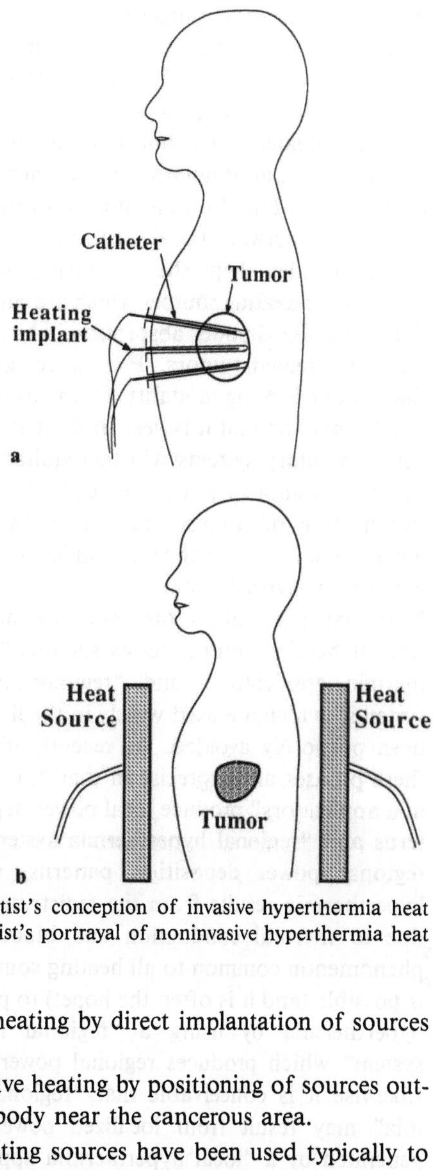

Fig. 2.2. a Artist's conception of invasive hyperthermia heat sources. **b** Artist's portrayal of noninvasive hyperthermia heat sources

1. invasive heating by direct implantation of sources or
2. noninvasive heating by positioning of sources outside the body near the cancerous area.

Invasive heating sources have been used typically to produce hyperthermia in a localized area (e.g., in the tumor) and therefore are generally referred to as local power deposition methods. Noninvasive heating sources have been used to produce hyperthermia in both localized areas as well as over large regions of the body (e.g., in the thorax) and commonly have been labeled as either local or regional power deposition methods. Generally, noninvasive heating sources are categorized as local power deposition methods when they are being used to treat superficially located tumors (<5 cm in depth from the body surface) whereas noninvasive heating sources are referred to as regional power deposition techniques when they are being used to treat deep-seated tumors (>5 cm in depth). Figure 2.2a, b shows conceptual drawings of invasive and noninvasive hyperthermia power sources.

Noninvasive heating sources have a certain natural appeal in that the therapy can be administered without a surgical procedure. The engineering challenges (especially for heating deep-seated tumor sites), however, are greater given that a successful noninvasive therapy device must not only deliver therapeutic doses to the tumor, but also must not overheat any normal tissue lying between the device itself and the tumor. Thus, the ideal hyperthermia system would utilize noninvasive heating sources which are capable of producing localized power absorption in both superficial and deep-seated tumors. Present research suggests that no one heating modality is superior to the others in all cases and that it is very likely that a number of complementary systems will be required to treat the variety of tumor sites encountered in the clinic. Effective heating of deep-seated tumors by noninvasive means remains one of the most difficult problems facing clinical hyperthermia.

Note that in the above discussion of the categorization of heating sources terms such as "local hyperthermia applicators" and "regional hyperthermia systems," which are used widely in the literature, have been purposely avoided. As recently discussed [86] these phrases are imprecise in that "local hyperthermia applicators" produce local power deposition patterns and "regional hyperthermia systems" produce regional power deposition patterns, whereas the hyperthermia results from the redistribution of heat due to thermal conduction and blood flow – a phenomenon common to all heating sources. Thus, it is possible (and it is often the hope!) to produce local hyperthermia by using a "regional hyperthermic system" which produces regional power absorption. Likewise it is conceivable that "regional hyperthermia" may result from localized power deposition generated by a "local hyperthermia applicator." The suggestion in [86] to substitute "local/regional power deposition (or absorption)" for "local/regional hyperthermia" when discussing hyperthermia delivery systems has been adopted herein.

The two heating sources that have been used most often to induce hyperthermia are electromagnetic and ultrasonic radiation. Classically, electromagnetic (EM) waves are known to dissipate energy as they propagate through a lossy medium such as tissue. The EM energy deposited at a point in tissue is proportional to the square of the magnitude of the electric field at that point. Mathematically, the instantaneous power absorbed per unit volume of tissue can be written as

$$Q_e = \sigma |\mathbf{E}|^2 \qquad (2.1)$$

where σ is the electrical conductivity and $\mathbf{E}$ is the electric field. Hence, knowledge of the EM field produced by a particular therapy system is needed in order to calculate its power deposition pattern. Similarly acoustic power is dissipated through the conversion of mechanical energy to internal energy as ultrasonic (US) waves propagate through tissue. The US power absorbed at a point in tissue is proportional to the intensity of the ultrasound wave at that point. Mathematically, the instantaneous power absorbed per unit volume of tissue from US radiation can be written as

$$Q_u = \alpha I \qquad (2.2)$$

where α is the absorption coefficient and I is the acoustic intensity. Thus, for US therapy devices, knowledge of the acoustic intensity is needed to calculate power absorption patterns within the body.

In general, the absorbed power whether generated by EM or US sources is a function of position and time; therefore, the electric field and acoustic intensity must be regarded as varying with space and time as well. However, most EM or US hyperthermia systems have time-harmonic sources such that the time variation of any wave can be represented by the complex exponential factor $e^{i\omega t}$ where ω is the angular frequency of the sinusoidal sources producing the wave. Under these conditions the propagation problem can be solved in a simplified form in which the time variation has been removed since only the steady-state power deposition pattern is of concern. When the power is controlled by pulse-width modulation, typically the controlling pulse width is long compared to the period of the EM or US waves and their transit times to steady-state, thus the use of the complex exponential factor represents no loss in generality [118]. In such cases, the steady-state power deposition pattern can be assumed during the "power on" cycle of the modulation.

As will be seen in the course of this chapter, one has the option of calculating the desired field quantities as either functions of time and space or as functions of space only. If both the time and space variations are explicit, the calculation will be considered as occurring in the *time-domain*. If, however, only the spatial variations are involved (i.e., the time variation has been removed via $e^{i\omega t}$), the computation will be regarded as taking place in the *frequency-domain*. Time and frequency-domain solutions representing time-harmonic waves are equivalent in such a way that the time-domain solution can be reconstructed from its frequency domain counterpart through the simple relationship $\mathbf{E}(x, t) = \mathrm{Re}\{\mathbf{E}(x) e^{i\omega t}\}$ where Re{ } denotes taking the real part of a complex quantity.

While wave equations can be used describe the propagation of electromagnetic and ultrasonic waves, electromagnetic and acoustic waves are very different in nature. One of the fundamental differences between these two types of waves is the speed at which they propagate. Since acoustic waves are linked to the propagation of mechanical vibrations which result in the displacement of tissue molecules whereas electromagnetic waves are associated with electric and magnetic fields produced from accelerating charges, sound waves propagate significantly slower in tissue than electromagnetic waves. It is this slower speed of sound in tissue that affords ultrasound hyperthermia devices several advantages over electromagnetic systems. Ultrasound wavelengths, for the same frequency of excitation, are much shorter than those of electromagnetic waves because of their (ultrasound's) slower propagation velocity. This shorter wavelength allows for greater focussing capabilities with ultrasound.

In the frequency range where suitable depths of penetration can be achieved (i.e., 1 – 10 MHz) wavelengths on the order of 1 mm are possible with ultrasound [5, 123]. These distances are approximately two orders of magnitude smaller than the corresponding wavelengths for electromagnetic waves. Further, the depth of penetration of ultrasound is greater than 10 cm at these frequencies, which is considerably larger than the few centimeters obtainable for EM fields at higher frequencies where some focussing can be achieved. While comparable conduction current penetration is possible at 1 – 10 MHz with electromagnetic devices, problems associated with excessive superficial heating are difficult to overcome, thus limiting their use at low frequencies [56]. Further, the velocity of sound and the acoustic impedance is relatively constant in most tissues except bone and air pockets; thus reflections at tissue interfaces are minimized in most cases. This is especially important at muscle-fat interfaces which can cause reflections that result in standing waves and excessive heating in the fat layer when EM devices are used.

While ultrasound appears to have many advantages over its electromagnetic counterpart, ultrasonic therapy devices are not without their own shortcomings. Specifically, the disadvantages of ultrasound center around

1. the high absorption coefficient of ultrasound in bone which can result in hot spots and patient pain in anatomical areas containing bone, and
2. the inability of ultrasound to penetrate gaseous spaces, hence making the therapeutic applications of ultrasound in the lung area of limited value.

Interestingly, electromagnetic hyperthermia does not appear to be particularly hindered by the presence of bones (which typically absorb very little power due to their low conductivity) and should be useful for applications in the lung where better penetration depths are possible [56]. Thus, a valid basis exists for considering ultrasonic and electromagnetic hyperthermia therapy systems as complementary rather than competitive in nature.

2.2.2 Governing Equations

Information about regional power deposition patterns is even more necessary than in the case of local power absorption. Since significantly more anatomical area, particularly normal tissue, is exposed to large field strengths when regional power deposition systems are used, more potential exists for damage of normal tissue from overheating. Further, temperature measurements currently cannot be made throughout the treatment field, thus increasing the risk of undetected overexposure of normal tissue. The calculation of fields produced in the body by external source arrangements (whether ultrasonic or electromagnetic) is an important step in determining the efficacy of any noninvasive heat delivery system and is especially important for devices which produce regional power depositions. Thus, a significant amount of the modeling work in the simulation of hyperthermia treatments has centered around the analysis of noninvasive systems, and the solution to this type of problem will form the focal point for much of the discussion to follow.

In order to make such a calculation, one must have a mathematical framework which represents the underlying physics. Unfortunately, the propagation of acoustic waves is highly nonlinear, but under certain assumptions a linear theory can be developed which is accurate enough to be useful [5]. In contrast, the propagation of electromagnetic waves is linear in most instances and a well-established linear mathematical framework is firmly in place. Since this is the case, the discussion in this section will center around the electromagnetic case. This will be true for most of the rest of the chapter as well, partly because of the relative simplicity that the linear nature of EM theory affords and partly because of the numerous applications of this work. Further, where the ultrasound equations have been linearized, their form mimics the electromagnetic equations and discussions concerning their solution and interpretation will be similar to the electromagnetic case.

The foundation of electromagnetic theory lies in four first-order partial differential equations known collectively as the Maxwell equations. With the aid of the constitutive relations for simple media [104] and the vector identity that the divergence of a curl of any vector is zero (i.e., $\nabla \cdot \nabla \times \mathrm{A} = 0$), one can show that only two of the four Maxwell equations are needed to define uniquely the electric and magnetic fields (provided that conservation of charge is maintained). Assuming a periodic time variation of $e^{-i\omega t}$, the two Maxwell curl equations, which relate the electric and magnetic fields, can be written in their differential form as

$$\nabla \times \mathbf{E} = i\omega\mu\mathbf{H} \tag{2.3 a}$$

$$\nabla \times \mathbf{H} = -i\omega\varepsilon^*\mathbf{E} \tag{2.3 b}$$

where **E** is the complex amplitude of the electric field, **H** is the complex amplitude of the magnetic field, μ is the magnetic permeability, $\varepsilon^* = \varepsilon + i\sigma/\omega$ is the complex permittivity, ε is the permittivity, σ is the electrical conductivity, ω is the radian frequency, and $i = \sqrt{-1}$.

While these equations are mathematically convenient, their physical interpretations can be more readily understood in terms of the integral forms of Eqs. 2.3 a and 2.3 b where the explicit time-dependence has been restored:

$$\oint_c \mathbf{E} \cdot \mathbf{dl} = -\frac{d}{dt} \int_s \mu\mathbf{H} \cdot \mathbf{ds} \tag{2.3 c}$$

$$\oint_c \mathbf{H} \cdot \mathbf{dl} = \frac{d}{dt} \int_s \varepsilon\mathbf{E} \cdot \mathbf{ds} + \int_s \sigma\mathbf{E} \cdot \mathbf{ds} \ . \tag{2.3 d}$$

For example, Eq. 2.3 c indicates that the net circulation (or rotation) of **E** around a closed contour is equal to the time rate of decrease of the magnetic flux through the surface bounded by that contour. Equations 2.3 c and 2.3 d show that changing magnetic fluxes produce electric field circulation while changing electric fluxes produce magnetic field circulation. Equations 2.3 a and 2.3 b merely represent mathematical statements of these phenomena at a fixed point. The interested reader may wish to consult an introductory electromagnetics textbook for more detailed discussions of the physical interpretations of the Maxwell equations (e.g., see [59]).

Equations 2.3 a and 2.3 b must be supplemented with certain boundary conditions at interfaces between different media (tissues in the present context) since the differential operations do not exist at such boundaries. At source-free boundaries (e.g., inside the body) the boundary conditions on the electric and magnetic fields are

$$\hat{\mathbf{n}} \cdot (\varepsilon_1^* \mathbf{E}_1 - \varepsilon_2^* \mathbf{E}_2) = 0 \tag{2.4 a}$$

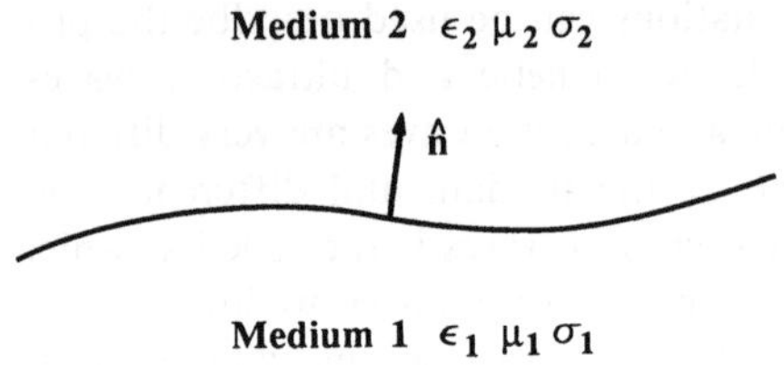

Fig. 2.3. Interface separating two electrically distinct regions and its associated normal direction

$$\hat{\mathbf{n}} \times (\mathbf{E}_1 - \mathbf{E}_2) = 0 \tag{2.4 b}$$

$$\hat{\mathbf{n}} \times (\mathbf{H}_1 - \mathbf{H}_2) = 0 \tag{2.4 c}$$

$$\hat{\mathbf{n}} \cdot (\mu_1 \mathbf{H}_1 - \mu_2 \mathbf{H}_2) = 0 \tag{2.4 d}$$

where the subscripts distinguish the two media types forming the interface and $\hat{\mathbf{n}}$ is a unit vector normal to the boundary. Figure 2.3 shows a conceptual drawing of a boundary separating two different regions and indicates the normal vector for the subscript convention in Eqs. 2.4. When sources are present on a boundary, Eqs. 2.4 a, c must be modified such that

$$\hat{\mathbf{n}} \cdot (\varepsilon_1^* \mathbf{E}_1 - \varepsilon_2^* \mathbf{E}_2) = \varrho \tag{2.5 a}$$

$$\hat{\mathbf{n}} \times (\mathbf{H}_1 - \mathbf{H}_2) = \mathbf{J} \tag{2.5 b}$$

where **J** and ϱ are the surface current and charge densities, respectively, residing on the boundary. The introduction of **J** and ϱ requires that conservation of charge be maintained through the continuity equation

$$\nabla \cdot \mathbf{J} = i\omega\varrho \ . \tag{2.5 c}$$

In the context of electromagnetically induced hyperthermia, μ is effectively constant, but σ and ε vary with tissue type as well as frequency. Hence, Eqs. 2.4 will have to be satisfied when making power deposition calculations. Equations 2.4 indicate that the magnetic field is continuous across all boundaries within the body while the electric field has a normal component (to the boundary) which is discontinuous by the ratio of the complex permittivities of the two tissues forming the boundary. Note that the tangential component of the electric field is continuous across all tissue boundaries like the magnetic field. These boundary conditions can play important roles in shaping power deposition patterns as is illustrated by the following simple example.

If one considers the instantaneous power absorbed on either side of a muscle-fat interface, then

$$Q_f = \sigma_f\,|\mathbf{E}_f|^2 = \sigma_f[(E_f^n)^2 + (E_f^t)^2] \tag{2.6 a}$$

$$Q_m = \sigma_m\,|\mathbf{E}_m|^2 = \sigma_m[(E_m^n)^2 + (E_m^t)^2] \tag{2.6 b}$$

where the m and f subscripts designate the muscle and fat sides of the interface and the n and t superscripts indicate the normal and tangential (to the boundary) components of the electric field. The ratio of the power deposited on the fat side to that on the muscle becomes

$$\frac{Q_f}{Q_m} = \frac{\sigma_f[(E_f^n)^2+(E_f^t)^2]}{\sigma_m[(E_m^n)^2+(E_m^t)^2]} = \frac{\sigma_f[(E_f^n)^2+(E_f^t)^2]}{\sigma_m\{[(\varepsilon_f^*/\varepsilon_m^*)E_f^n]^2+(E_f^t)^2\}} \tag{2.6c}$$

in light of the boundary conditions on the electric field which must be satisfied. In the extreme cases where the electric field is either perfectly normal (i.e., $E^t = 0$) or perfectly tangential (i.e., $E^n = 0$) to the boundary, this ratio varies from

$$\frac{Q_f}{Q_m} = \frac{\sigma_f}{\sigma_m}\left(\frac{\varepsilon_m^*}{\varepsilon_f^*}\right)^2 \approx 10 \quad \text{to} \quad \frac{Q_f}{Q_m} = \frac{\sigma_f}{\sigma_m} \approx 0.075 \tag{2.6d}$$

for typical values of muscle and fat electrical properties. Thus one can conclude that it is this jump discontinuity in the normal component of the electric field which contributes to the excessive heating in the fat layer that has been observed with some electromagnetic heating devices [29, 56]. In accordance with Eq. 2.6c, such devices often produce electric fields that are predominantly perpendicular to the body's subcutaneous muscle-fat interface.

Since the task is to calculate power deposition patterns, and power absorption is directly related to the electric field, two choices seem clear: (1) compute the electric field directly or (2) compute the magnetic field directly and then take its curl (i.e., apply Eq. 2.3b to obtain **E**). To isolate **E**, divide Eq. 2.3a by $i\omega\mu$, take the curl of Eq. 2.3a, and substitute Eq. 2.3b. The magnetic field can be isolated in a similar manner by dividing Eq. 2.3b by $i\omega\varepsilon^*$, taking the curl of Eq. 2.3b, and substituting 2.3a. Performing these operations results in the following second-order partial differential equations in the quantity of interest – either **E** or **H**:

$$\nabla\times\frac{1}{i\omega\mu}\nabla\times\mathbf{E}+i\omega\varepsilon^*\mathbf{E} = 0 \tag{2.7a}$$

$$\nabla\times\frac{1}{i\omega\varepsilon^*}\nabla\times\mathbf{H}+i\omega\mu\mathbf{H} = 0\ . \tag{2.7b}$$

Since μ is constant in hyperthermia applications, Eq. 2.7 can be rewritten as

$$\nabla\times\nabla\times\mathbf{E}-k^2\mathbf{E} = 0 \tag{2.8a}$$

$$\nabla\times\frac{1}{k^2}\nabla\times\mathbf{H}-\mathbf{H} = 0 \tag{2.8b}$$

where $k^2 = \omega^2\mu\varepsilon^*$. One of these two equations, in conjunction with any required boundary conditions, needs to be solved in order to calculate power deposition.

At a glance, it may seem that solving Eq. 2.8b for the magnetic field is a simpler route since **H** is continuous across all boundaries inside the body and hence the boundary conditions can be applied as a natural consequence of the formulation. Under some circumstances (as will be indicated later) this turns out to be true; however, the apparent ease of solving Eq. 2.8b (relative to Eq. 2.8a) due to the simplicity of its associated boundary conditions is counterbalanced by the extra work required to obtain **E** from Eq. 2.3b. In fact, whether one solves Eq. 2.8a for the electric field directly (in which case the less appealing boundary conditions on **E** are obviously needed) or solves for **H** and then calculates **E**, the boundary conditions on **E** must be satisfied in either case unless one is content to avoid computing **E** on the boundaries when **H** is calculated first.

Two convenient classifications for electromagnetic field configurations are transverse magnetic (TM) and transverse electric (TE). If one considers the x–y plane as the plane of analysis, then the TM electromagnetic field configuration implies that the magnetic field is confined to the transverse or analysis plane while the electric field is everywhere perpendicular to this plane (i.e., in the z direction). Conversely, the TE electromagnetic field configuration has the electric field lying in the analysis plane while the magnetic field is everywhere perpendicular to it. These classifications will be used to refer to such EM field configurations as they arise in the following sections. Note that in the TM case, a two-dimensional calculation in the x–y plane requires no special consideration at the interface between tissues since **E** can only be tangential to any such interface and H is continuous under the assumption that μ is constant. In the TE case, however, **E** is in the analysis plane and its normal-direction discontinuity must be observed at tissue boundaries.

When acoustic wave theory is linearized a wave equation can be written in terms of the acoustic pressure

$$\nabla^2 P+k^2 P = 0 \tag{2.9}$$

where k is a complex wavenumber whose real part is approximately $2\pi/\lambda$ (λ is the wavelength in tissue) at the frequencies of interest in hyperthermia and whose imaginary part is the attenuation coefficient in the medium [5, 118, 123]. Equation 2.9 is a scalar version of Eq. 2.8a for the electric field. For example, when the TM case is considered and the x–y plane is assumed to be the transverse plane, then $\mathbf{E} = E_z\hat{\mathbf{z}}$ and $\nabla\times\nabla\times\mathbf{E}$ collapses to $-\nabla^2 E_z$ in which case Eq. 2.8a is rewritten as

$$\nabla^2 E_z + k^2 E_z = 0 \; . \tag{2.10}$$

Thus, the same solution techniques that apply to Eq. 2.8a or its scalar version Eq. 2.10 will also be applicable to the linearized ultrasound theory expressed by Eq. 2.9.

The acoustic intensity, which is needed to calculate the ultrasonic power deposition, is proportional to the magnitude squared of the acoustic pressure. Mathematically the relationship between the instantaneous acoustic intensity and the acoustic pressure at a point in tissue can be expressed as

$$I = \frac{|P|^2}{Z} \tag{2.11}$$

where Z is the acoustic impedance. The acoustic impedance is the product of the medium density and velocity of propagation of sound in the medium [5, 123]. Recall that the propagation velocity is relatively constant in many tissues (with a few notable exceptions which are very important) and likewise the densities of many tissues are also quite similar. Hence reflections (i.e., boundary conditions) can be ignored for many types of interfaces, making the problem basically a calculation in homogeneous media. However, in the presence of interfaces between muscle and bone or muscle and air, the impedance mismatches cannot be ignored and suitable boundary conditions must be applied. Under such circumstances the mismatch is so great that almost all of the energy is reflected, which results in additional and potentially excessive heating. Care must be exercised to account for these boundaries and knowledge of their location can be especially important.

Wave equations in linear form can also be written in terms of particle displacement. The quantities of primary interest, the acoustic pressure and the particle velocity, can then be expressed in terms of the particle displacement. Finally, it is interesting to note that the attenuation of the medium has been neglected in a large portion of the studies where fields have been calculated for ultrasonic transducers. This assumption has been acceptable to the medical diagnostic community, where the field patterns of different sizes and shapes of transducers are of interest and the attenuation is of secondary concern [118]. Clearly, this is not the case for hyperthermia applications. In terms of the calculation of acoustic pressure, accounting for medium attenuation requires considering the wavenumber as a complex rather than purely real quantity.

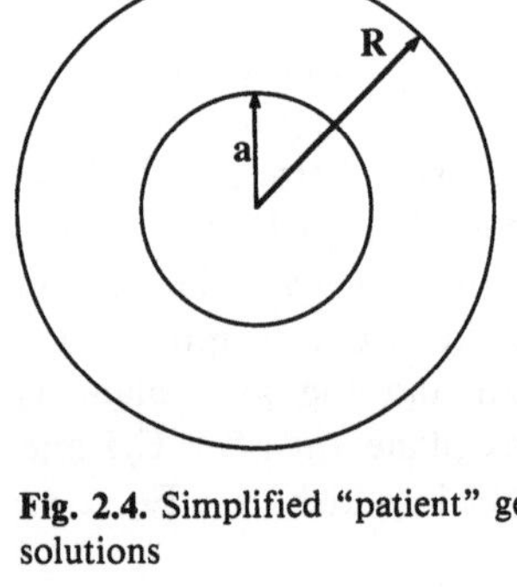

Fig. 2.4. Simplified "patient" geometry amenable to analytical solutions

2.2.3 Solution Techniques

Thus far the basic equations that need to be solved in order to calculate power deposition patterns have been discussed and the task of arriving at solutions to these equations must now be considered. At this point, it is important to keep in mind the intended purposes of any calculations to be made. If power deposition calculations are being made as an initial step in thermal dosimetry simulations and the resulting simulations are intended to fall within one of the four categories of hyperthermic dosimetry previously outlined – comparative, prospective, concurrent, or retrospective – then there must be some accounting for irregular boundaries and inhomogeneous tissue properties which suggests that numerical techniques are in order. If the purpose of the power deposition calculations is to illuminate some basic physical principles then analytical solutions under simplified, but representative, circumstances, may be the best way to gain insight into the problem. Since this chapter is primarily concerned with calculations having the former purpose in mind, the emphasis here will be on numerical methods. However, analytical solutions have important roles in hyperthermia modeling such as providing checks on numerical computations and illustrating first-order analysis of complicated problems and should not be ignored. In fact, one possibility that has yet to be investigated fully is the use of an analytical solution or analytical approximation in lieu of a full-blown numerical computation only for the power deposition part of the thermal dosimetry problem. These results would then be used with a numerical method to solve for temperature distributions. Such an approach may be critical for the near future success of three-dimensional patient treatment planning in the clinic given that detailed three-dimensional power deposition calculations in realistic patient geometries are currently too computer intensive for routine clinical use. This is particularly true for the electromagnetic problem which, because of its vector nature, consists of a set of three coupled scalar equations (i.e., three equations and three unknowns at each calculation point). Whether a quasi-analytical approach is viable for accurate simulation of hyperthermia treatments remains to be seen.

One of the simplest, but most useful, analytical solutions is that of infinite concentric cylinders where either the electric or magnetic field is specified at the outer cylinder boundary and is directed perpendicularly to the cylinder cross-section. The analytical solution in the ith layer, where each concentric cylinder contains different tissue properties, is

$$E_z(r) = A_i J_0(k_i r) + B_i Y_0(k_i r) \tag{2.12}$$

for the electric field case where J_0 is the Bessel function of the first kind order zero, Y_0 is the Bessel function of the second kind order zero, $k = \omega\sqrt{\mu\varepsilon^*}$, z is the direction of infinite extent, r is the radial coordinate and A_i and B_i are determined from the boundary conditions. The geometry for two concentric cylinders is shown in Fig. 2.4. In this case, A_i and B_i (i = 1 to 2) must not only satisfy the conditions imposed on the boundary of the outer cylinder, but also must ensure continuity of E_z and $\frac{\partial E_z}{\partial r}$ at the boundary of the inner cylinder. These boundary conditions provide the system of equations

$$\begin{bmatrix} -J_0(k_1\alpha) & J_0(k_2\alpha) & Y_0(k_2\alpha) \\ -k_1 J_1(k_1\alpha) & k_2 J_1(k_2\alpha) & k_2 Y_1(k_2\alpha) \\ 0 & J_0(k_2 R) & Y_0(k_2 R) \end{bmatrix} \begin{Bmatrix} A_1 \\ A_2 \\ B_2 \end{Bmatrix} = \begin{Bmatrix} 0 \\ 0 \\ E_0 \end{Bmatrix} \tag{2.13}$$

where J_1 is the Bessel function of the first kind order one, Y_1 is the Bessel function of the second kind order one, α is the radius of the inner cylinder, R is the radius of the outer cylinder, and E_0 is the imposed electric field at R, which can be solved by any convenient method to obtain the coefficients in Eq. 2.12. This solution or its counterpart for the magnetic field has served many purposes in hyperthermia research. It has been used as a simple verification or comparison for numerical algorithms (e.g., see [73]) and as a means of providing some initial analysis of magnetic induction and annular array applicators [17, 142]. Figure 2.5 shows a typical example where an analytical and a numerical solution are compared for the purpose of verifying the accuracy of a numerical algorithm.

Another common application of analytical solutions in calculating power deposition patterns in hyperthermia is to use classical expressions for basic electromagnetic source elements such as point sources or

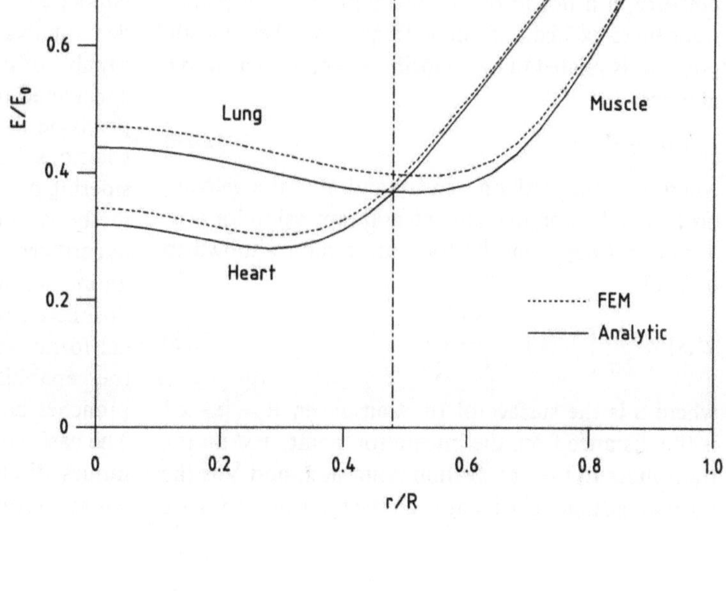

Fig. 2.5. Sample comparison of analytical and numerical solutions on the geometry in Fig. 2.4 for the purpose of verifying a numerical algorithm. The inner cylinder radius is shown by the *dashed vertical line* and the tissues contained in each cylinder are indicated

infinitesimal dipoles or some other idealized fundamental radiator. The actual applicator or array of applicators that are being simulated are then considered to be represented by a collection of these fundamental EM source elements. The total electric field is found by integrating over the surface of the applicator and vectorially adding the contributions from each elemental source. This method has been used to analyze power deposition patterns produced by a variety of different hyperthermia applicators [2, 46, 64, 135]. A related analytical method for calculating source fields is the gaussian beam model, which not only accounts for the finite size of apertures, but also accommodates simple interfaces between different media [3].

The approach described above is often considered to be a numerical calculation in that the resulting expression (usually an integral over the source surface) for the desired field quantity cannot be evaluated explicitly and some kind of numerical integration must be implemented. In many cases, assumptions must be made about the field distributions on the source surface to keep the problem a numerical integration or summation of known quantities as compared with an integral equation, where unknowns also occur in the integrand. This type of technique has been considered here to be an analytical method for two reasons:

1. to distinguish it from numerical techniques to be discussed later which require matrix equation solutions or iteration schemes, and
2. because the quantity of interest can be represented in a closed form which contains entirely known (or assumed to be known) quantities.

The basic approach has also been used in acoustic field calculations [21, 38, 123]. As an example of the general method, consider the calculation of acoustic pressure in a nonabsorbing medium due to a planar transducer excited at a single frequency. The acoustic pressure is related to the velocity potential in a simple manner:

$$P = i\omega\varrho\Psi \tag{2.14}$$

where ϱ is the medium density and Ψ is the velocity potential. An approximate integral expression for ψ at a point x away from the transducer can be shown to be [123]

$$\Psi(x) = \frac{1}{2\pi} \int_S V(x') \frac{e^{-ikR}}{R} dS \tag{2.15}$$

where S is the surface of the transducer, $R = |x-x'|$ is the distance from the integration point at x' on the transducer to the observation point at x, and V is the normal particle velocity at x' on the transducer. Figure

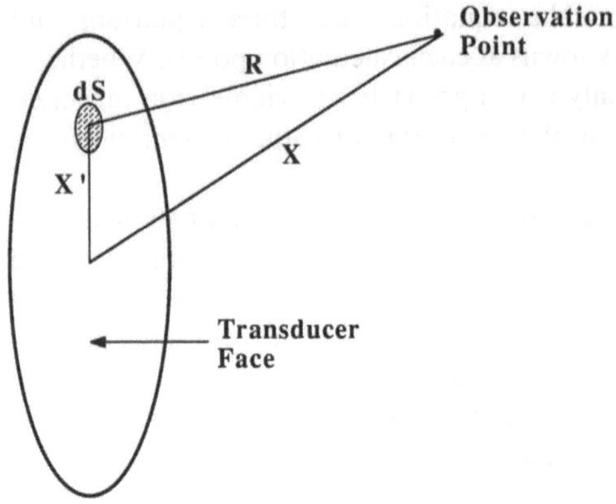

Fig. 2.6. Integration of known quantities over the face of a transducer in order to obtain the field at an observation point some distance away

2.6 shows the relevant geometry. Note that Eq. 2.15 results from the integration via Green's theorem of a scalar wave equation in Ψ where certain approximations have been made.

Provided that the normal particle velocity is known over the transducer face, Eq. 2.15 becomes an integration that cannot be done analytically but which can be performed numerically by dividing the transducer surface into a discrete set of incremental areas. This type of method for calculating the field quantities needed to compute power absorption patterns has been classified as analytical in nature even though a numerical procedure is required to obtain a solution. Note that in these types of approaches the medium is taken to be homogeneous – a significant limitation for clinical problems which normally have irregular boundaries and heterogeneous tissue properties. In order to account for these kinds of details numerical methods are generally required.

Numerical computation is a valuable form of present-day analysis because high-speed computers are capable of carrying approximations, which were once considered to be of little use, to such high degrees of precision that they are essentially as accurate as exact solutions. This idea is especially important when considering problems that are not solvable with analytical methods such as those routinely faced in clinical hyperthermia. In order for numerical analysis to have an impact on understanding/predicting hyperthermic dosimetry, robust mathematically defensible numerical formulations combined with a keen awareness of the capabilities and limitations of the numerical approaches are required.

The basic strategy behind the numerical solution techniques discussed herein is to reduce the functional equation into an algebraic equation or matrix of algebraic equations that can then be solved with standard techniques such as matrix equation solvers which are readily available on most computers as subroutines in user-accessible libraries. As a starting point for understanding this basic concept, consider a physical process (in the present context, e.g., the propagation of electromagnetic waves in tissue) which can be described by the mathematical expression

$$Lu = g \qquad (2.16)$$

where L is an operator which is differential, integral, or integro-differential, u is the unknown physical quantity to be determined, and g is some known source or excitation. Only deterministic problems are of concern, that is, problems which are unique in that only one u is possible for a given g. Once Eq. 2.16 has been reduced into an acceptable matrix of algebraic equations, it will be assumed solved since standard techniques (e.g., matrix inversion) can be employed. If a residual, R(u), is defined as

$$R(u) = Lu - g \qquad (2.17)$$

then, if the exact solution, u, were known, R(u) could be multiplied by any spatial function W(x) and this result integrated over the problem domain would be identically zero given that R(u) = 0 everywhere u is known exactly, i.e.,

$$\langle R(u)\, W(x)\rangle = 0 \qquad (2.18)$$

where $\langle\,\rangle$ denotes integration over the problem domain. In general u is not known (if it were, there would be no need for a numerical method!); however, u can be approximated by $\hat{u}$ as the sum of some unknown coefficients, u_j, multiplied by some known basis functions, b_j:

$$\hat{u} = \sum_{j=1}^{N} u_j\, b_j(x)\ . \qquad (2.19)$$

Then L operating on $\hat{u}$ is no longer equal to g; hence $R(\hat{u}) \neq 0$. The idea for reducing the functional Eq. 2.16 into a matrix of algebraic equations is to force $R(\hat{u}) = 0$ "on average" over the problem domain (recall the exact solution would have $R(u) = 0$ everywhere over the problem domain) by using N independent functions, W_i, such that for each i:

$$\langle R(\hat{u})\, W_i\rangle = 0\ . \qquad (2.20)$$

Equation 2.20 provides a simple recipe for generating N equations in N unknown coefficients $u_i, i = 1, 2, \ldots N$. This technique is known as the weighted residual method [32, 47] and the W_i's are referred to as the weighting functions (another name for this approach is method of moments [47], although this name is used almost exclusively to refer to the case where the operator, L, in Eq. 2.16 has an integral form). In matrix form, the weighted residual approximation to Eq. 2.16 can be written as

$$[\mathscr{L}]\,\{\mathscr{U}\} = \{\mathscr{G}\} \qquad (2.21)$$

where $\{\mathscr{U}\}$ = column vector of coefficients, $u_1, u_2 \ldots u_N$, $\{\mathscr{G}\}$ = column vector of elements $\langle g\, W_i\rangle$, and $[\mathscr{L}]$ = square matrix of elements $\langle L(b_j)\, W_i\rangle$. Note that the elements of the column matrix, $\mathscr{G}$, and the square matrix, $\mathscr{L}$, in Eq. 2.21 simply comprise domain integrations of completely known functions, and standard numerical integration techniques such as gaussian quadrature can be used.

A host of mathematical considerations surround the convergence of Eq. 2.21 and the relationship between $\hat{u}$ and u. Analysis of such is usually embedded in the concepts of Hilbert space operator theory, which is beyond the intended scope of this chapter. The interested reader may wish to consult [28] for a brief summary of the fundamental issues involved in establishing convergence. From a practical standpoint, the operators to be discussed in this chapter often have well-known properties and convergence of the numerical approximations have either been established mathematically (e.g., see [113]) or shown numerically.

In order to compute the elements of these matrices, appropriate basis and weighting functions must be chosen. A number of factors including solution accuracy, degree of difficulty in evaluating individual matrix elements, and the sparseness and invertibility of the resulting matrix need to be considered. Further, the type of operator that L represents is important. For example, if L symbolizes the operation of second-order differentiation, the choice of a pulse as a basis function would not be allowed since it is not considered to be in the domain of L. In practical terms, there would be no way to evaluate the elements in the matrix $\mathscr{L}$ in this case. Thus, some care is required in the choice of basis and weighting functions for a particular problem.

Fortunately, a great deal of experience has been accumulated concerning the appropriate selection of these functions and for most problems of interest such choices have been more or less standardized. Some commonly used basis and weighting functions are:

$$b_i(x) = \delta(x - x_i) \qquad (2.22\,a)$$

$$b_i(x) = 1 \qquad (2.22\,b)$$

$$b_i(x) = \text{polynomial}\ . \qquad (2.22\,c)$$

Typically Eqs. 2.22a and 2.22b are used when L is an integral operator since they simplify the integrations

that need to be performed whereas Eq. 2.22c is often used for differential operators because of the simplicity in differentiating polynomials (linear and quadratic functions are the most widely used). When Eq. 2.22a is used as the weighting function, this choice is known as "point-matching" since the residual in Eq. 2.20 is set equal to zero at a discrete number of points throughout the problem domain. Note that if the basis and weighting functions are selected to be identical, this is referred to as Galerkin's method [61].
For problems involving complicated domains (i.e., domains having an inhomogeneous, irregular geometry) a common strategy is the use of basis functions (and weighting functions) that exist only over a subregion of the domain. Such basis functions are often referred to as having local support in that they only influence a localized region of the problem domain (note that basis/weighting functions which have influence over the entire problem domain are said to have global support). Thus $\hat{u}$ at a given point in the problem domain will only be the sum of a few of the unknown coefficients multiplied by the appropriate basis functions, since only the basis functions in the immediate vicinity of where $\hat{u}$ is to be calculated are involved. In this case the number of terms in the summation of Eq. 2.19 is typically much less than N, depending on the extent of the local influence of b_j.
The use of basis functions which exist only over a subsection of the problem domain necessitates the adoption of some strategy for dividing up the domain and prescribing the functional behavior of the basis functions over a piece of local geometry. The result of a domain that has been divided into such subregions is called a *grid* or *mesh*. Typically the subregions within the grid are referred to as *elements* (or cells) while the points of interconnection of the elements are called *nodes*. In many cases the governing equations are enfoced at the nodes, and the unknown coefficients, once computed, represent the numerical solution at these nodal points. In other situations the element center is the position where each equation is assembled and the computed coefficients are considered to be the value of the solution at these locations. Figure 2.7 shows an example of a basic mesh

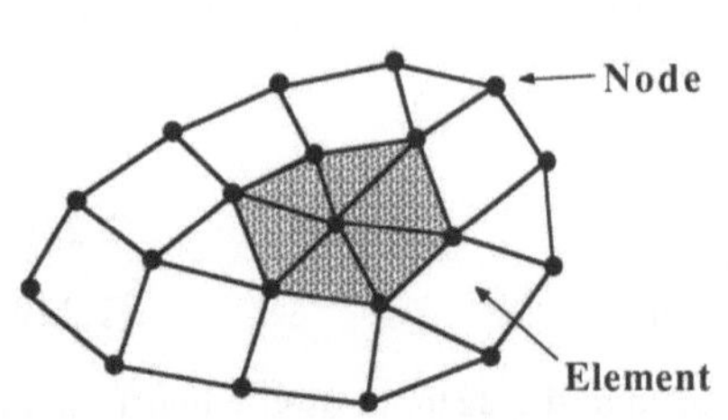

Fig. 2.7. The concept of a mesh

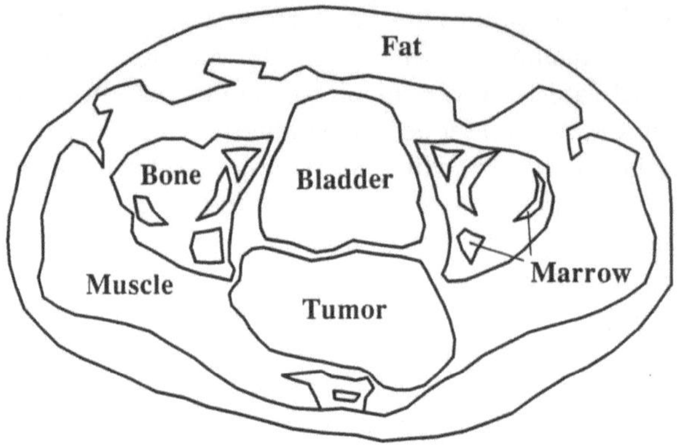

Fig. 2.8. Patient anatomy obtained from a CT scan

where an element and a node have been labeled to illustrate these concepts. Within the grid, a functional variation of the basis functions which is localized in nature can be used. A typical choice, for example, would be a piecewise linear dependence such that the basis function for a given node in Fig. 2.7 would vary linearly over all elements containing the node and would be zero in any other element in the entire grid. The shaded region in Fig. 2.7 indicates the portion of the grid over which the basis function associated with the center node has local support – it varies linearly in this example. Outside of this localized region the basis function for this particular node has no influence (i.e., it can be considered to be zero). Each node within the mesh is considered to have this type of behavior and the entire problem domain of interest is represented by such an interconnection of nodes and elements. Higher-order elements (i.e., elements over which the basis functions have higher degrees of polynomial variation, for example, quadratic) and lower-order elements are also possible. Note that if a function with the same type of localized influence is also used for the weighting function, the resulting algebraic equation at each node consists of only a few unknowns (this is provided that L in Eq. 2.16 does not contain operations that are global in extent). This produces a matrix structure in Eq. 2.21 which is sparse and, as a result, leads to computer memory and run time economies.
To illustrate a mesh in the context of calculating power deposition patterns in hyperthermia, Figs. 2.8 and 2.9 have been included. Figure 2.8 shows a drawing of a typical patient geometry where the boundaries of the tissues and organs of interest have been delineated. Figure 2.9 shows the grid which has been constructed from the anatomy of the cancer patient displayed in Fig. 2.8. This mesh consists of a set of linear elements and associated nodes for the problem domain. After computation of the field variable being

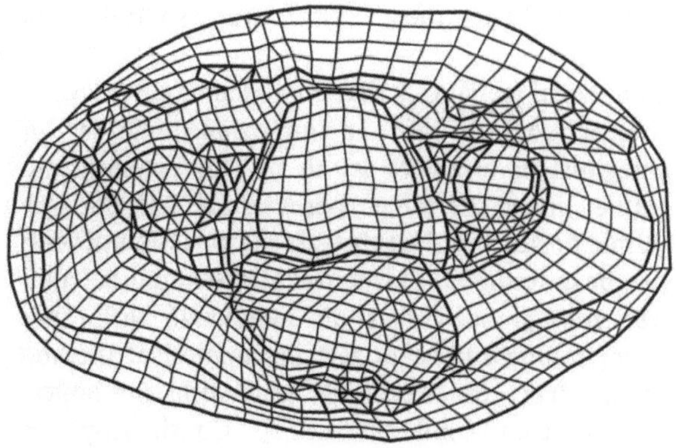

Fig. 2.9. Grid based on the geometry of Fig. 2.8

sought, the solution is known at each node within the grid. The field variable can then be found at any point within the problem domain that does not coincide with a node in the mesh by invoking Eq. 2.19. For example, if the solution is desired at the point (x_0, y_0), which does not fall on any particular node, but which must then be contained within a given element, Eq. 2.19 would become $\hat{u}(x_0, y_0) = u_1 b_1(x_0, y_0) + u_2 b_2(x_0, y_0) + u_3 b_3(x_0, y_0)$ for a triangular element composed of nodes 1 through 3 with corresponding basis functions, b_1, b_2, and b_3. Note that only three terms in the summation of Eq. 2.19 are involved in this case since typical basis functions only have local support as illustrated in Fig. 2.7.

Two types of elements

1. domain elements or
2. boundary elements

can comprise a mesh depending on the numerical techniques being implemented. As the names suggest, domain elements are used to subdivide the entire problem space whereas boundary elements are used only to subdivide the boundaries of the problem. Hence in three dimensions domain elements represent small volumes and in two dimensions they consist of incremental areas. Likewise, boundary elements correspond to pieces of surface area on a three-dimensional object and degenerate into contours in the two-dimensional case. In many situations, the same two-dimensional and one-dimensional domain elements can be used as three-dimensional and two-dimensional boundary elements, respectively. This economy

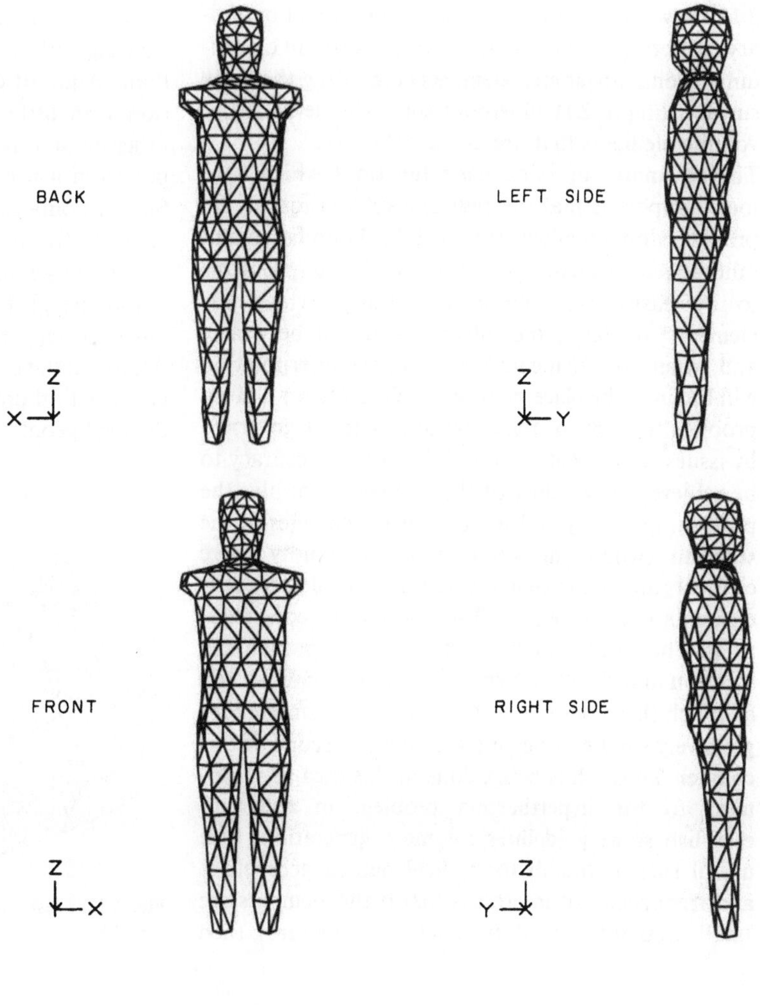

Fig. 2.10. Three-dimensional grid constructed from boundary elements

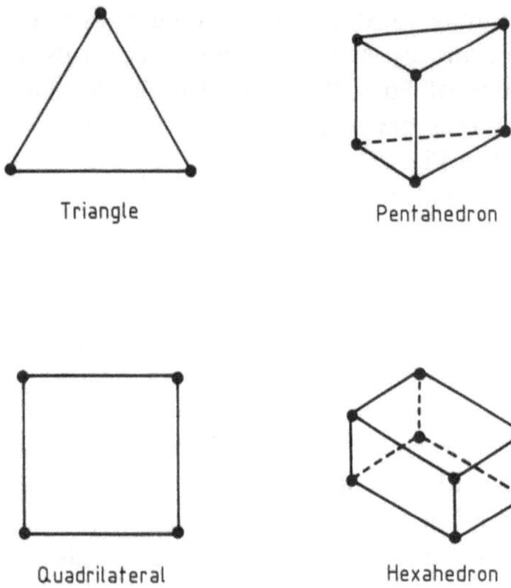

Fig. 2.11. Simple area and volume elements

in terms of both numbers of elements and their ease of construction which results from the reduction in problem dimension makes boundary elements attractive from the grid generation point of view. Figure 2.10 shows four views of a three-dimensional boundary element grid which consists of a collection of two-dimensional linear area elements composing the body surface. Figure 2.11 illustrates some simple area and volume elements that are commonly used.

The advantage of using basis functions which have local support is that the requisite subdivision of the problem domain allows the irregular boundaries and inhomogeneous tissue properties of clinical problems to be easily accommodated. Clearly, where the elements are large, the interpolation will be coarse and, where the elements are small, the interpolation will be fine. The placement of the elements for a given problem in terms of their size and shape is governed by issues which center around the desired accuracy to be achieved. The ability of the elements to resolve the problem geometry and to account for changes in the solution (where the solution varies rapidly more elements are often needed, where it varies slowly fewer elements may be required) are important considerations. The correspondence between the approximated solution and the unknown exact solution and the rate at which they converge as the elements are made progressively smaller is beyond the intended scope of this chapter. Research is being done in this area as it pertains to the hyperthermia problem in order to establish some guidelines for mesh generation. One useful rule of thumb for typical patient geometries and frequencies of interest is that if the elements are small enough to resolve the anatomical features, then acceptable (better then 5%) accuracy should result [73].

If numerical techniques that are based on dividing the problem domain into an interconnecting set of subregions or elements are to be incorporated into routine clinical use for purposes of predicting hyperthermic dosimetry, then the grid construction process must be automated. This automation should be complete enough such that an individual with little understanding of the underlying numerical method can construct an acceptable grid with anatomical detail derived from CT scans. Considering the geometrical detail shown in Fig. 2.8, this task, while essential, is nontrivial. Further, since the size of the elements within the grid directly impacts the accuracy of the resulting solution, rules of thumb about nodal spacings like the one described above must also be developed. Figure 2.12 shows a grid that has been constructed with an automatic mesh generation scheme where the user has control over the maximum element size [75]. This grid is based on the same set of boundaries from which the mesh in Fig. 2.9 was also developed. The difference is in the time and effort required to arrive at the mesh in Fig. 2.12 as compared with that of Fig. 2.9. With the automatic grid generation algorithm, Fig. 2.12 was constructed using less than 10 min of CPU time on a Micro Vax II workstation with little user intervention. Figure 2.9 on the other hand took many hours of interactive graphic input from a user skilled in grid generation concepts. Such automated algorithms are now becoming available and will bring the routine use of numerical techniques closer to the clinic. An example of another automatic grid generation program for clinical use has been reported in [25].

Although the use of variable element sizes in the mesh construction provides the flexibility needed to resolve detailed geometries, the complexity of generating this

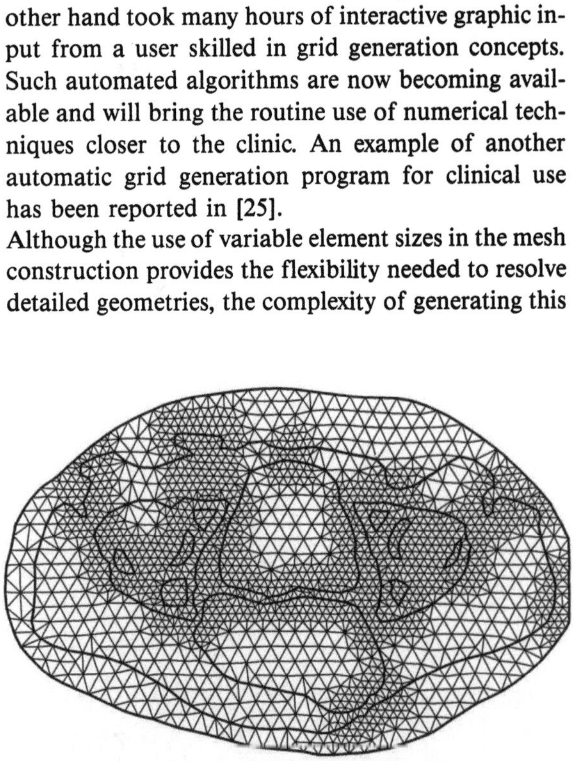

Fig. 2.12. Mesh automatically generated from the geometry in Fig. 2.8

kind of grid by hand or developing automated procedures for doing the same has been problematic. As a result, numerical approaches which rely on grids with uniform spacing throughout the problem domain have a certain appeal in terms of the simplified data input. In a uniform grid, an indexing system can easily be used such that the indices of each node designate its coordinates. Further, for some numerical approaches, the uniform mesh spacing provides computationally attractive features that would be lost if nonuniform spacing were used (these economies will be discussed later in the chapter). The price paid for the inherent simplicity of a uniformly spaced grid is in terms of the inability of such a mesh to resolve curved boundaries. Figure 2.13 shows an example of the "stair-stepping" effect that results when a uniform grid is used to discretize a curved boundary. Of course, the effect of this "stair-casing" can be reduced by decreasing the grid spacing; however, in a uniform grid this requires decreasing the nodal spacing throughout the entire problem domain and hence can cause excessive detail in regions of less importance. This meshing inefficiency is the primary argument against the use of uniform grids. The availability of nonuniform automatic mesh generation, at least in two dimensions, makes the variable-sized-element mesh the grid of choice for problems of interest in clinical hyperthermia. Hence, numerical methods which can readily accommodate variable nodal spacing within a grid are to be preferred in this context. Note that the computational economies associated with some methods, when uniform grids are used, are significant and must also be considered in such a choice of one numerical technique over another. These topics will be taken up further at a latter point in this chapter.

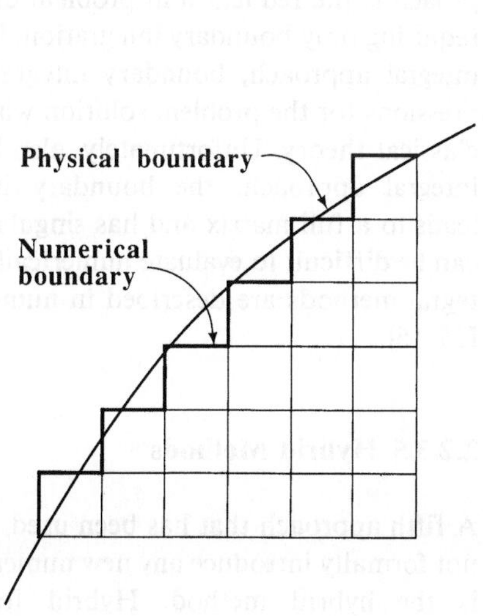

Fig. 2.13. Curved boundary discretized with uniform elements

In three dimensions, the choice of a nonuniform mesh of domain elements should also be favored over a uniformly spaced grid; however, the current lack of automated grid generation algorithms which can handle the complex three-dimensional shapes of tissues and organs makes the uniform mesh very practical. Further, the same indexing approach can still be used in three dimensions with a uniform grid and the simplicity in the data input it affords is even more magnified in the three-dimensional case. This is partly responsible for the early success of three-dimensional numerical calculations that are based on methods which exploit uniform grid spacing [121]. A potentially competing three-dimensional grid which utilizes nonuniform nodal spacing is a boundary element grid. Such a grid (e.g., see Fig. 2.10) can be constructed by connecting a series of two-dimensional contours, consisting of simple one-dimensional domain elements, in the remaining third dimension (thus creating an interconnection of two-dimensional domain elements that resolve the surface of a three-dimensional object). The relative ease of constructing this type of grid, which has the advantages of nonuniform spacing for resolving complex geometrical shapes, will make methods that use boundary elements attractive options in three dimensions, at least as far as data input is concerned.

Having discussed the concept of a grid, which basically supplies the input information concerning the problem domain, attention is now turned to particular techniques for generating an algebraic representation of Eq. 2.16. Any method whereby a functional equation is reduced to a matrix equation can be interpreted in terms of the method of weighted residuals [47]; hence the foregoing discussions of basis/weighting functions apply in general. While the methods have varied, the starting point is generally the same: a second-order partial differential equation (PDE) in the quantity of interest. With this starting point, four approaches have been used most extensively. Below a brief overview of these methods is given in terms of the electromagnetic problem. The intent here is a survey whereas at a latter point in the chapter (Sect. 2.4) each method is discussed in a more illustrative, albeit mathematical, manner.

2.2.3.1 Domain Integrals

In domain integral solutions, the EM sources are treated as inhomogeneous terms in the governing second-order PDE. An analytical form of the solution to the inhomogeneous PDE, which is based on the unbounded-space Green's function, is then numerically implemented. The approach is attractive for problem formulation given that the EM sources are easily handled as inhomogeneous terms in the PDE, and that the Green's function solution is an exact solution firmly embedded in classical theory. In effect, these calculations represent the superposition of point source solutions where the boundaries are located at infinity. The approach is unattractive numerically because the singular Green's function can be difficult to evaluate, and the kernels of the domain integrals have global influence which leads to a full matrix requiring inversion. The use of domain integral approaches in electromagnetics has been well described in the literature [47, 79, 81].

2.2.3.2 Finite Elements

In finite elements, the solution to the governing second-order PDE is piecewise approximated by a simple function upon which the differential operations are carried out exactly. Typically, the EM sources are handled through boundary integrals which arise from the integration by parts of the second-order differentiation. The finite element method requires domain integration, but in contrast to the domain integral approach the boundaries are closed and finite. Also, unlike the domain integral approach, the exact solution has to be approximated by an expansion of an incomplete basis. This feature, however, leads to the numerical attractiveness of finite elements since the integrations that must be performed are carried out on simple, regular functions which lead to a sparse matrix that is effectively inverted by LU decomposition. Further, geometrical irregularity as well as regional heterogeneity are easily handled with finite elements. One drawback is that knowledge of the source is required around the boundary of the entire domain of interest. Since many electromagnetic problems are fundamentally unbounded, this requirement can be limiting, and explains in part why integral equations have dominated numerical electromagnetics. Finite element applications in electromagnetics can be found in [23, 106].

2.2.3.3 Finite Differences

In finite differences, an exact solution is obtained for operators which approximate those contained in the governing PDE. Typically, the first-order differential Maxwell equations relating the electric and magnetic fields have been used in the time-domain. With this formulation, an explicit time-stepping scheme can be employed which leads to the desirable feature that no matrix solutions are needed. This makes the finite difference time-domain approach particularly attractive for large-scale EM problems (three dimensions), but can be counterbalanced by the required iteration procedure through time. As with finite elements, the application of finite differences is limited in unbounded problems, and requires that additional assumptions be made in such cases to terminate the problem domain. Further complications occur when the problem domain has highly irregular geometrically detailed boundaries which, if represented accurately, require the use of variable grid spacings throughout the mesh or excessive detail in regions of less importance (for a uniform grid). Examples of the use of finite differences in EM problems can be found in [125, 141].

2.2.3.4 Boundary Integrals

Boundary integral statements are derived by employing Green's theorem [58, 114] on the governing second-order PDE. In this case, integrations are performed only around the boundaries of homogeneous, source-free domains; hence, all EM sources must reside on these boundaries. After the set of boundary equations is assembled and solved, calculation of interior fields can be made as the appropriate weighting of the known boundary values. In direct contrast to finite elements, boundary integrals are ideal for homogeneous, unbounded problems. For inhomogeneous media, this approach suffers from the additional complexity of either the inclusion of domain integration or the creation of multiple interior boundaries enclosing homogeneous subdomains. One of the most appealing features of the boundary integral approach is the reduction in problem dimension via its requiring only boundary integration. Like the domain integral approach, boundary integrals are exact expressions for the problem solution which are based in classical theory. Unfortunately, also like the domain integral approach, the boundary integral method leads to a full matrix and has singular kernels which can be difficult to evaluate numerically. Boundary integral methods are described in numerous textbooks [15, 16].

2.2.3.5 Hybrid Methods

A fifth approach that has been used, but which does not formally introduce any new numerical techniques, is the hybrid method. Hybrid formulations are numerical methods which combine two or more of the preceding approaches. For example, a hybrid element technique has been established to couple the advantages of finite and boundary element methods while avoiding the inherent weaknesses of each method when used alone [74]. As discussed above, the finite element method is best suited for problems with geometric irregularity and region heterogeneity which are confined by a finite boundary that completely contains the problem domain and on which known boundary conditions can be applied. The major weakness of the finite element method is that, in general, it cannot be used in cases where portions of the problem domain extend to infinity without additional assumptions and approximations. On the other hand, the boundary element method is ideally suited for problems containing large homogeneous regions which can extend to infinity. It is weakened for problems with domains having severe heterogeneity by globally influential, singular kernels which must be integrated over the increased number of boundaries. Hence, in the present context, the hybrid element method employs the finite element method in regions of heterogeneity (i.e., inside the patient) and the boundary element method in regions of unbounded homogeneity (such as the background medium containing the patient as well as the electromagnetic source). The finite element method effectively treats the variation of tissue electrical properties with the use of simple piecewise linear basis functions which can be integrated easily and which lead to sparse sets of algebraic equations. The boundary element method is used to couple the finite element equations to the remote source and the surrounding infinite domain by removing the requirement that known boundary conditions be applied at all finite element boundaries. Hence, the hybrid element method provides a formal approach to the problem of a heterogeneous body irradiated by a detached source.

2.2.4 Sample Results

At this point, it is instructive to consider some typical electromagnetic source configurations that have been used to induce hyperthermia. The intent of this section is to illustrate the types of calculations that can be made and to show the kind of treatment planning and equipment design information that can be obtained from such calculations. Three noninvasive EM source arrangements

1. magnetic induction coils,
2. annular arrays of apertures, and
3. capacitive heating systems

are taken as examples. Representative calculations of the field distributions theoretically produced by these types of devices are shown and briefly discussed below.

Magnetic induction, where tissue is heated by power deposited from eddy currents induced by magnetic fields, has been widely used to induce hyperthermia. A typical configuration is to place the body section to be treated inside a single-turn concentric coil. An alternating current ($\approx 10-30$ MHz) is impressed on the copper sheet and a time-varying magnetic field is created which circulates around the coil down its long axis. This magnetic field results in eddy currents (i.e., an induced electric field) that tend to be confined to the transverse planes of the coil.

Figure 2.14 shows a two-dimensional calculation of the electric field produced by a magnetic induction coil inside the body cross-section of Fig. 2.8 and the space between the body and the coil itself. The vectors plotted in this figure represent the direction of the imaginary component of **E** and their lengths are proportional to the strength of this quantity. The imaginary component of **E** is basically in a clockwise direction, but the heterogeneity within the patient creates considerable variation in both the strength and direction of the field. However, nowhere does the **E** circulation confine itself to a single tissue type or region. A general decrease in the vector lengths is clear as the

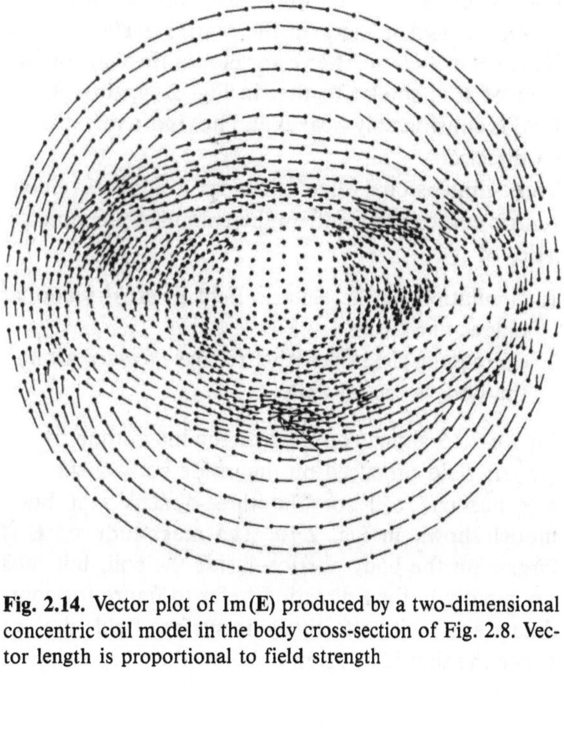

Fig. 2.14. Vector plot of Im(**E**) produced by a two-dimensional concentric coil model in the body cross-section of Fig. 2.8. Vector length is proportional to field strength

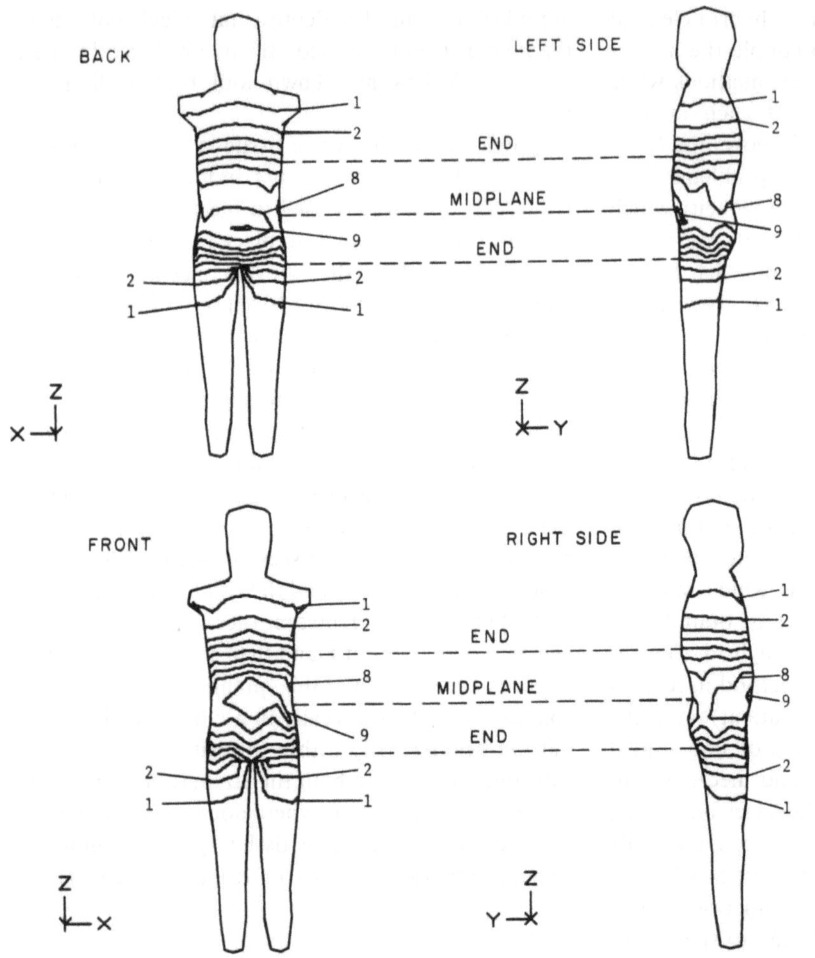

Fig. 2.15. Contours of |**E**| produced by a concentric coil on the inside surface of the three-dimensional body model in Fig. 2.10. Contours are scaled to a maximum of ten

body's central axis is approached, representing a decrease in field strength in the central portion of the body cross-section. The vector plot of the real component of **E** is similar to that in Fig. 2.14, though the field is considerably weaker and has more variation in its direction.

Three-dimensional calculations for a single-turn concentric coil further confirm these dominant characteristics of

1. circulation of the electric field in cross-sectional planes and
2. decrease in field strength effectively to zero around the body's central axis.

Figure 2.15 shows contours of the magnitude of the electric field produced on the inside body surface by a concentric coil for the three-dimensional body model shown in Fig. 2.10. The magnitude of **E** is largest on the body portion inside the coil, but falls off rapidly in the z direction (refer to figure for coordinate axes) with effectively no surface fields present above the shoulder region or below the midportion of the thighs when the coil is positioned for treatment of the lower abdomen. These contour lines are fairly uniform around the body above and below the coil where the body diameter is relatively constant, but show some circumferential variation inside the coil where the body surface is radially less uniform.

Contours of |**E**| can also be drawn for the outside body surface since the electromagnetic boundary conditions require discontinuity in the normal component of **E** at the interface between two electrically distinct regions (air and muscle in this simulation), thus resulting in two sets of electric field distributions at the body surface. The contours equivalent to those in Fig. 2.15 for the air side of the body surface are quite similar in shape, but slightly larger in magnitude and extend somewhat further in the z direction. Multiplying the contour levels in Fig. 2.15 by 0.95 results in a scaling to the maximum |**E**| on the outside body surface. The degree of similarity between the magnitude distributions on either side of the body surface indicates that the electric field is mainly tangential to the body surface, and, therefore, continuous at the body surface despite the three-dimensional geometrical variation of the body contour.

Based solely on these three-dimensional surface contours of $|\mathbf{E}|$, one might conclude that the single-turn concentric coil produces a desirable electric field distribution for inducing hyperthermia – the magnitudes of **E** are largest inside the coil, which is the region where the most intense exposure is desired, but fall off rapidly outside the coil in the areas which are not part of the treatment field. Unfortunately, this desirable surface distribution of $|\mathbf{E}|$ does not result in desirable $|\mathbf{E}|$ patterns inside the three-dimensional body. Figure 2.16 shows contours of $|\mathbf{E}|$ in transverse slices through the body. The number below each plot in this figure indicates the distance away from the midplane of the coil with the positive direction being toward the head. The coil itself is 35 cm in length; hence, a label of *−17.5 cm* on a plot in Fig. 2.16 would designate a transverse slice through the body at the edge of the coil closest to the feet. This figure not only shows the decrease in the electric field magnitude toward the center of the patient which was observed in the two-dimensional calculation of Fig. 2.14, but it also shows that this behavior is dominant regardless of where the transverse section is taken relative to the coil. Also note that only very small electric fields exist inside the patient 10 cm beyond the ends of the coil.

Figures 2.15 and 2.16 suggest that three-dimensional simulations of the field distributions produced by a single-turn magnetic induction coil should not dramatically alter the conclusions drawn from two-dimensional models. This would seem to be particularly true because the electric fields remained largely tangential to the body surface and parallel with transverse slices through the body regardless of the three-dimensional geometry. Thus, the behavior of the three-dimensional electric field distribution would not be expected to be altered significantly by the presence of longitudinal tissue variations which cannot be accounted for with cross-sectional models.

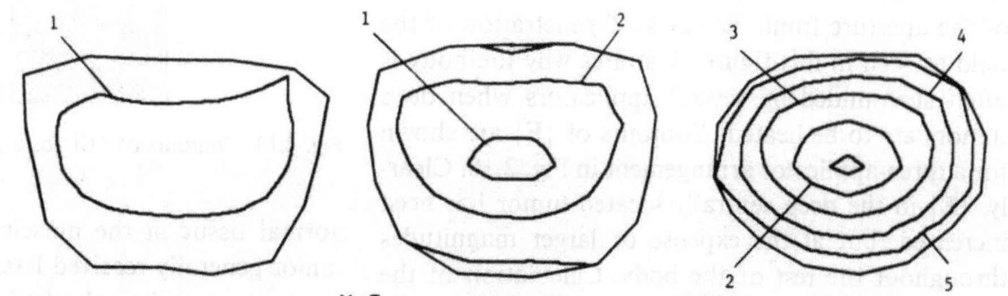

Fig. 2.16. Contours of $|\mathbf{E}|$ produced by a concentric coil in transverse slices through the three-dimensional body model in Fig. 2.10. The number below each plot indicates the distance of the slice from the midplane of the coil

Another class of noninvasive systems which have been used to produce deep-seated heating via regional power deposition patterns consists of multiple rf or microwave applicators arranged in an array placed around the diseased body section. These types of devices are fundamentally different from the inductive coil in that they contain multiple sources which produce an electric field that is oriented predominantly parallel rather than transverse to the longitudinal axis of the patient. A two-dimensional model can be constructed where the transverse slice through the device and the patient consists of a tumor-bearing body cross-section surrounded by a ring of sources. The electric field is assumed to be everywhere perpendicular to this analysis plane, and, hence, tangential and continuous at tissue interfaces.

Figure 2.17 shows contours of the magnitude of **E** produced by a single 70-MHz applicator in a pelvic body cross-section containing a centrally located tumor. The electric field distribution across the front of the aperture is assumed to be a half-wavelength cosine function whose peak value occurs at the center of the aperture front. The lack of penetration of the field as seen in this figure illustrates why the body is often surrounded by several applicators when deep tumors are to be heated. Contours of $|\mathbf{E}|$ are shown for a three-applicator arrangement in Fig. 2.18. Clearly, $|\mathbf{E}|$ in the deep centrally located tumor has been increased, but at the expense of larger magnitudes throughout the rest of the body. Calculation of the heating rate for this three-applicator system indicates that the maximum absorbed power occurred in the

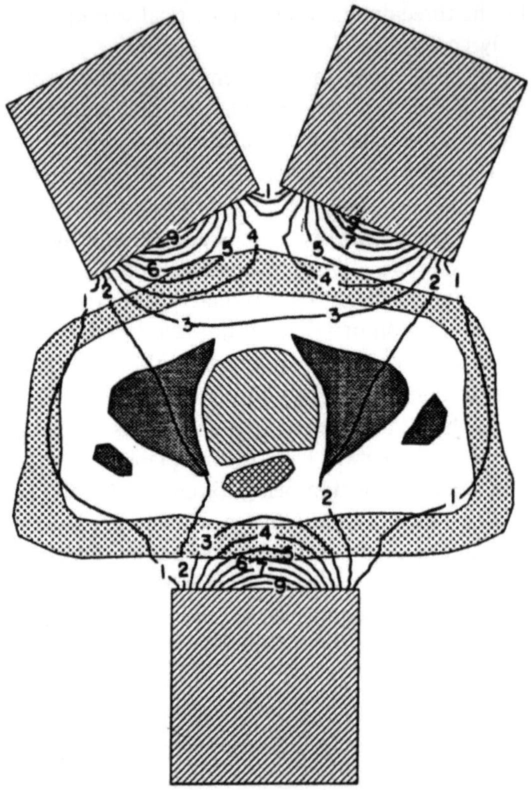

Fig. 2.18. Contours of $|\mathbf{E}|$ for a three-applicator arrangement

normal tissue at the muscle-fat interface, while the tumor generally received less than 50% of this maximum. Surrounding the body by an annular ring of eight apertures further improves the situation. Contours of constant heating rate for this case are shown in Fig. 2.19. Now a sizable portion of the tumor has received better than 60% of the overall maximum; however, the maximum heating rate still occurs in the normal tissue at the muscle-fat interface. Whether further improvements can be made by adjusting the relative amplitude and phases of the signal driving each applicator is a question that is now under investigation. Further, the optimum number and placement of applicators for a given tumor site is being studied. However, for the deep centrally located tumor of Fig. 2.19, one would expect that the inphase arrangement (as shown) would produce the "best case" results for this type of device in this situation. Three-dimensional calculations for an annular array of applicators yield some interesting field patterns that would not be predictable with two-dimensional cross-sectional models. Figure 2.20 shows contours of the magnitude of the electric field on the inside body surface. Like the concentric coil model, the magnitude of the surface electric fields is largest on the body portion inside the applicator, but, unlike the

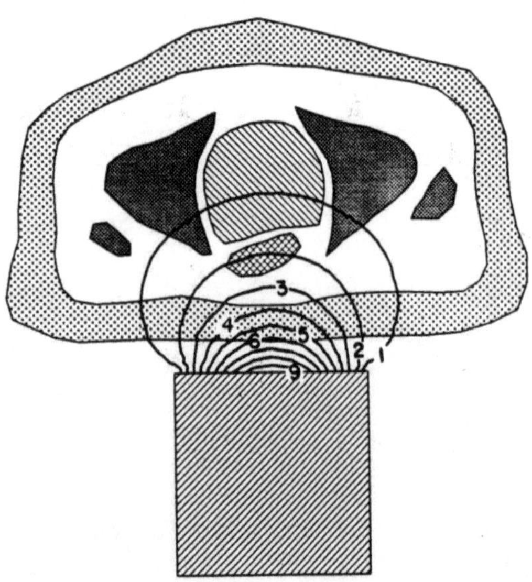

Fig. 2.17. Contours of $|\mathbf{E}|$ produced by a single 70-MHz applicator in a pelvic cross-section with a centrally located tumor

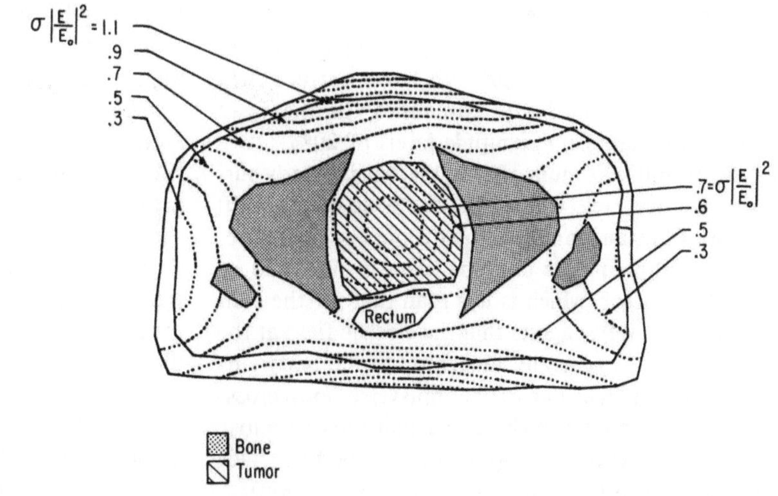

Fig. 2.19. Contours of heating rate for an annular ring of eight applicators

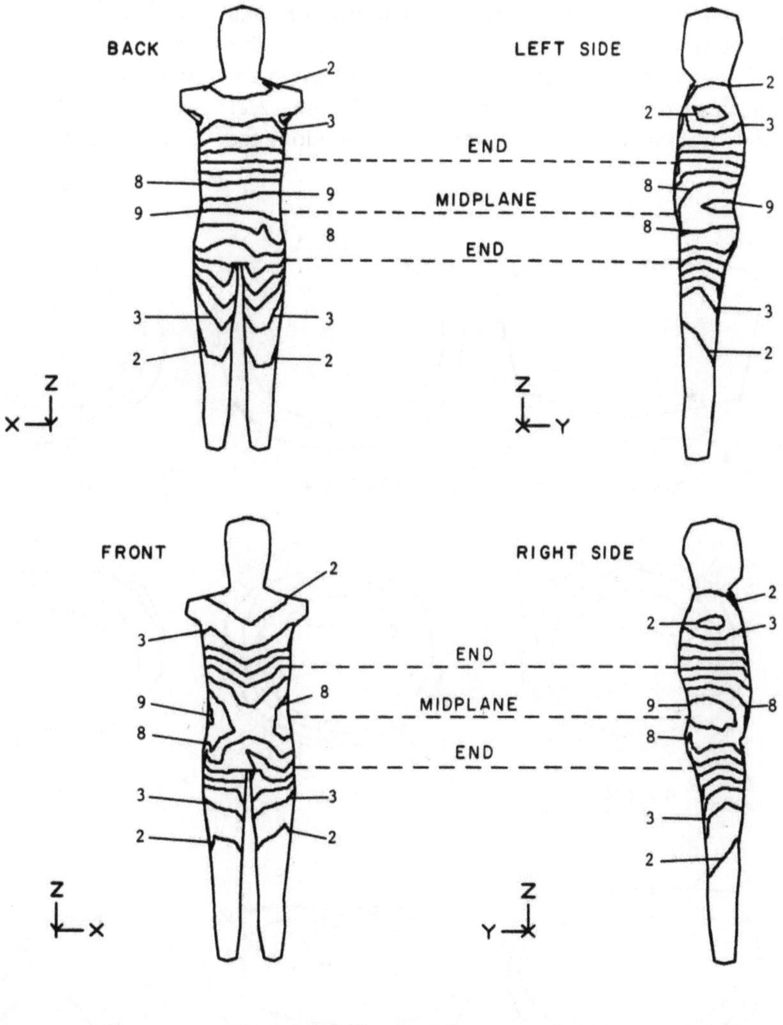

Fig. 2.20. Contours of |E| produced by an annular array of applicators on the inside surface of the three-dimensional body model in Fig. 2.10. Contours are scaled to a maximum of ten

concentric coil, the magnitude of these fields falls off much less rapidly in the z direction. Surface electric field magnitudes of 10%–20% of the overall maximum are readily found above the shoulders and below the knees. As in Fig. 2.15 for the concentric coil, the contour lines in Fig. 2.20 are more uniform around the body toward the ends of the applicator where the body diameter is relatively constant, but show circumferential variation near the applicator center where the body surface is radially less uniform.

Contours of $|\mathbf{E}|$ on the outside body surface have been found to show even greater spreading of the contour lines in the z direction with larger surface field magnitudes on the body extremities. In the head region, for example, magnitude levels of 20% – 30% of the overall maximum $|\mathbf{E}|$ on the outside body surface have occurred. Converting the scale of Fig. 2.20 to that of the maximum $|\mathbf{E}|$ on the outside surface requires multiplying the contour levels in Fig. 2.20 by 0.85. This factor (which is less than that for the concentric coil case) suggests that the electric field at the body surface is generally tangential to the body surface (but perpendicular to the transverse body cross-section), though not to the extent that the concentric coil electric fields are tangential to the body surface (but parallel to the transverse body cross-section). Inspection of the $|\mathbf{E}|$ in cross-sectional slices through the body brings to light the positive aspects of this EM source relative to that of magnetic induction for inducing deep-seated hyperthermia. Figure 2.21 shows transverse contours at various z levels along the body length. As before, the numbers below each plot indicate the distance away from the midplane of the applicator with the positive direction toward the head. As shown in Fig. 2.21, $|\mathbf{E}|$ is relatively constant over large sections containing the center of each transverse slice, and, in fact, over these portions $|\mathbf{E}|$ is generally greater than 60% of the overall maximum within the slice. Furthermore, the body center received 50% or more of the maximum $|\mathbf{E}|$ on the inside surface of the body for more than 20 cm (approximately two-thirds of the applicator length) in the longitudinal direction. However, one cannot ignore the extension of $|\mathbf{E}|$ in the z direction above and below the applicator. As indicated by Fig. 2.21, three-dimensional modeling may be critical for understanding the capabilities of an annular array of applicators given the longitudinal influence of the electric field. Further, whether depositing 50% – 60% of the overall maximum power absorbed is enough to heat deep-seated tumors to therapeutic levels without overheating superficial normal tissue is a question that can on-

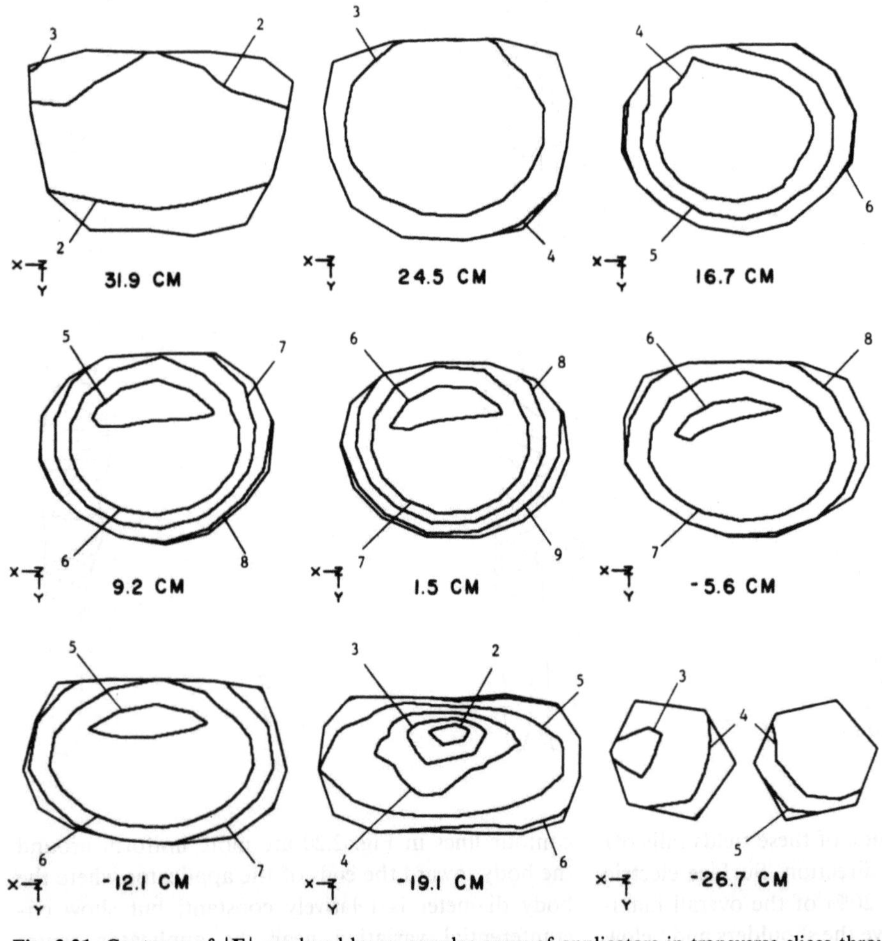

Fig. 2.21. Contours of $|\mathbf{E}|$ produced by an annular array of applicators in transverse slices through the three-dimensional body model in Fig. 2.10

ly be answered by considering the bioheat transfer aspects of the hyperthermia simulation problem.

Capacitive hyperthermia systems typically consist of a pair of flat-plate or circular electrodes upon which an alternating current ($\approx 1-10$ MHz) is impressed. Such systems have been considered to cause excessive heating in the body's superficial fat layer. This shortcoming has been attributed to the fact that this type of device produces an electric field which is predominantly perpendicular to the body surface, and, therefore, to any subcutaneous muscle/fat interface. As discussed earlier, the electromagnetic boundary conditions in such a case require that the power deposited on the fat side be many times larger than that absorbed on the muscle side of the interface.

A two-dimensional model of a parallel-plate capacitive heating system based on a transverse slice through the device with the patient positioned for treatment can be used to investigate the type of field pattern produced. Figure 2.22 shows the electric field distribution for two parallel plates excited at 10 MHz in free space (i.e., with the body removed). The dominant characteristics in this field distribution are clear

1. the direction of the field is largely perpendicular to the plates in the region between the electrodes and
2. the field strengths are largest near the ends of the plates where the patterns "fringe" from the electrode ends (fringing fields).

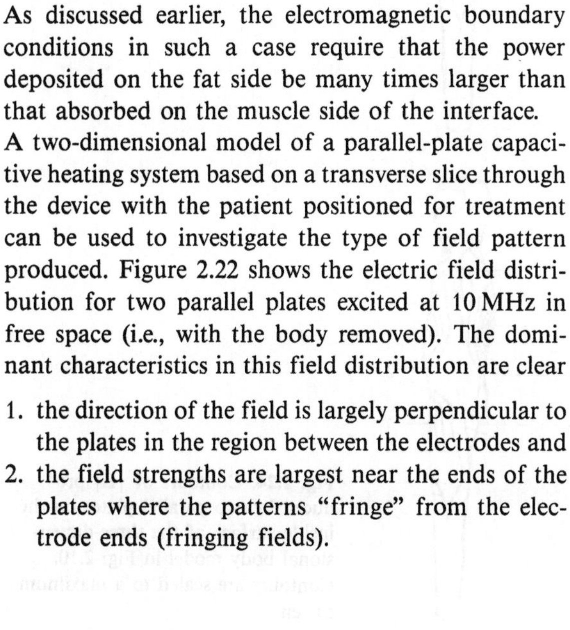

Fig. 2.23. Vector plot of **E** produced by two parallel plates in the body cross-section of Fig. 2.8

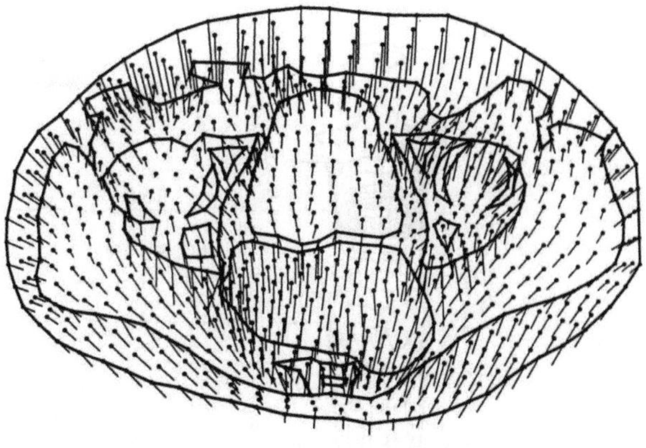

Fig. 2.22. Vector plot of **E** for two parallel plates energized at 10 MHz. Vector length is proportional to field strength

Figure 2.23 contains a vector plot when the body cross-section of Fig. 2.8 is placed between the energized plates. The fields outside the body are not plotted since they are quite large relative to those internal, which are mainly of interest. Figure 2.23 shows that the field patterns become quite complicated (relative to Fig. 2.22) due to the presence of tissue heterogeneities and the associated electromagnetic boundary conditions that must be enforced. One can appreciate the degree of complexity of this problem by realizing that each internal boundary can be represented by an equivalent surface charge which produces the same electric field but in homogeneous space (like Fig. 2.22), and then envisioning the electric field produced by such a complicated charge distribution. This example illustrates one reason why simulations are so valuable – the computer accounts for all the boundary conditions (or equivalent charge distributions) that are too numerous for one's mind to assimilate at once.

Figures 2.24 and 2.25 show some three-dimensional results for parallel plates energized at 8 MHz. Contours of $|\mathbf{E}|$ on the inside body surface are plotted in Fig. 2.24. These contours are quite different than their counterparts for the other two source arrangements. In contrast to Figs. 2.15 and 2.20, large surface field magnitudes occurred near the ends of the applicators while the portion of the body contained within the electrodes showed reduced levels of surface $|\mathbf{E}|$. This distribution of surface electric field magnitudes seems attributable to a combination of the highly variable distance of the body from the parallel plates and the electromagnetic boundary conditions that must be applied at the body surface. The back of the body is an especially acute example of the variable body contour: the back is closest to the plate at the edge nearest the head, and increases in its distance from the electrode until a maximum extent is reached at the lower

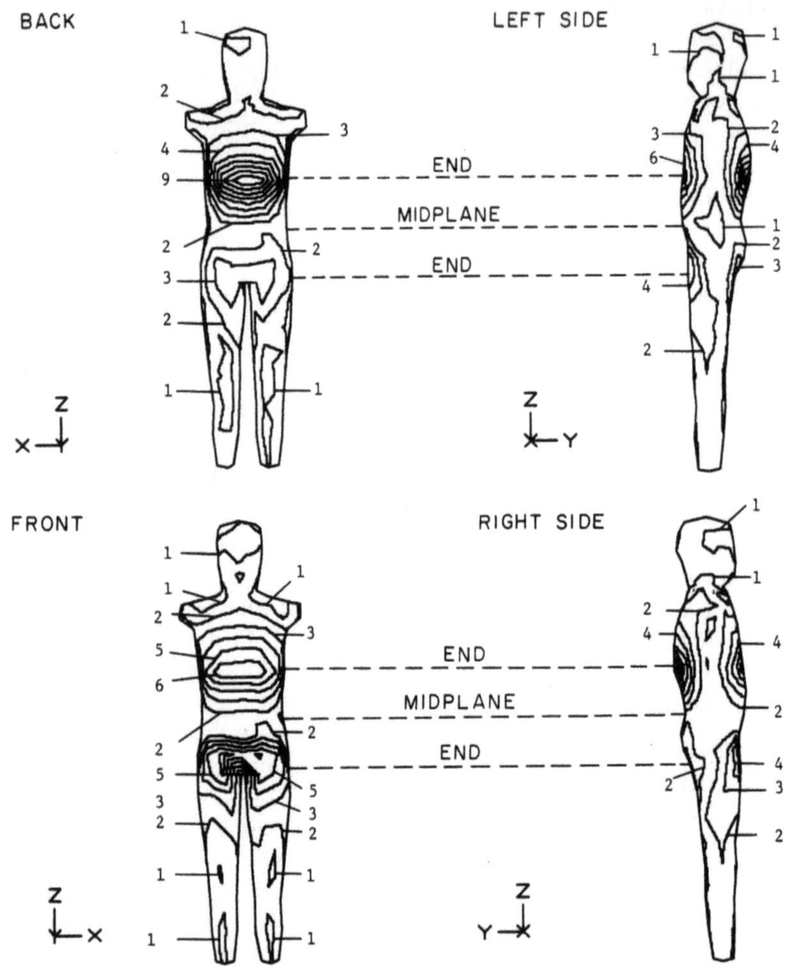

Fig. 2.24. Contours of |**E**| produced by two parallel plates on the inside surface of the three-dimensional body model in Fig. 2.10. Contours are scaled to a maximum of ten

back at which point the distance from the plate begins to decrease again with the bulging of the buttocks. The contours of |**E**| on the outside body surface follow suit with the changing distance from the plate in that a peak occurs at the electrode edge nearest the head, then a valley followed by another peaking of the surface |**E**| as one moves in the negative z direction across the plate. The same sort of surface contour can be followed on the front of the body beginning with the bulge in the stomach through the depression of the pelvic front and ending in the extension of the upper thighs.

The impact of this variable distance of the body surface from the plates is further illustrated in Fig. 2.25. Now contours of |**E**| on the outside surface of the body are shown when the separation distance between electrodes has been increased. In this case the variations in the body contour are made much smaller relative to the distance of the body from the plates. Figure 2.25 demonstrates the longitudinal smoothing of the magnitude levels through the applicator section of the body. The peaking of the |**E**| contours on the inside body surface at the ends of the electrodes are also reduced, but not to the extent shown in Fig. 2.25. This result indicates that the electromagnetic boundary conditions also play a significant role in creating the type of distribution shown in Fig. 2.24. For the parallel-plate source, the electric field is generally normal to the body surface, resulting in a high degree of discontinuity in its magnitude at the body surface. Examination of the contours of |**E**| on the outside body surface reveal that the contours in Fig. 2.24 have to be multiplied by 0.4 in order to be scaled to the maximum outside surface |**E**| (as compared with the factors of 0.95 and 0.85 for the concentric coil and annular array cases), reflecting the impact of the discontinuous normal electric field component. The longitudinal spreading of the |**E**| contours also indicates the importance of considering these electromagnetic boundary conditions.

While the surface |**E**| contours are like the annular array model in that levels of unity or greater were

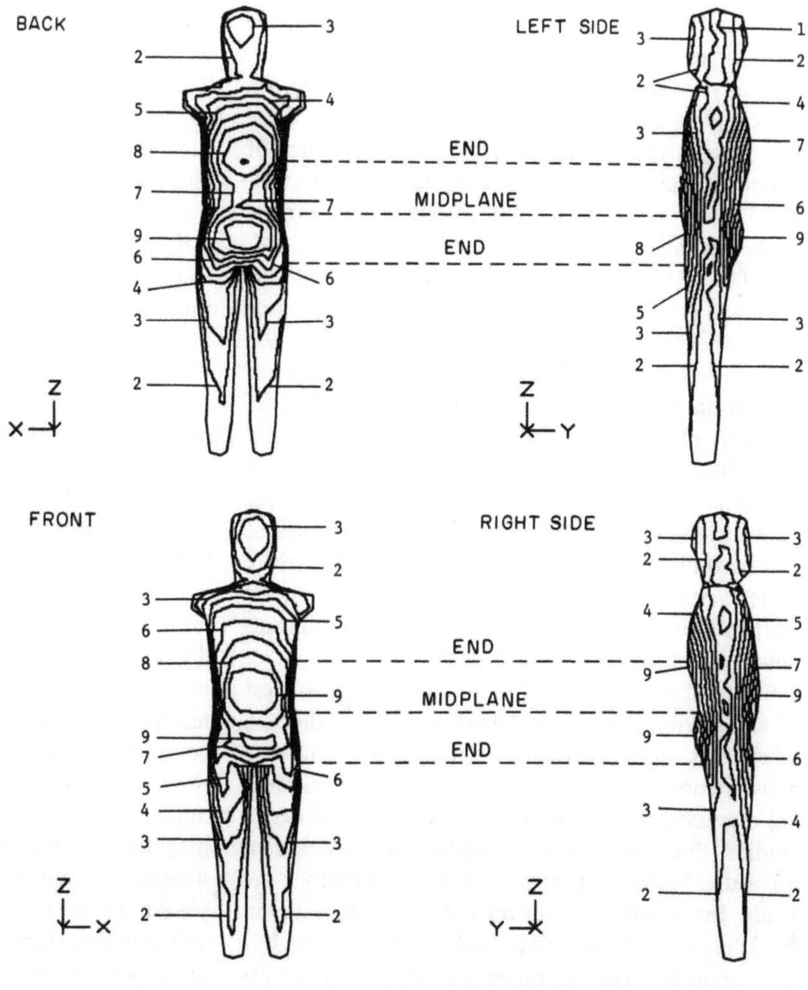

Fig. 2.25. Contours of |**E**| produced by two parallel plates on the outside surface of the three-dimensional body model in Fig. 2.10 where the separation distance between the plates has been increased to 50 cm

found throughout the body from the top of the head to the bottom of the legs, transverse slices through the body show contours which are more similar to those produced by the concentric coil model. Like the concentric coil model, the electric field magnitude shows little penetration depth with large portions of the body center containing levels of 20% or less of the overall maximum. Further, this type of distribution appears throughout the z direction regardless of where the body slice is taken relative to the midplane of the electrodes.

It is important to keep in mind that the above results and discussion are based on theoretical models that have been idealized in many respects. While the dominant characteristics described in these calculations have, to a large extent, been observed either directly or indirectly in the clinic and in phantom measurements, electric field distributions and power deposition patterns of actual physical devices may be significantly different. Nonetheless, this kind of analysis of generic types of hyperthermia systems helps to provide a quantitative comparison of potentially competing electromagnetic source configurations.

2.3 Modeling Progress

2.3.1 Current Status

Prior to 1980, little interest in numerical modeling existed in the field of hyperthermia; however, in the last several years numerical simulation of hyperthermia treatments has become one of the major areas of interest to hyperthermia researchers [117, 118]. The success of recent numerical models in predicting the performance of certain therapy devices prior to the accumulation of significant quantities of clinical data has demonstrated the impact that numerical simulation can have on the evaluation of these systems. For example, two noninvasive hyperthermia applicators which produce regional power deposition patterns are the Annular Phased Array [133] and the Magnetrode [110] magnetic induction coil. These devices are commercially available and have received widespread clinical attention. This attention naturally made these two electromagnetic applicators the focus of much of the numerical simulation work to date (e.g., see [45, 51, 57, 89, 120]). Now that a number of clinical studies of these systems have been completed [36, 87, 99, 100], the opportunity exists for comparing the predicted performance to the clinical performance of these devices. Qualitative comparisons [89, 96, 97, 120] as well as quantitative comparisons with limited clinical data [120] suggest that numerical models accurately predicted the dominant capabilities and limitations of the annular array applicator and magnetic induction coil. Specifically, the modeling gave insight into the types of thermal distributions that might be seen in the clinic, showed regions where these systems may have difficulty in achieving good temperature distributions, and showed the importance of knowledge of blood perfusion.

This initial success has led to an increased awareness of and interest in numerical analysis of hyperthermia treatments. In this section the advances in calculating power deposition patterns for hyperthermic treatment are discussed. The progress is charted by pointing to studies that have been presented in the current literature. While a number of literature citations are made, the intent is to illustrate the current status in modeling capabilities and to point to areas where further research is needed, rather than to provide an exhaustive review of the recent literature.

In general, two types of emphasis have emerged in the studies which calculate power absorptions

1. initial analysis of complicated problems based on simplified models and
2. detailed power deposition calculations using complex models where as much information as is possible (e.g., patient anatomy, source type, and location) is included.

There has been a natural evolution from the first type of emphasis to the second as the fundamental understanding of power deposition in hyperthermia has grown and as the need has increased for solving clinical problems where irregular boundaries and tissue heterogeneities are the norm.

As an example of this natural progression from simplified to more complex models, consider the modeling evolution that has taken place for a single-turn magnetic induction coil. The first papers that were aimed at theoretically studying this type of hyperthermia applicator reported analytical solutions on azimuthally symmetrical cylinders [14, 142]. Several investigators have used an approximate analytical expression for the power deposition produced in cylindrical or spherical body models by the concentric coil in order to calculate resulting temperature distributions [18, 35, 45, 115]. The theory indicated that under reasonable physiological assumptions about blood flow, tumors near the body's central axis would not elevate to therapeutic temperatures. At that time the results from these simple theoretical models were not in agreement with some of the experimental and clinical data reported [109, 111, 112]. This prompted the development of increasingly more complex models from two-dimensional inhomogeneous elliptical body geometries to two-dimensional heterogeneous cross-sections based on CT scans to three-dimensional models [4, 51, 88, 89]. The conclusions from these computations were essentially the same as those reached through the simple one-dimensional analysis. At the same time, in-depth experimental and clinical evaluation of a magnetic induction coil was carried out [85, 87] and the observations from these studies agreed with the conclusions reached through modeling. Interestingly, the more complete models did not add a great deal of additional insight into the understanding of this type of applicator. However, for other kinds of devices this may not prove to be the case. Further, one cannot necessarily know *a priori* whether simple models will yield the same insight that more sophisticated models will produce; hence, increasing model complexity is an important step in the modeling process. Similar histories of modeling evolution can be traced for other types of hyperthermia systems such as annular phased arrays and capacitive heating devices.

The evolution toward increasingly more complex simulations does not imply that the role of simplified models is obsolete in hyperthermia research. For example, as new applicators are investigated, the initial analysis afforded by simplified models is not only appropriate, but often preferred for illuminating basic physical principles. Further, verification of theory with experiment and complicated theories with simplified ones are often best performed when experimental setups and models can be easily constructed and interpreted.

A current topic of study which illustrates that valuable contributions are still being made with simple models (here "simple" refers to the idealization of the problem geometry) is the focussing of power absorption at a predefined target. Solutions based on analytical expressions for the fields inside concentric cylinders have been presented and used to examine the ability of multiple concentric antennae to focus power inside this idealized geometry [39, 138, 139]. Other recent examples can be found where analytical expressions for the field values of interest are integrated over various source arrangements. Rather than using a confined region such as a cylinder as the simplified patient model, these approaches typically assume an unbounded region of homogeneous tissue (usually muscle). This type of unbounded "patient" is often used when analyzing local power deposition patterns from superficial applicators [34, 46, 84, 135] or interstitial antennae [129, 130, 134].

In the focussing context, successful calculations have been made of power deposition patterns produced by a planar array of 16 surface applicators using an unbounded region approach along with an analytical integral over the radiating faces of the applicator configuration [46]. Likewise, the phasing of interstitial microwave antennae have been examined by assuming an unbounded region of homogeneous tissue and integrating over the source distribution to find the fields produced. These results have then been incorporated into thermal calculations where heterogeneous tissue models have been used [119]. A similar strategy where the region of interest is assumed electrically homogeneous, but thermally heterogeneous (especially in terms of blood flows), has been used in the simulation of other interstitial techniques such as RF needles and ferromagnetic seeds [19, 78, 116, 119]. Also in ultrasound calculations the assumption of an unbounded region of acoustically homogeneous tissue (which is used for the calculation of power deposition patterns) has been coupled to heterogeneous thermal models with success [21, 98]. Typically, the thermal models, though heterogeneous, have been idealized by regularly shaped tumors and surrounding normal tissues.

While a natural classification between those simulations which undertake analysis on simplified models and those which provide detailed power deposition calculations exists, hyperthermia treatment simulation studies can also typically be categorized as technique- or application-oriented. Technique-oriented works have tended to be demonstrative presentations where the emphasis has been placed on the formulation of the numerical method and how it can be applied to hyperthermia (e.g., [33, 52, 57, 73, 74]). Often a few illustrative examples of interest are provided, but no in-depth analysis of a hyperthermia problem is undertaken. In contrast, application-oriented studies spend little effort outlining the techniques employed, but rather apply the methods to examine the details of a particular clinical situation (e.g., [41, 89, 90, 96, 97]). To date, most of the applications work has consisted of studies where a range of clinical parameters are considered in order to explore the limits pertinent to hyperthermic treatment. Clearly, the clinical applications of methods for simulating hyperthermia treatments are of most interest to hyperthermia researchers; however, the undertaking of such studies would not be possible if the techniques and methods, themselves, were not being developed. Most application-oriented or parametric analyses based on model simulations have considered the power deposition problem only as an intermediary step in the calculation of temperature distributions and have not studied the power deposition problem in isolation. This approach is appropriate from the standpoint that tissue temperature is the fundamental quantity of interest. Further, parametric studies based solely on power deposition calculations may result in misleading conclusions since the thermal redistribution of heat can produce temperature profiles which are significantly different than their corresponding power absorption patterns. Thus, most parametric studies of this type are performed better in terms of temperature distributions and have been discussed elsewhere in this volume (see Chap. 3). They will only be mentioned in passing here as the discussion permits. The emphasis, instead, will be on the techniques that are being developed for making the power deposition calculations which allow these application-oriented studies to be performed.

The majority of numerically calculated power absorption patterns that have been reported to date are based on two-dimensional approximations; hence, the two-dimensional models which have been developed and implemented will be discussed first. In terms of the five numerical methods outlined in the previous section

1. domain integrals,
2. finite elements,
3. finite differences,
4. boundary integrals, and
5. hybrid techniques

the domain integral approach has been used most often among investigators calculating fields in biological tissue. The details of this approach in the biological context has been outlined in complete three-dimensional form [24].

While posed in three dimensions, a number of investigators have made simplifying assumptions to reduce the three-dimensional formulation to a two-dimensional problem in order to obtain the kind of computational resolution that is needed for making detailed power deposition calculations. If the z direction is taken to be the long axis of the patient, the incident field is assumed to be along this axis, and no variation in geometry, electrical properties, or source characteristics is allowed in the z dimension, then the calculation of the electric field in the plane transverse to the z direction is a scalar problem. Further, the dyadic Green's function of three-dimensional problems reduces to a scalar Green's function for the scalar Helmholtz equation. These assumptions have been used to calculate electric fields in two-dimensional body cross-sections where the geometry and electrical properties have been preserved via CT-scan information (e.g., see [27, 57, 136]). In these studies the body was assumed to be surrounded by various electromagnetic source arrangements which collectively produced an incident electric field polarized in the z direction. In some cases, subsequent calculations were performed to determine temperature rise based on the numerically calculated electric field [27, 136]. Domain integrals have also been used to calculate the electric field in a two-dimensional, symmetrical, ellipsoidal model of a body cross-section containing a tumor [51, 52]. In this study the field calculations were two dimensional, but the components present were assumed to be in the plane of analysis. Certain low-frequency assumptions were made to facilitate the numerical implementation and were justified on the basis of attempting to simulate low-frequency magnetically induced hyperthermia.

The use of finite elements in hyperthermia power deposition problems, while not as prevalent as the use of the domain integral approach, has increased substantially over the past several years. A Galerkin finite element formulation of the Maxwell equations for calculating power deposition patterns has recently been reported [73]. In this work, several clinical devices have been modeled as boundary value problems, in which case the finite element method with simple linear and bilinear elements has been used to solve the governing equations. The details of the patient interior have been preserved by generating finite element grids from CT scans of actual cancer patients. All of the calculations in realistic body models have been based on two-dimensional approximations where both the transverse magnetic and transverse electric cases have been studied. The use of finite element methods in the simulation of electromagnetically induced hyperthermia has recently been reviewed and extended [120]. Other examples of finite element use in electromagnetic hyperthermia include [48, 94], and finite elements have been used in ultrasonic simulations as well [60]. All of the above computations were based on frequency-domain solutions to the Maxwell equations, but the finite element method has also been used in the time-domain in the context of computing power deposition patterns for hyperthermia [75].

Finite differences have been used in the simulation of hyperthermia treatments largely to make the thermal calculations involved in the modeling process. As such, these studies will not be addressed here (see Chap. 1). In the frequency-domain, there has been little use of finite differences in order to make power deposition calculations. An impedance formulation which is essentially a finite difference treatment of the Maxwell equations where displacement currents have been assumed negligible has been reported [4, 33]. The impedance technique is basically a low-frequency method (<30 MHz) and has been used to compute electrical fields for magnetically induced hyperthermia in realistic body cross-sections. Finite differences have been implemented in the time-domain and this finite difference time-domain (FDTD) approach has recently been used to make three-dimensional power deposition calculations in models containing very large numbers of elements [65, 66, 121]. The application of this FDTD method to three-dimensional hyperthermia problems will be discussed further below.

Boundary integral equations (or boundary elements) have appeared in simulations of power deposition patterns through hybrid formulations [74] and in three-dimensional computations (which will be addressed below) [90]. A number of clinical settings of interest result in electromagnetic problems which are fundamentally unbounded. For these simulations a hybrid method has been devised where finite elements, which are used inside the patient, are coupled to boundary elements, which are used on the patient surface and detached source. This technique provides a formal solution to the problem of an electromagnetic source which delivers energy to a highly heterogeneous body embedded in an infinite medium. As illustrative examples of unbounded electromagnetic problems of interest in hyperthermia, two-dimensional models of a capacitive heating system and an array of radiating applicators which do not completely surround the patient have been posed and sample calculations have been shown [74].

While the two-dimensional models described above have led to studies which have been informative and agree qualitatively with clinical observations, three-dimensional numerical models of hyperthermia therapy systems are needed. In some cases, the two-dimensional models are too crude to be used for patient-specific treatment planning and have shown poor correlation with clinical results. Thus, three-dimensional calculations must be obtained to establish the extent of the validity of the assumptions which have led to the simpler two-dimensional models. Further, phenomena such as resonances in the body extremities or tissue variations in the direction normal to the two-dimensional model plane, which may play important roles in understanding the capabilities of electromagnetic therapy devices, must be addressed with three-dimensional simulations. Clearly, since the physical problem of interest is truly three-dimensional due to the vector nature of the EM field, the arbitrary tissue variation in all directions, and the comparatively equal sizes of the longitudinal and cross-sectional dimensions, the most realistic and accurate simulations will result from three-dimensional models.

Studies have been reported where electrical fields induced in three-dimensional block models of man have been calculated in the context of potential health hazards due to electromagnetic radiation [24, 42, 71]. These works have relied on the domain integral equation formulation in order to make the necessary computations. More recently, this same three-dimensional approach has been used in hyperthermia applications to analyze the heating of tissue between parallel capacitive plates [50], and the absorption of energy in the body outside the area of direct treatment exposure [41]. While these studies are based on fully three-dimensional calculations which were pioneering in nature, the models of man that were used were intended to study gross effects rather than detailed energy deposition patterns. The computational resolution required for making detailed electromagnetic field calculations inside the body has forced most investigators using the domain integral equation approach to implement simplifying assumptions which reduce the problem to a two-dimensional calculation.

However, studies are beginning to emerge where detailed energy deposition patterns are being calculated inside inhomogeneous three-dimensional models of the body [65, 121]. This work is based on the finite difference time-domain (FDTD) method which requires a large number of elements for good resolution, but is reasonably straightforward to program. Further, this technique has an advantage over frequency-domain methods because large matrices do not need to be stored and inverted. While the stepping through time to steady-state tends to increase computational time, the decreased storage at least makes these detailed three-dimensional problems solvable on high-speed computers whereas the corresponding frequency-domain solution often becomes impossible due to the massive matrix storage requirements. Three-dimensional FDTD results have been obtained which show good agreement with experimental measurements for a simple radiative applicator [66].

An alternative formulation to the Maxwell equations which has been applied to hyperthermia problems is based on boundary elements. This approach is expected to require considerably fewer unknowns than the FDTD method, but it leads to a more computationally complex solution [90]. Three-dimensional frequency-domain formulations of the finite and hybrid element methods have also been developed and implemented for application to problems of interest in hyperthermia modeling [91]. To date only three-dimensional calculations on simple homogeneous and heterogeneous cylindrical geometries have been attempted in this work. The drawback, at the moment, seems to be the extremely large amounts of memory required for large-scale problems. A finite element time-domain method (FETD) which should possess the same economies in storage requirements that accompany the FDTD method, but which can readily be implemented on nonuniform meshes, has recently been discussed [75]. To date, only two-dimensional calculations have been attempted in the hyperthermia context with this formulation. Further work will be required to explore the advantages and disadvantages of these and other approaches in three dimensions. It can be expected that these techniques will expand and improve in the near future as more investigators start solving increasingly realistic three-dimensional problems.

For all studies, whether technique or application oriented, whether based on simplified or complex models, or whether two or three dimensional, an important, but often ignored, consideration is how well the theoretical predictions compare to the phantom experiments and the patients they are intended to simulate. Once again most of the comparisons of experiment with theory have been done through the quantity of temperature (e.g., see [120, 137]) and will not, as such, be discussed here. However, the topic of experimental verification of theoretical calculations is an important one if modeling of hyperthermia treatments is to have a continued impact on clinical hyperthermia; hence, it is mentioned briefly below.

Comparisons between numerical and experimental SAR patterns have been reported for interstitial techniques embedded in homogeneous phantoms [134, 140]. The agreement between theory and experiment has been good, which is an important result for establishing the validity of the theoretical model. These studies provide excellent examples of the type of comparisons which need to be done more often. Comparisons of theoretical and experimental regional power deposition patterns have been more sparse. When regional SAR comparisons have been performed, they typically have been presented as single isolated cases included in technique-oriented studies in order to add some additional credibility to the method being described (e.g., see [50, 57]). While this kind of comparison is also important, more studies are needed where the comparison aspects are the main focus of the work rather than secondary to the numerical technique, itself, as has often been the case to date. It is not surprising that theoretical versus experimental comparisons have been presented most rigorously for interstitial heating applications since they are easier to study both theoretically and experimentally than most of their superficial or regional counterparts largely due to the smaller size and more homogeneous nature of the heated tissue.

2.3.2 Future Directions and Summary

While advancements, as described in the preceding pages, have been made in the field of computer simulation of hyperthermia, this research area is still in its incipient stages and a number of fundamental questions remain unanswered. Several gaps in the state of existing knowledge, which are basic to the continued clinical impact of numerical simulation, exist:

1. the effects of detailed three-dimensional numerical calculations on the evaluation, design, and development of hyperthermia therapy devices and
2. the extent to which numerical models can predict specific power deposition patterns and resultant temperature distributions.

Clearly, the general problem to be solved is three dimensional and most of the numerical formulations discussed herein have been posed as such. The major limitation of two-dimensional models is precisely their two-dimensional nature. Some of the ramifications of this shortcoming are being discussed in the current literature [40]. Cases where two-dimensional models are inadequate have been shown both numerically [41] and experimentally [132]. Typically, the cross-sectional dimensions in a clinical setting are on the order of the longitudinal dimension and the extent of the errors introduced in two-dimensional models by ignoring the "end effects" has not been carefully quantified. While three-dimensional calculations which have the resolution necessary to account for the details of the body anatomy are beginning to appear, their use in routine analysis of clinical problems may take a number of years of further research. This leaves one with the question of what is the role of two-dimensional analysis in simulating hyperthermia treatments. Should two-dimensional models be regarded as worthless due to flaws in their basic assumptions or do they have some intrinsic merit in predicting hyperthermia dosimetry which should be exploited?

One view would be that the simpler plane calculation represents a "best case" analysis since treatments which fail to produce satisfactory heating patterns in two dimensions would not be expected to perform better in three dimensions. At a minimum, then, the plane analysis could be use as a screening mechanism to reduce (or even avoid) the computing in the third dimension where solutions are not only more expensive, but also more difficult to display and interpret. The extent to which three-dimensional performance correlates with two-dimensional performance remains an open question that needs to be addressed with more research. A main thrust of future two-dimensional modeling should then be directed toward establishing the propriety of the two-dimensional assumptions.

This kind of study can take place in two forms:

1. comparisons of two-dimensional numerical results with phantom and clinical measurements and
2. comparisons of two-dimensional numerical calculations with planar results generated from full three-dimensional computations.

Generally, the comparisons of numerical versus experimental results that have been published have been intended to lend some further credibility to the numerical models that were being developed, and as such were not the main focus of the study. In contrast to this approach, studies are needed that will make these comparisons of primary interest in order to investigate under what conditions the numerical results are, or are not, in agreement with measured data, and, when agreement is lacking, to determine the cause of such disagreement (i.e., boundary conditions, inappropriate equations, or assumptions). If a range of validity of a model can be established, then the degree of this validity and how often the conditions under which the model is valid occur in clinical problems will ultimately decide its utility. This same sort of protocol which has an emphasis on rigorously testing a model for conditions of both validity and invalidity is also needed for comparing three-dimensional predictions with experiments.

A possible outcome of such work may be that two-dimensional models will fail miserably, but this failure needs to be quantified along with how often conditions of certain failure arise in the clinic. Such an outcome would be an important result; however, it would not necessarily predicate that two-dimensional models are useless clinical tools given that the redistribution of thermal energy due to heat conduction and blood flow may smooth out inaccuracies in predicted power deposition patterns. In fact, a very useful piece of information would be the degree of accuracy required in the power deposition pattern to obtain a reasonable prediction of the temperature distribution. Further, two-dimensional numerical simulations may be valuable tools for routine clinical treatment planning if they can consistently provide qualitative or semiquantitative predictions of treatment outcome. This may be all that can be expected, even from three-dimensional models, given the current lack of knowledge concerning blood flow which appears to be the dominant parameter in shaping calculated thermal distributions.

The foregoing discussion on the role of two-dimensional models is in no way intended to suggest that two-dimensional models are adequate or to diminish the importance of three-dimensional calculations. The fact that three-dimensional computations are more difficult both to make as well as to interpret provides no scientific basis to prefer two-dimensional models over three-dimensional ones. Three-dimensional models are essential to the future success of simulating hyperthermia treatments and the major emphasis in hyperthermia modeling should be directed toward such three-dimensional calculations. Further, their impact on the evaluation, design, and development of hyperthermia therapy devices is still relatively unknown and may provide new insights that will improve hyperthermia delivery systems. It seems clear that, as future applications call for more detailed and accurate calculation of power deposition patterns, numerical modeling techniques will be required that account for the full three-dimensional effects within realistic body anatomies.

In summary, the modeling efforts in hyperthermia have evolved from simple analytical solutions to one-, two-, and even three-dimensional calculations. All of these models, from analytical to three-dimensional numerical, have important roles to fulfill in hyperthermia research. Analytical solutions provide the crucial checks on numerical algorithms and the avenue for initial analysis of complicated problems that is particularly useful for illuminating basic principles. One- and even two-dimensional numerical models can also provide these kinds of simplified results which are generally easier to interpret but which lead to greater physical intuition. Two-dimensional models may perform a screening function such that three-dimensional computations can be avoided in cases which show little promise in two dimensions. They may also be of use in routine clinical practice if they are able to provide consistently qualitative or semiquantitative treatment information which can be used to produce more effective heat delivery. Further, two-dimensional models may assist in developing relative rankings for hyperthermia systems based on simulated performance for similar types of tumors. Three-dimensional models can provide information about all "end effects"; thus they will be the most realistic and accurate prediction tools capable of supplying the detailed information needed for sophisticated treatment planning and control. Three-dimensional calculations are also needed as a standard against which the validity of any simplifying assumptions, including those that may lead to models of lower dimensionality, can be compared. That is, three-dimensional calculations can be used to determine the extent to which good three-dimensional performance can be extrapolated from good two-dimensional performance. Issues can then be addressed as to whether two-dimensional analysis consistently represents the best case, and under what conditions the best case is most likely to occur.

Increases in model complexity in terms of the irregular boundaries and tissue heterogeneities found in clinical problems have likewise progressed from homogeneous cylinders, to heterogeneous cylinders and ellipses, to body models based on CT scans of actual patients. Simple homogeneous and symmetrically layered tissue models play a similar role to that discussed above for analytical solutions. In general, they are useful in initial stages of analysis where the goal is to understand the basic mechanisms of complicated processes, and they provide a foundation upon which more complex body models can be implemented. Further, this level of model complexity (i.e., homogeneous or symmetrically layered) allows for comparisons of theory and experiment under controlled and interpretable circumstances which can readily be constructed in the laboratory. As with increases in model dimensionality, increases in anatomical detail will be the only way to account for the effects caused by such irregularities and heterogeneities and are needed in modeling where this level of detail is essential to the accuracy or interpretation of the computed results.

Finally, the emphasis of future work in the development of algorithms and methods for simulating hyperthermia treatments should be toward three-dimensional numerical models which account for tissue heterogeneity and irregular geometry. Coupled with this research, special attention should be paid to comparison between experiment and theory. These comparisons are appropriate in both two and three dimensions and must be performed with the intent of thoroughly examining the range and extent of model validity in representative clinical settings rather than presenting isolated situations of agreement. Numerical simulations have had a positive impact on clinical hyperthermia to date and can continue to do so provided the future studies which are needed support a scientific basis for the clinical applicability of numerical simulation in hyperthermia dosimetry problems.

2.4 Numerical Methods

In this section each of five numerical methods

1. domain integral equations,
2. finite elements,
3. finite differences,
4. boundary elements, and
5. hybrid formulations

will be considered in more detail. The strengths and weaknesses of the methods will be discussed and some of the issues impacting the selection of one of these numerical strategies over another for solving power deposition problems of interest in clinical hyperthermia will be addressed. All discussion will take place in the context of power absorption for the electromagnetic case.

Numerical electromagnetics has a long history and its progress can be charted through many monographs which survey various approaches, past and present (e.g., [23, 47, 79, 81, 106]). However, the hyperthermia electromagnetic problem has several distinct features which makes it somewhat nonclassical in terms of the types of problems that numerical electromagnetics has traditionally addressed. The aspects of the hyperthermia electromagnetic problem which place extra burdens on numerical formulations include

1. the region of interest is heterogeneous and lossy, and interfaces between electrically distinct portions have pronounced effects,
2. the frequency and electrical properties are typically such that neither conduction nor displacement currents can be ignored, and
3. the body is in the near-field of the source.

It is important to keep these features in mind when applying classical formulations which may not have been developed with such concerns in mind.

If hyperthermia treatment simulation is to be a useful tool for routine clinical analysis, the numerical models developed will have to be run on computers which are readily available in the hospital environment. This limitation in computer resources must be considered as one contemplates the relative merits of one numerical method over another. Because of the rapidly changing computer industry, today's supercomputers will be tomorrow's workstations, and one must also realize that increasing computer capabilities will continue to be found at decreasing costs. For the purpose of the ensuing discussion, however, a standard is needed and the following will be adopted and should be kept in mind as one proceeds through this section. A "large" computer will be considered to be an upper end "VAX" style machine such as a VAX-8600, and "moderate-sized" computing capabilities will be regarded as a typical workstation similar to a Micro VAX II.

2.4.1 Domain Integral Equations

In terms of the previous discussion of the method of weighted residuals as a general technique for reducing a functional equation into an algebraic one, the domain integral equation approach can be cast in this light where the operator, L, in Eq. 2.16 involves integration over the entire problem space. The basic mathematical framework is set up by considering the electric field as the sum of an incident and scattered component

$$\mathbf{E} = \mathbf{E}^{i} + \mathbf{E}^{s} \; . \tag{2.23}$$

The incident field, $\mathbf{E}^{i}$, is defined to be the field radiated by the sources in the absence of the body. The scattered field, $\mathbf{E}^{s}$, then can be viewed as the difference between the total field and the incident field; that is, the field that results as a consequence of the presence of the body (or scatterer). Figure 2.26 shows a conceptualization of the incident and scattered fields. In this figure, an object (the body in the hyperthermia context) is impinged upon by the incident field which in turn gives rise to the scattered field. Incident and scattered fields do not exist physically (i.e., only the left side of Eq. 2.1 can be directly measured in the lab); however, the decomposition of the electric (and magnetic) field into these components is a con-

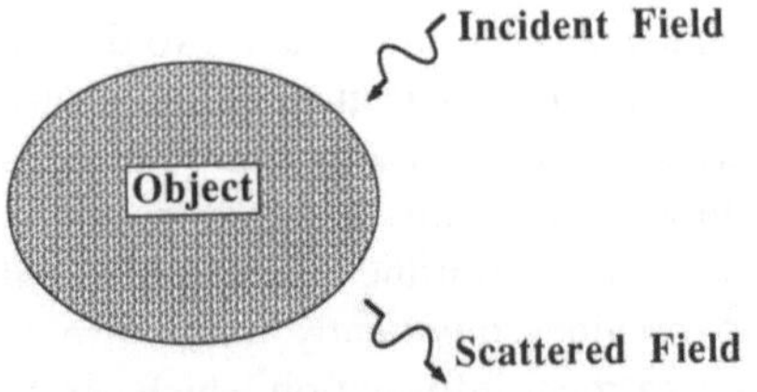

Fig. 2.26. Incident and scattered fields

struct which facilitates the mathematics and its interpretation as follows.

Assume that an electromagnetic field is produced by time-harmonic radiating currents, **J**, located in the free-space external to the body. In this case, the Maxwell curl equations can be written as

$$\nabla \times \mathbf{E} = i\omega\mu_0 \mathbf{H} \qquad (2.24\,a)$$

$$\nabla \times \mathbf{H} = -i\omega\varepsilon^* \mathbf{E} + \mathbf{J} \qquad (2.24\,b)$$

where ε^* is a function of position inside the body and equal to the free-space value, ε_0, outside. If the same currents radiate in the absence of the body, then ε^* is everywhere constant and equal to ε_0, such that Eqs. 2.24 become

$$\nabla \times \mathbf{E}^i = i\omega\mu_0 \mathbf{H}^i \qquad (2.25\,a)$$

$$\nabla \times \mathbf{H}^i = -i\omega\varepsilon_0 \mathbf{E}^i + \mathbf{J} \qquad (2.25\,b)$$

where the fields produced by **J** are distinct from those in Eqs. 2.24 and are referred to as the incident fields. Since the scattered fields constitute the difference between the quantities in Eqs. 2.24 and 2.25, one can write

$$\nabla \times \mathbf{E}^s = i\omega\mu_0 \mathbf{H}^s \qquad (2.26\,a)$$

$$\nabla \times \mathbf{H}^s = -i\omega(\varepsilon^* - \varepsilon_0)\mathbf{E} - i\omega\varepsilon_0 \mathbf{E}^s \qquad (2.26\,b)$$

by subtracting Eqs. 2.25 from their counterparts in Eq. 2.24. By defining an equivalent current as

$$\mathbf{J}_e = -i\omega(\varepsilon^* - \varepsilon_0)\mathbf{E} \qquad (2.27)$$

Eq. 2.26 b can be cast in the form

$$\nabla \times \mathbf{H}^s = -i\omega\varepsilon_0 \mathbf{E}^s + \mathbf{J}_e\ . \qquad (2.28)$$

Combining Eqs. 2.26 a and 2.28 in order to isolate the scattered electric field gives

$$\nabla \times \nabla \times \mathbf{E}^s - k_0^2 \mathbf{E}^s = i\omega\mu_0 \mathbf{J}_e \qquad (2.29)$$

where $k_0^2 = \omega^2\mu_0\varepsilon_0$. Thus, the electrical inhomogeneities (i.e., tissues) act like sources of the scattered field. In other words, an equivalent problem to the one of computing the electric field inside a lossy object irradiated by an external source (i.e., combining Eqs. 2.24 such that $\nabla \times \nabla \times \mathbf{E} - k^2\mathbf{E} = i\omega\mu_0\mathbf{J}$) is to replace the object by an equivalent current in free-space which results in the same calculated field distribution (i.e., combining Eqs. 2.25 to isolate $\mathbf{E}^i$ and solving for $\mathbf{E}^i$ along with $\mathbf{E}^s$ in Eq. 2.29). Figure 2.27 shows a schematic of the equivalence of these two approaches where in the latter case the effects of the inhomogeneous scatterer are replaced by equivalent current distributions residing in free-space.

Proceeding along the lines of the equivalent problem approach, the solution to Eq. 2.29 for the scattered fields can be written as

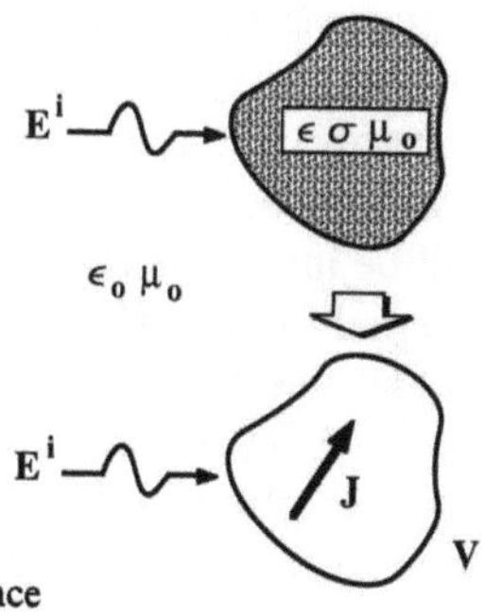

Fig. 2.27. The notion of equivalence

$$\mathbf{E}^s(x) = i\omega\mu_0 \int_V \mathbf{J}_e(x') \cdot \mathscr{G}(x,x')\,dv' \qquad (2.30)$$

where x is the observation point, x′ is the source point, and the integration is over the volume containing the equivalent current distribution, $\mathbf{J}_e$. $\mathscr{G}$ is a dyadic Green's function satisfying, in unbounded space, the equation

$$\nabla \times \nabla \times \mathscr{G} - k_0^2 \mathscr{G} = I\delta(x-x') \qquad (2.31)$$

where I is the unit dyad. Equation 2.31 consists of nine scalar equations which reflect the nine combinations of three source directions producing any one of three response directions. The solution of Eq. 2.31 results in a 3×3 matrix of functions, $\mathscr{G}$, the rows of which contain the response, in each of three coordinate directions, of an impulse pointed in one of each of these directions.

Likewise, the combination of Eqs. 2.25 which isolates $\mathbf{E}^i$ produces

$$\nabla \times \nabla \times \mathbf{E}^i - k_0^2 \mathbf{E}^i = i\omega\mu_0 \mathbf{J} \qquad (2.32)$$

and its solution can also be written in terms of a dyadic Green's function

$$\mathbf{E}^i(x) = i\omega\mu_0 \int_V \mathbf{J}(x') \cdot \mathscr{G}(x,x')\,dv' \qquad (2.33)$$

where the integration is now over the volume containing **J**, the known external source distribution. Since **J** is known and $\mathscr{G}$ can be found from Eq. 2.31, $\mathbf{E}^i$ can be considered known and plays the role of the source or excitation, g, in Eq. 2.16 of the weighted residual approach. A particularly convenient choice for the location of the source currents, **J**, is far from the scattering body in which case $\mathbf{E}^i$ becomes the field of a plane wave; however, this convenience is of little help in hyperthermia applications where the body is near the source.

Combining Eqs. 2.23, 2.27, and 2.30 results in an integral equation

$$\mathbf{E}(x) - k_0^2 \int_V (\varepsilon_r^* - 1)\mathbf{E}(x') \cdot \mathscr{G}(x,x')\,dv' = \mathbf{E}^i(x) \qquad (2.34)$$

where $\varepsilon_r^* = \varepsilon^*/\varepsilon_0$, the integration is over the volume containing the body, $\mathbf{E}$ is the unknown to be determined, and $\mathbf{E}^i$ is known through Eq. 2.33. Note that since one is interested in calculating the electric field inside the body, the observation points, x, in Eq. 2.33 will be inside the body, but the source points, x′, are external to the body; hence, x is never equal to x′ and $\mathscr{G}$ does not become singular. However, this is not the case in Eq. 2.30 (which is also contained in Eq. 2.34) since the source locations, x′, are those of the equivalent currents which are inside the body; hence, the evaluation of Eq. 2.30 is complicated by the singularity in $\mathscr{G}$ when $x = x'$. Generally, this kind of integral results in the evaluation of a principal value plus an extra source term [7, 71]. The principal value integral is found by choosing a smaller volume (or area in two dimensions) that excludes the singularity, but which in the limit approaches the original volume. Under some circumstances, the extra source term vanishes and the principal value integral can be computed analytically by approximating volume elements with spheres of equivalent size (or area elements with a circle of equal area) [7, 93].

To carry out the weighted residual approach and thereby transform Eq. 2.34 into a matrix algebra statement, the body is subdivided into numerous small elements (or cells) which are electrically homogeneous. Thus, the body is thought of as a collection of tiny scattering elements, each of which can be replaced by an equivalent current distribution (depending on its electrical properties) existing in free-space. Hence, the scattered field at a point in the body is the superposition of the fields produced by all these equivalent current distributions which collectively comprise the entire body. Typically, the electric field is expanded in terms of a simple basis function such as a pulse which is constant over an element since the integral in Eq. 2.34 is already difficult enough to perform. The most common choice for the weighting function is the delta function centered at each element. This also greatly simplifies the construction of the matrix $\mathscr{L}$ in Eq. 2.21 since one of the double integrals (double because L, itself, is an integral) can be performed analytically, the result being that the residual is forced to zero at a discrete number of points within the domain (i.e., Eq. 2.34 is enforced at the location of each delta-weighting function).

While these choices of basis and weighting functions simplify the task of numerically assembling the matrix, $\mathscr{L}$, they can lead to some nonphysical consequences in the resulting solution. These consequences center around the inability of pulse functions to account correctly for the boundary conditions between adjacent element interfaces since pulse functions are everywhere constant within an element. For example, at the boundary between two elements having the same electrical properties, all components of the electric field should be continuous (since there is no physical boundary in terms of changing electrical properties); however, this continuity can never be preserved with pulse functions at such element boundaries regardless of how small the individual element sizes are made. In effect, the discontinuity enforced by the use of pulse functions at nonphysical boundaries within the mesh (i.e., at interfaces between individual elements where no change in electrical properties occur) introduces a surface charge which does not exist, but which nonetheless becomes a source of the fields to be calculated. Further, at physical boundaries where changes in electrical properties do indeed exist, pulse basis functions cannot ensure continuity in the tangential component of the electric field at the interface, nor is there any guarantee that the required discontinuity in the normal component will be accounted for correctly.

The inaccuracies of using pulse functions as bases appears to be exacerbated when combined with cubical elements (or square elements in two dimensions) which cannot accurately resolve an interface where electrical properties change abruptly. Thus, in combination (i.e., when pulse bases are used with cubical elements) not only are the numerical boundary conditions nonphysical, but the numerical boundaries, themselves, do not readily conform to their physical counterparts (e.g., see Fig. 2.13). Recently, these issues have been discussed in the literature [13, 43, 44] and formulations of domain integral equations using linear basis functions have been reported [131]. Hence it appears that polyhedral (or polygonal) elements conforming to the physical boundaries of the problem in conjunction with at least linear basis function expansions will be required in order to achieve consistently accurate results (which will be needed for detailed hyperthermia simulations) with the domain integral equation approach. Unfortunately, this significantly complicates the assembly of the $\mathscr{L}$ matrix in Eq. 2.21 when L has a domain integral form.

An alternative domain integral equation formulation (e.g., see [47, 101]), which has the attractive feature that it avoids the dyadic Green's function in Eq. 2.34, is based on using vector and scalar potentials. In this case the scattered field is written as

$$\mathbf{E}^s = i\omega\mathbf{A} - \nabla\Phi \tag{2.35}$$

where $\mathbf{A}$ and Φ are the vector and scalar potentials, respectively. These potentials can be shown to obey inhomogeneous Helmholtz wave equations under the Lorentz condition [104] and their solutions are well-known:

$$\mathbf{A}(x) = \mu_0 \int_V \mathbf{J}_e(x')G(x,x')dv' \quad (2.36a)$$

$$\Phi(x) = \frac{1}{\varepsilon_0} \int_V \varrho_e(x')G(x,x')dv' \quad (2.36b)$$

where the integration is over the equivalent source distribution and G is the unbounded-space Green's function satisfying the scalar Helmholtz equation with singularity at $x = x'$. The equivalent current and charge density distributions which replace the effects of the inhomogeneities within the body are related by the continuity equation

$$\nabla \cdot \mathbf{J}_e = i\omega\varrho_e \,. \quad (2.37)$$

Combining Eqs. 2.35, 2.36, and 2.37 along with 2.23 and 2.27 produces the integral equation

$$\mathbf{E}(x) - k_0^2 \int_V (\varepsilon_r^* - 1)\mathbf{E}(x')G(x,x')\,dv' - \nabla \int_V \nabla' \cdot [(\varepsilon_r^* - 1)\mathbf{E}(x')]G(x,x')dv' = \mathbf{E}^i(x) \quad (2.38)$$

which is in terms of the unknown electric field inside the body. As before, the incident field is assumed known and formally may be calculated from

$$\mathbf{E}^i(x) = i\omega\mu_0 \int_V \mathbf{J}(x')G(x,x')dv' - \frac{1}{i\omega\varepsilon_0} \nabla \int_V \nabla' \cdot \mathbf{J}(x')G(x,x')dv' \quad (2.39)$$

where **J** is the known source current external to the body. In cases where the sources are far from the body, the incident field becomes a plane wave.

Direct assembly of Eq. 2.34 (or Eq. 2.38) results in a matrix which is full; that is, none of its entries can be assumed to be zero. This feature is dictated by the global nature of the Green's function kernel. The algebraic matrix is of size N^2 where N is the number of unknowns and its inversion requires operations of order N^3. The straightforward solution of Eq. 2.34 by the weighted residual approach is thus burdened by the large matrix storage requirements and operations count when finely discretized problem domains are required. This is especially true in three dimensions as is evidenced by the fact that typically only a few hundred domain elements have been possible with direct matrix solutions of domain integral equations [24, 41, 42].

However, several possible alternatives to storing and inverting the complete N^2 matrix have been devised and implemented for domain integral equations, thereby improving their utility [10, 12, 13, 62, 122]. Most of these approaches are based on the observation that the integral in Eq. 2.34 had a convolutional form. Hence, in the spectral domain, Eq. 2.34 can be written as

$$\tilde{\mathbf{E}} = i\omega\mu_0\tilde{\mathbf{J}}_e\,\tilde{\mathscr{G}} + \tilde{\mathbf{E}}^i \quad (2.40)$$

where ~ indicates a three-dimensional Fourier transform on the position vector, x. An iterative procedure which alternates between the spatial and spectral domains can then be established as follows. An initial guess for $\mathbf{J}_e$ consisting of a set of discrete values in the spatial domain is transformed (along with $\mathbf{E}^i$, which is, of course, already known) into the spectral domain. The electric field in the spectral domain is computed from the algebraic Eq. 2.40 and is then inverse transformed back into the spatial domain, where a new set of values for $\mathbf{J}_e$ is calculated through the algebra in Eq. 2.27. The new value of $\mathbf{J}_e$ is compared with the old value and the procedure is repeated until some sort of stopping criterion has been met and convergence obtained. The transformations to and from the spectral domain are performed by using FFT (Fast Fourier Transform) algorithms to speed up the computations. This technique is known as the K-space method [10], and has the advantage that it does not require the storage and inversion of an N^2 matrix; however, convergence can be problematical [13].

A number of variations of this basic approach aimed at improving convergence have been successfully implemented [12, 13]. When the domain integral equation approach is formulated on a uniform mesh with pulse basis functions and delta weighting functions, the discretized form of Eq. 2.34 amounts to the convolution of two sequences that can be efficiently computed with the FFT [13]. Because the linear matrix algebra has inherited the convolutional form of the integral Eq. 2.34, matrix multiplies can be performed via an FFT with an operations count proportional to $N \log_2 N$ rather than the traditional N^2. This efficient computation of a matrix product is then coupled with an iterative solution technique for linear systems (such as conjugate gradients) which involves these kinds of products (or conjugate transposes which have the same convolutional features). Further, storage requirements scale proportionally to N (compared to N^2) with this method. Thus, the linear system of equations can be solved iteratively with the aid of the FFT algorithm requiring only order N storage and order $N \log_2 N$ operations per iteration. However, these savings are only afforded when the grid spacing is constant and are lost when nonuniform meshes are used since the discretized linear system no longer exhibits the convolutional form of the integral equation.

The foregoing presentation of the domain integral equation approach has centered around frequency-domain analysis; however, time-domain formulations are also possible. Detailed discussions of numerical solutions of time-domain integral equations in general electromagnetic or acoustic contexts can be found in [11, 49, 68, 128]. The main advantage from a computational viewpoint that time-domain methods can have over their frequency-domain counterparts is the removal of the matrix storage and inversion requirements associated with frequency-domain methods. The basic strategy in time-domain techniques is to obtain an explicit projection of discrete values of the quantity of interest (e.g., **E**) at time $t+\Delta t$ based solely on values at previous times $(t, t-\Delta t, \ldots)$. Clearly, the storage requirements begin to increase the farther back in time the method must reach in order to obtain the solution at the next future time level, $t+\Delta t$.

Unfortunately, the domain integral representation in the time-domain possesses two complicating features:

1. the spatial integration is still global in nature (similarly to the frequency-domain) such that the solution at one point in the mesh is influenced by all other points in the problem domain, and
2. the projection of the solution to a new time level requires past histories determined by the finite speed of wave propagation, thus involving knowledge of the solution at many previous time levels.

Typically, nodal spacing is chosen such that in one time-step a wave can propagate from one node to the next, i.e., $c = \Delta x/\Delta t$ where Δx is the mesh spacing and Δt is the time step. Hence, the number of time-steps into the past that the solution at the new time level involves is proportional to the number of nodal spacings across the largest mesh dimension. Further, because of the global spatial integrations, each node has such a set of previous time histories that must be remembered. This storage burden tends to nullify any gains over frequency-domain matrix storage requirements for geometrically irregular, heterogeneous problem domains. This global nature is to be contrasted with the local structure of both the space and time derivatives in time-domain differential formulations (to be discussed in Sects. 4.2, 4.3) where typically only a few neighboring points in space are involved and only one or two previous time levels are required. Thus, time-domain differential formulations, at least presently, appear to be more promising for hyperthermia treatment simulation than their domain integral equivalents.

In summary, one of the most desirable features of the domain integral equation approach is its ability to satisfy exactly the radiation boundary condition at infinity, thus making it an attractive method for unbounded electromagnetic problems. Further, by separating the electric field into its incident and scattered components, source terms can be implemented through the incident field, and this is particularly convenient when the sources are far from the scattering body of interest. If uniform grids are used to discretize the problem domain, the resulting algebraic system can be efficiently solved with the FFT coupled to an iteration scheme such as conjugate gradient or steepest decent methods.

While the radiation condition at infinity is exactly satisfied as part of the formulation of the integral equation, interfacial boundary conditions within the electrically inhomogeneous body cause problems for this method on two fronts. First, the use of simple pulse basis functions cannot provide a solution that is capable of satisfying boundary conditions either at nonphysical boundaries between adjacent elements with identical electrical properties or at physical boundaries where the electrical properties change abruptly. Second, the use of cubical or square elements does not permit the construction of numerical boundaries which conform to the physical boundaries of the problem. The resolution of this deficiency is to use higher order basis/weighting functions (e.g., linear), which significantly complicates the assembly of the $\mathscr{L}$ matrix in Eq. 2.21 due to its double integral form, and to employ polyhedral or polygonal elements to conform the numerical boundaries to the physical ones. If these remedies are accommodated in order to represent accurately the physical boundaries and to satisfy exactly the interfacial boundary conditions, the resulting discretized integral equation loses its convolutional form and the solution economies associated with the FFT are lost. This leaves one with the computational burden of storing and inverting a full matrix (order N^2 storage and N^3 operations) or using an iterative solution scheme (order N^2 storage and N^2 computations per iteration) which can be slow to converge. Further, the interaction of the scattered field with the source is generally ignored in the formulation. While this is not a concern in many electromagnetic problems where the source is assumed far from the scattering body, it is critical in hyperthermia. Since far-field problems were the main application when this type of integral equation approach was initially formulated, care must be exercised in its adoption or adaptation to the near-field situation in hyperthermia.

Translating the above considerations in terms of calculating power deposition patterns for hyperthermia, where irregular boundaries, tissue heterogeneities, near-field external sources, and unbounded fields are often the norm, one concludes that several trade-offs must be acknowledged when domain integral equations are used. Clearly, the irregular boundaries and tissue heterogeneities of clinical problems call for accurate boundary representation and boundary condition implementation, which suggests the use of nonuniform meshes and linear basis/weighting functions. Using such may make the domain integral equation approach to the problem untractable on moderate-sized computers because of the computational overhead associated with dense matrices. Thus, model detail and accuracy may have to be compromised in order to make domain integral equation solutions possible when computer resources are limited. As a result, only problems containing unbounded fields should be considered as candidates for domain integral equation formulations. Bounded problems in hyperthermia are much better suited for differential equation methods such as finite elements (to be discussed in Sect. 4.2). However, in unbounded problems one must recognize that the computation of the incident field is made more difficult in hyperthermia because the body is typically located in the near-field of the source and the usual plane wave assumptions are inappropriate. Further, the interaction of the scattered field with the nearby hyperthermia source needs to be included.

2.4.2 Finite Element Method

The finite element solution of Eqs. 2.7 presented in this section is based on the weighted residual statements

$$\left\langle \left(\nabla\times\frac{1}{\mathrm{i}\omega\mu}\nabla\times\mathbf{E}\right)\phi_{\mathrm{i}}\right\rangle+\langle \mathrm{i}\omega\varepsilon^{*}\mathbf{E}\phi_{\mathrm{i}}\rangle=0 \qquad (2.41\,\mathrm{a})$$

$$\left\langle \left(\nabla\times\frac{1}{\mathrm{i}\omega\varepsilon^{*}}\nabla\times\mathbf{H}\right)\phi_{\mathrm{i}}\right\rangle+\langle \mathrm{i}\omega\mu\mathbf{H}\phi_{\mathrm{i}}\rangle=0 \qquad (2.41\,\mathrm{b})$$

where $\langle\,\rangle$ indicates integration over the volume and ϕ_{i} is a scalar function. Here, ϕ_{i} is to be considered a simple function with the properties – $\phi_{\mathrm{i}}=1$ at node i, $\phi_{\mathrm{i}}=0$ at all other nodes, and ϕ_{i} varies linearly over all elements containing node i. More detailed discussions of such functions may be found in most standard finite element textbooks [106, 143]. An integral theorem [58] can be used on the first term in equations (41) producing

$$\left\langle \left(\frac{1}{\mathrm{i}\omega\mu}\nabla\times\mathbf{E}\right)\times\nabla\phi_{\mathrm{i}}\right\rangle+\langle \mathrm{i}\omega\varepsilon^{*}\mathbf{E}\phi_{\mathrm{i}}\rangle$$
$$=-\oint \hat{\mathbf{n}}\times\left(\frac{1}{\mathrm{i}\omega\mu}\phi_{\mathrm{i}}\nabla\times\mathbf{E}\right)\mathrm{d}s \qquad (2.42\,\mathrm{a})$$

$$\left\langle \left(\frac{1}{\mathrm{i}\omega\varepsilon^{*}}\nabla\times\mathbf{H}\right)\times\nabla\phi_{\mathrm{i}}\right\rangle+\langle \mathrm{i}\omega\mu\mathbf{H}\phi_{\mathrm{i}}\rangle$$
$$=-\oint \hat{\mathbf{n}}\times\left(\frac{1}{\mathrm{i}\omega\varepsilon^{*}}\phi_{\mathrm{i}}\nabla\times\mathbf{H}\right)\mathrm{d}s \qquad (2.42\,\mathrm{b})$$

where $\hat{\mathbf{n}}$ is the outward-pointing unit normal to the surface containing the volume. The motivation for performing this operation is to expose $\hat{\mathbf{n}}\times\mathbf{H}$ as the natural boundary condition for the electric field, and in the dual problem to expose $\hat{\mathbf{n}}\times\mathbf{E}$ as the natural boundary condition for the magnetic field. By substituting Eqs. 2.3 into the surface integrals on the right-hand sides of Eq. 2.42, these boundary conditions become apparent:

$$\left\langle \left(\frac{1}{\mathrm{i}\omega\mu}\nabla\times\mathbf{E}\right)\times\nabla\phi_{\mathrm{i}}\right\rangle+\langle \mathrm{i}\omega\varepsilon^{*}\mathbf{E}\phi_{\mathrm{i}}\rangle$$
$$=-\oint \hat{\mathbf{n}}\times\mathbf{H}\phi_{\mathrm{i}}\,\mathrm{d}s \qquad (2.43\,\mathrm{a})$$

$$\left\langle \left(\frac{1}{\mathrm{i}\omega\varepsilon^{*}}\nabla\times\mathbf{H}\right)\times\nabla\phi_{\mathrm{i}}\right\rangle+\langle \mathrm{i}\omega\mu\mathbf{H}\phi_{\mathrm{i}}\rangle$$
$$=\oint \hat{\mathbf{n}}\times\mathbf{E}\phi_{\mathrm{i}}\,\mathrm{d}s\;. \qquad (2.43\,\mathrm{b})$$

It is interesting to note that in accordance with classical theory [114] Eq. 2.43 a indicates that, if $\hat{\mathbf{n}}\times\mathbf{H}$ is known on some closed surface, then $\mathbf{E}$ is uniquely determined everywhere inside the volume contained by that surface. A similar statement can be made regarding $\hat{\mathbf{n}}\times\mathbf{E}$ and $\mathbf{H}$.

In the context of electromagnetically induced hyperthermia where μ is constant, Eqs. 2.43 can be simplified to

$$\langle(\nabla\times\mathbf{E})\times\nabla\phi_{\mathrm{i}}\rangle-\langle k^{2}\mathbf{E}\phi_{\mathrm{i}}\rangle=-\mathrm{i}\omega\mu\oint \hat{\mathbf{n}}\times\mathbf{H}\phi_{\mathrm{i}}\,\mathrm{d}s \qquad (2.44\,\mathrm{a})$$

$$\left\langle \left(\frac{1}{k^{2}}\nabla\times\mathbf{H}\right)\times\nabla\phi_{\mathrm{i}}\right\rangle-\langle\mathbf{H}\phi_{\mathrm{i}}\rangle$$
$$=-\frac{1}{\mathrm{i}\omega\mu}\oint \hat{\mathbf{n}}\times\mathbf{E}\phi_{\mathrm{i}}\,\mathrm{d}s \qquad (2.44\,\mathrm{b})$$

where $k^{2}=\omega^{2}\mu\varepsilon^{*}$. The finite element solution presented here is based on the Galerkin form of Eq. 2.41 where the quantities $\mathbf{E}$ and $\hat{\mathbf{n}}\times\mathbf{H}$ in Eq. 2.44 a are expanded in terms of the basis function, ϕ_{j}, such that

$$\mathbf{E}=\sum_{\mathrm{j}=1}^{N}\mathbf{E}_{\mathrm{j}}\phi_{\mathrm{j}}(x) \qquad (2.45\,\mathrm{a})$$

$$\hat{\mathbf{n}}\times\mathbf{H}=\sum_{\mathrm{j}=1}^{N}(\hat{\mathbf{n}}\times\mathbf{H})_{\mathrm{j}}\phi_{\mathrm{j}}(x)=\sum_{\mathrm{j}=1}^{N}\mathbf{F}_{\mathrm{j}}\phi_{\mathrm{j}}(x)\;. \qquad (2.45\,\mathrm{b})$$

If a direct solution for the magnetic field is sought, **H** and $\hat{\mathbf{n}}\times\mathbf{E}$ in Eq. 2.44b can be expanded in the same manner. Hence, the numerical discretization is completed with the enforcement of Eq. 2.44a for i = 1 through N. Substitution of Eqs. 2.45 into Eq. 2.44a results in the matrix statement

$$[A]\{E\} = \{b\} \tag{2.46}$$

where A, E, and b comprise the complex submatrices

$$A_{ij} = \begin{bmatrix} \left\langle \frac{\partial\phi_j}{\partial y}\frac{\partial\phi_i}{\partial y} + \frac{\partial\phi_j}{\partial z}\frac{\partial\phi_i}{\partial z} - k^2\phi_j\phi_i \right\rangle & \left\langle -\frac{\partial\phi_j}{\partial x}\frac{\partial\phi_i}{\partial y} \right\rangle & \left\langle -\frac{\partial\phi_j}{\partial x}\frac{\partial\phi_i}{\partial z} \right\rangle \\ \left\langle -\frac{\partial\phi_j}{\partial y}\frac{\partial\phi_i}{\partial x} \right\rangle & \left\langle \frac{\partial\phi_j}{\partial x}\frac{\partial\phi_i}{\partial x} + \frac{\partial\phi_j}{\partial z}\frac{\partial\phi_i}{\partial z} - k^2\phi_j\phi_i \right\rangle & \left\langle -\frac{\partial\phi_j}{\partial y}\frac{\partial\phi_i}{\partial z} \right\rangle \\ \left\langle -\frac{\partial\phi_j}{\partial z}\frac{\partial\phi_i}{\partial x} \right\rangle & \left\langle -\frac{\partial\phi_j}{\partial z}\frac{\partial\phi_i}{\partial y} \right\rangle & \left\langle \frac{\partial\phi_j}{\partial x}\frac{\partial\phi_i}{\partial x} + \frac{\partial\phi_j}{\partial y}\frac{\partial\phi_i}{\partial y} - k^2\phi_j\phi_i \right\rangle \end{bmatrix},$$

$$E_j = \begin{Bmatrix} E_{x_j} \\ E_{y_j} \\ E_{z_j} \end{Bmatrix}, \quad b_i = -i\omega\mu \begin{Bmatrix} \sum_{j=1}^{N} F_{x_j} \oint \phi_j\phi_i\, ds \\ \sum_{j=1}^{N} F_{y_j} \oint \phi_j\phi_i\, ds \\ \sum_{j=1}^{N} F_{z_j} \oint \phi_j\phi_i\, ds \end{Bmatrix}$$

with i and j running from 1 to N. The dual matrix formulation for the magnetic field can be obtained with a similar set of substitutions beginning with Eq. 2.44b.

In the two-dimensional situation where TM and TE field configurations are considered, Eqs. 2.42a in the TM case and 2.42b in the TE case collapse to the simple scalar forms

$$\left\langle \frac{1}{i\omega\mu} \nabla E_z \cdot \nabla\phi_i \right\rangle + \langle i\omega\varepsilon^* E_z\phi_i \rangle = \oint \frac{1}{i\omega\mu} \nabla E_z \cdot \hat{\mathbf{n}}\phi_i\, ds \tag{2.48a}$$

$$\left\langle \frac{1}{i\omega\varepsilon^*} \nabla H_z \cdot \nabla\phi_i \right\rangle + \langle i\omega\mu H_z\phi_i \rangle = \oint \frac{1}{i\omega\varepsilon^*} \nabla H_z \cdot \hat{\mathbf{n}}\phi_i\, ds \tag{2.48b}$$

which become

$$\langle \nabla E_z \cdot \nabla\phi_i \rangle - \langle k^2 E_z\phi_i \rangle = \oint \nabla E_z \cdot \hat{\mathbf{n}}\phi_i\, ds \tag{2.48c}$$

$$\left\langle \frac{1}{k^2} \nabla H_z \cdot \nabla\phi_i \right\rangle - \langle H_z\phi_i \rangle = \oint \frac{1}{k^2} \nabla H_z \cdot \hat{\mathbf{n}}\phi_i\, ds \tag{2.48d}$$

if μ is assumed constant. These statements are weighted residual forms of the Helmholtz equation. Solution of matrix Eq. 2.46 requires that either $\hat{\mathbf{n}}\times\mathbf{H}$ or **E** be specified over the closed boundary containing the finite element mesh. When **E** is given, the Galerkin equation at the boundary node is removed from the algebraic system in favor of the known boundary condition. Once **E** has been computed, the discarded Galerkin equations become a vehicle for computing $\hat{\mathbf{n}}\times\mathbf{H}$ on the boundary everywhere **E** was originally specified. When $\hat{\mathbf{n}}\times\mathbf{H}$ is known, its boundary integral in Eq. 2.44a is assembled directly and becomes the right-hand side of matrix Eq. 2.46 as shown, thus closing the algebraic system. If all the Galerkin equations are used (either directly in the matrix or subsequently to compute $\hat{\mathbf{n}}\times\mathbf{H}$), this finite element formulation can be shown to conserve energy exactly [73]. Thus, when $\hat{\mathbf{n}}\times\mathbf{H}$ is given, the computed **E** on the boundary is that field which would have to exist in order to sustain the given $\hat{\mathbf{n}}\times\mathbf{H}$ in the presence of the load (i.e., the body). Likewise, when **E** is specified, the required $\hat{\mathbf{n}}\times\mathbf{H}$ needed to maintain the given **E** with the load in place can be computed.

This approach is somewhat different from that of dividing the field into its incident and scattered components. In the above scheme, either **E** or $\hat{\mathbf{n}}\times\mathbf{H}$ must be specified assuming the load in place, and its counterpart that would be needed is computed as part of the solution. This can be used as a design tool, such that if the imposed **E**, for example, results in an unrealistic requirement for $\hat{\mathbf{n}}\times\mathbf{H}$ (due to the presence of the load), a new **E** distribution can be tried until the resulting $\hat{\mathbf{n}}\times\mathbf{H}$ is more physically realizable. While not ideal in that an initial guess or measurement of the boundary conditions with the load in place is required, this strategy may be better than using the incident/scattered approach for hyperthermia applications because the interactions of the scattered field with the nearby source cannot be readily accounted for. Thus, the sum of the incident and scattered field at the location of the source will not accurately reflect the value of the total **E** nor the total $\hat{\mathbf{n}}\times\mathbf{H}$ (because the scattered field, in effect, does not "see" the source) when the source is near the scatterer (i.e., the body). At least by directly applying the boundary conditions on the total fields, a self-consistent, although not necessarily practical, set of quantities (i.e., **E** and $\hat{\mathbf{n}} \times \mathbf{H}$) will result from the solution process.

The interfacial boundary conditions (see Eqs. 2.4) also need to be accounted for during the assembly of matrix Eq. 2.46. Conceptually, a cut in the finite element grid is made along an interface between two tissues as shown in Fig. 2.28. The Galerkin equation for a node located on such an interface contains contributions from elements on either side, and, hence, the interface node is split into two nodes which represent the two unknowns that exist on either side of the interface. The relationships between these unknowns, which are necessary to close the algebraic system, can be obtained by expressing Eqs. 2.4a and 2.4b in a Cartesian coordinate system, and solving for the electric field on one side of the boundary in terms of its components on the other side:

$$E_{x_2} = \left(n_x^2 \frac{\varepsilon_1^*}{\varepsilon_2^*} + n_y^2 + n_z^2\right) E_{x_1} + n_x n_y \left(\frac{\varepsilon_1^*}{\varepsilon_2^*} - 1\right) E_{y_1} + n_x n_z \left(\frac{\varepsilon_1^*}{\varepsilon_2^*} - 1\right) E_{z_1} \tag{2.49a}$$

$$E_{y_2} = n_x n_y \left(\frac{\varepsilon_1^*}{\varepsilon_2^*} - 1\right) E_{x_1} + \left(n_x^2 + n_y^2 \frac{\varepsilon_1^*}{\varepsilon_2^*} + n_z^2\right) E_{y_1} + n_y n_z \left(\frac{\varepsilon_1^*}{\varepsilon_2^*} - 1\right) E_{z_1} \tag{2.49b}$$

$$E_{z_2} = n_x n_z \left(\frac{\varepsilon_1^*}{\varepsilon_2^*} - 1\right) E_{x_1} + n_y n_z \left(\frac{\varepsilon_1^*}{\varepsilon_2^*} - 1\right) E_{y_1} + \left(n_x^2 + n_y^2 + n_z^2 \frac{\varepsilon_1^*}{\varepsilon_2^*}\right) E_{z_1} \tag{2.49c}$$

where the unit normal vector $\hat{\mathbf{n}} = (n_x, n_y, n_z)$. Similar expressions can be written for the magnetic field with μ taking the place of ε^* in Eqs. 2.49. Note that Eqs. 2.49 collapse to the correct expressions when the interface is aligned along either the x, y, or z axis, or the problem domain is confined to two dimensions.

In practice, only a single node is used to represent a point on a tissue interface. Prior to matrix assembly one of the unknowns at the interface is selected to be retained in the algebraic system, say the tissue 1 unknowns in Fig. 2.28. Matrix assembly over elements in tissue 1 proceeds directly since these unknowns are part of the matrix algebra. However, during assembly of elements in tissue 2, the unknowns on this side of the interface are not represented in the column vector of unknowns to be determined, but

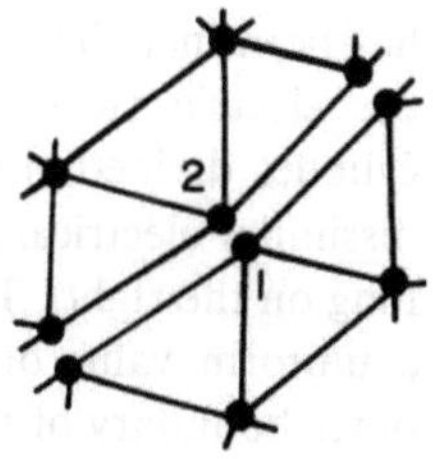

Fig. 2.28. Conceptual cut in the finite element grid along an interface dividing two electrically distinct tissues

their contributions to the matrix can be included by expressing them in terms of the tissue 1 unknowns via Eqs. 2.49 (for the electric field case).

The contribution from an interface node to the left-hand side of a given Galerkin equation can be written as $[C_1]\{E_{j1}\} + [C_2]\{E_{j2}\}$, where C is a 3×3 coefficient matrix having the form of A in Eq. 2.46 for a given i or j and the numeric subscript indicates the two regions forming the interface (the given Galerkin equation will have similar contributions from several other interface nodes). Equations 2.49 can be written as the matrix statement $\{E_{j2}\} = [A']\{E_{j1}\}$; hence substituting for $\{E_{j2}\}$ gives $[C_1]\{E_{j1}\} + [C_2][A']\{E_{j1}\}$ leaving only $\{E_{j1}\}$ as part of the matrix algebra.

To provide a more visual demonstration of the exact satisfaction of these interfacial boundary conditions where electrical properties change abruptly, Fig. 2.29

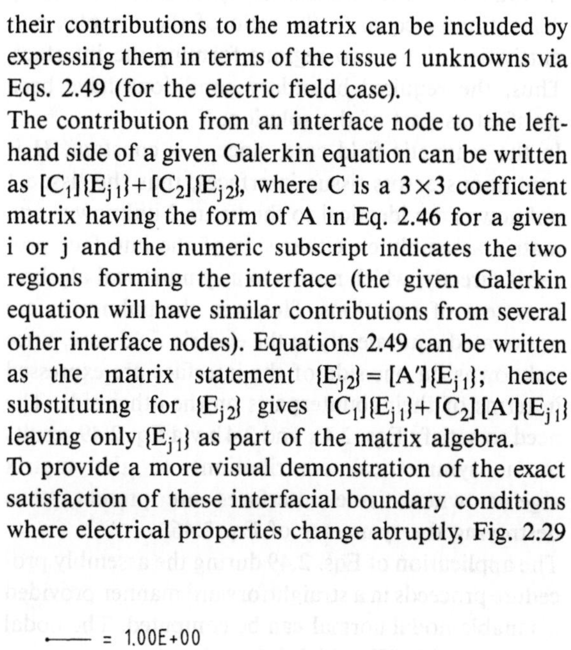

Fig. 2.29. Exact satisfaction of interface boundary conditions along the y-axis with the finite element method. Re(**E**) is plotted with its strength proportional to the vector length

has been included. This figure shows the real part of the electric field calculated in a two-dimensional cylinder divided along its y-axis into two regions of dissimilar electrical properties (muscle on the left and lung on the right). To close the problem algebraically, a uniform value of $\hat{\mathbf{n}}\times\mathbf{H}$ has been imposed at the outer boundary of the cylinder. Two vectors are plotted at the interface along the y-axis – one for either side of the boundary. The point illustrated is that the tangential components of these vectors are continuous while their normal components have a jump discontinuity equal to the ratio of the complex permittivities of the two regions forming the interface. Thus, the required boundary conditions have been satisfied as part of the solution.

In the magnetic field case, since μ is constant, $\mathbf{H}$ is continuous across tissue interfaces, thus the tissue 1 unknowns are identical to the tissue 2 unknowns and matrix assembly on either side of the interface proceeds directly, which results in a symmetrical algebraic system of equations. However, the unknowns are not treated equivalently in the electric field case, since unknowns on one side of the interface are expressed in terms of their counterparts on the other side. The need to satisfy Eqs. 2.4a and 2.4b via Eq. 2.49 results in nonsymmetrical contributions to the matrix algebra when tissue interfaces are present, thus destroying the symmetry of Eq. 2.46.

The application of Eqs. 2.49 during the assembly procedure proceeds in a straightforward manner provided a suitable nodal normal can be computed. The nodal normal in [30, 37], which is based on mass conservation principles, is used. In three dimensions the nodal normal, $\hat{\mathbf{n}}_i = (n_x, n_y, n_z)$, can be computed on finite elements as

$$n_x = \frac{1}{n}\left\langle\frac{\partial\phi_i}{\partial x}\right\rangle, \quad n_y = \frac{1}{n}\left\langle\frac{\partial\phi_i}{\partial y}\right\rangle, \quad n_z = \frac{1}{n}\left\langle\frac{\partial\phi_i}{\partial z}\right\rangle \tag{2.50}$$

where

$$n = \left[\left\langle\frac{\partial\phi_i}{\partial x}\right\rangle^2 + \left\langle\frac{\partial\phi_i}{\partial y}\right\rangle^2 + \left\langle\frac{\partial\phi_i}{\partial z}\right\rangle^2\right]^{1/2},$$

and $\langle\,\rangle$ indicates domain integration only over the tissue region for which the normal is being computed. Direct assembly of matrix Eq. 2.46 (including interfacial boundary conditions) results in a matrix algebra that is sparse due to the local nature of the basis and weighting functions. Thus, associated with direct solution of a finite element system of equations is the notion of a bandwidth [20]. If adjacent nodes are numbered close together, then in a standard square matrix representation all of the nonzero coefficients will occur in a band about the diagonal. By "turning" the diagonal upright and only storing out to the edge of this band (the half-bandwidth) on either side of the diagonal, a banded matrix storage scheme can be achieved. Compared with conventional matrix inversion techniques which require order N^2 storage and order N^3 operations count (where N is the number of unknowns), the banded matrix solvers have storage and algebraic operations on the order $2NL$ and NL^2, respectively, where L is the half-bandwidth. A typical first-order estimate of the half-bandwidth would be $L \approx \sqrt{N}$ in two dimensions and $L \approx N^{2/3}$ in three dimensions for N degrees of freedom (these estimates are obtained by considering a simple square area or cubic volume containing N nodes). Thus, for large N and small L, the savings in computer resources can be substantial with banded matrix solvers compared with full matrix solution routines. However, the effective use of banded matrix solvers requires bandwidth reduction routines which automatically renumber the nodes in order to reduce the bandwidth, thus keeping the analyst free of such node-numbering concerns during the grid construction process. This is particularly critical for hyperthermia problems where mesh generation involves detailed anatomical information which can require successive refinements. Examples of bandwidth reduction algorithms can be found in [26].

In three dimensions, the bandwidth grows approximately as $N^{2/3}$ and the banded structure of the matrix is diminished. In fact, direct solution can become impractical because of this large bandwidth and resulting matrix sizes which exceed computer memory capabilities. Even though the bandwidth grows quite large, the algebraic finite element equations are still quite sparse, with many zero coefficients contained within the band, and the advantage of the sparseness of the finite element system of equations is not fully realized in terms of its reduced storage requirements. Iterative methods, such as conjugate gradients, appear to provide an answer to the storage problem. With this type of approach, only nonzero entries in the system of equations are stored, which represents a substantial reduction in memory. For illustrative purposes, consider a three-dimensional scalar problem (i.e., one degree of freedom per node) with 10000 nodes. Using the estimates given above, one can expect $L \approx 464$, which requires storing roughly 9.28×10^6 double precision numbers or about 74 Megabytes of memory for direct banded matrix solution – beyond the capabilities of many computer systems and most found in the hospital environment. Assuming a relatively uniform grid of bilinear hexahedrons, one can estimate that 27 nodes, and hence coefficients, will be involved with each of the 10000

Galerkin equations. If an iterative solution scheme which only requires storing the nonzero coefficients is used, 2.7×10^5 double precision numbers or approximately 2 Megabytes need to reside in memory – a substantial saving. The trade-off is, of course, in terms of the convergence of a given iterative solution method, and the speed of its convergence, both of which are issues that must be considered. Note that in the frequency-domain electromagnetic case, the storage requirements are actually much worse than that described above, since in typical three-dimensional problems three degrees of freedom are needed at each node, and the unknowns are represented as complex numbers (i.e., a total of six double precision variables per node are present). Other solution techniques, such as frontal methods [53, 55], have been used to reduce main memory storage burdens. In the frontal scheme, once an equation has been assembled and manipulated it is written to disk and later recalled during the back substitution phase of the gaussian elimination process. This strategy is possible because matrix assembly occurs at the element level. Its effectiveness requires that the neighboring elements be close in number (analogously to node numbering in banded matrix storage) and "frontwidth" reduction algorithms, which attempt to optimize element ordering, are available (e.g., see [108]).

Since **E** is needed to determine the energy deposited in tissue, one convenient approach to calculating **E** is to solve numerically for **H** first, then to differentiate this solution according to Eq. 2.3b. This approach eliminates the need for directly applying the interface conditions (since **H** is continuous across all tissue boundaries), and also preserves the symmetry of the matrix formulation leading to storage economies. Two problems arise by calculating **E** from a numerical **H**:

1. the increased grid resolution needed due to lower order convergence resulting from the differentiation of **H**, and
2. the discontinuous nature of the **E** solution across all element boundaries – a nonphysical result.

The discontinuity of the **E** solution can be removed via a Galerkin treatment of Eq. 2.3b [74]:

$$\langle \mathbf{E}\phi_i\rangle = -\left\langle\left(\frac{1}{i\omega\varepsilon^*}\,\nabla\times\mathbf{H}\right)\phi_i\right\rangle \tag{2.51}$$

where **E** is interpolated according to Eq. 2.45a. After **H** is obtained via Eq. 2.44b, Eq. 2.51 becomes

$$[\langle\phi_i\phi_j\rangle]\{E_j\} = \{\mathbf{R}_i\} \tag{2.52}$$

where $\mathbf{R}_i$ is known and represents the right-hand side of Eq. 2.51. Matrix inversion of $\langle\phi_i\phi_j\rangle$ is avoided by "integral lumping" [72], where the quadrature points are placed coincident with nodal positions, such that $\langle\phi_i\phi_j\rangle = 0$ for $i\neq j$; hence

$$\mathbf{E}_i = \frac{\mathbf{R}_i}{\langle\phi_i\phi_i\rangle}\ . \tag{2.53}$$

At tissue boundaries, the interface conditions on **E** can be met by employing Eqs. 2.49 during the assembly of $\langle\phi_i\phi_j\rangle$. For the ith tissue boundary node, Eq. 2.51 can be written as

$$\langle\phi_i\phi_i\rangle_1\mathbf{E}_{i_1} + \langle\phi_i\phi_i\rangle_2\mathbf{E}_{i_2} = \mathbf{R}_{i_1} + \mathbf{R}_{i_2} \tag{2.54}$$

where the numerical subscripts indicate the two regions forming the interface. Since the tangential electric field, E_t, is continuous and the normal electric fields are related by $\varepsilon_1^* E_{n_1} = \varepsilon_2^* E_{n_2}$, then

$$E_{t_1} = E_{t_2} = \frac{(\mathbf{R}_1+\mathbf{R}_2)\cdot\hat{\mathbf{t}}}{A_1+A_2} \tag{2.55 a}$$

$$E_{n_1} = \frac{(\mathbf{R}_1+\mathbf{R}_2)\cdot\hat{\mathbf{n}}}{A_1+(\varepsilon_1^*/\varepsilon_2^*)\,A_2} \tag{2.55 b}$$

$$E_{n_2} = \frac{(\mathbf{R}_1+\mathbf{R}_2)\cdot\hat{\mathbf{n}}}{(\varepsilon_2^*/\varepsilon_1^*)\,A_1+A_2} \tag{2.55 c}$$

where $A_1 = \langle\phi_i\phi_i\rangle_1$ and $A_2 = \langle\phi_i\phi_i\rangle_2$. On the finite element mesh boundary E_t as calculated above is discarded in favor of $\hat{\mathbf{n}}\times\mathbf{E}$, which is either specified as a natural boundary condition on **H**, or, if **H** is known on the boundary, calculated from the right-hand side of Eq. 2.44b after its solution has been obtained.

In many electromagnetic problems of interest in clinical hyperthermia the source does not completely surround the problem domain, and application of appropriate boundary conditions around the outer boundary of the finite element mesh can be problematical. In general, the finite element method cannot be used in cases where portions of the problem boundary extend to infinity and the lack of a definitive boundary condition that can be applied to finite boundaries, as an approximation to infinite boundaries, has been a significant limitation in the use of finite elements for such unbounded problems. A variety of strategies such as truncating the mesh at some large, but finite, distance, which can then be considered an effective infinity, matching to analytical far-field solutions, and global and local mappings of the exterior domain or infinite elements have been suggested [8, 9, 83, 105, 107, 144]. Most of these approaches can be expensive, particularly in three dimensions, because of increased grid sizes due to the extended region, which is typically of less interest, but which must be added onto the actual problem domain in order to keep the given infinite domain approximation from degrading the solution in the interior region. Infinite element strategies seem to have the most promise and a number of different schemes have been proposed [8, 9, 144]. The basic idea behind the method of infinite elements is to use a finite element which is extended to infinity by using shape functions and integration schemes having a reciprocal behavior that decays to zero at infinity. The uncertainties that surround the use of infinite elements involve capturing the correct decay order of the solution for a given positioning of the infinite element relative to the source location. This is especially important in hyperthermia applications where the body and source are in close proximity.

While the above discussion has presented finite element analysis for electromagnetic problems in the frequency-domain, one has the option of numerically working in the time-domain. Numerical frequency-domain analysis is an elegant extension of classical work, but can require large matrix storage requirements, especially in three dimensions (as discussed above), which tends to limit its utility on present-day computer workstations, unless special efforts are made to exploit the sparse matrix structure. Time-domain approaches, however, can be formulated such that no matrix inversion is necessary. Finite element time-domain methods have been posed for general electromagnetic problems (e.g., see [22]) as well as for problems of specific interest in hyperthermia [75].

The governing equations are the time-domain analogs of Eq. 2.3

$$\nabla \times \mathbf{E} = -\mu \frac{\partial \mathbf{H}}{\partial t} \tag{2.56a}$$

$$\nabla \times \mathbf{H} = \varepsilon \frac{\partial \mathbf{E}}{\partial t} + \sigma \mathbf{E} \ . \tag{2.56b}$$

The conventional time-domain approach has been to discretize both Eqs. 2.56 and solve them alternately for **E** and **H** at half-time step intervals. This tactic is discussed more fully in the context of finite differences in the next section. Instead, in [75], the second-order wave equation for **E** alone is solved

$$\varepsilon \frac{\partial^2 \mathbf{E}}{\partial t^2} + \sigma \frac{\partial \mathbf{E}}{\partial t} = -\nabla \times \left(\frac{1}{\mu} \nabla \times \mathbf{E} \right) \tag{2.57}$$

which is obtained by differentiating Eq. 2.56b with respect to time and substituting Eq. 2.56a. Equation 2.57 allows for the solution of **E** without explicitly involving **H** and can be spatially implemented in either finite element or finite differences form. Further, the second-order equation eliminates a parasitic mode at the mesh scale which otherwise contaminates the solution on equal-order interpolation elements [72]. Control of this parasite may be achieved in finite difference models by use of a space-staggered mesh, an option with no direct analog in the finite element realm. Numerical implementation of Eq. 2.57 is free of this problem at the start.

As in the frequency-domain analysis, the weighted residual form of Eq. 2.57 is constructred

$$\left\langle \varepsilon \frac{\partial^2 \mathbf{E}}{\partial t} \phi_i \right\rangle + \left\langle \sigma \frac{\partial \mathbf{E}}{\partial t} \phi_i \right\rangle = \left\langle \nabla \phi_i \times \left(\frac{1}{\mu} \nabla \times \mathbf{E} \right) \right\rangle + \oint \hat{\mathbf{n}} \times \frac{\partial \mathbf{H}}{\partial t} \phi_i \, ds \tag{2.58}$$

where as before ⟨ ⟩ indicates integration over the problem domain and $\oint$ denotes integration over its enclosing surface. The use of the expansion in Eq. 2.45a completes the spatial discretization and results in a set of coupled ordinary differential equations in time

$$\sum_{j=1}^{N} \langle \varepsilon \phi_i \phi_j \rangle \frac{d^2 \mathbf{E}_j}{dt^2} + \sum_{j=1}^{N} \langle \sigma \phi_i \phi_j \rangle \frac{d\mathbf{E}_j}{dt} = \sum_{j=1}^{N} \left\langle \frac{1}{\mu} \nabla \phi_i \times \nabla \phi_j \right\rangle \mathbf{E}_j + \oint \hat{\mathbf{n}} \times \frac{\partial \mathbf{H}}{\partial t} \phi_i \, ds \ . \tag{2.59}$$

If the integral lumping technique is used, where the quadrature points and nodes coincide, the left-side matrices in Eq. 2.59 become diagonal, which forms the basis for a completely explicit time-stepping scheme. A three-level time discretization can be employed [75], where the right-hand side of Eq. 2.59 is evaluated at time t, and second-order correct time differences centered at t are used for the left side. This produces an explicit expression for nodal values of **E** at time $t + \Delta t$ in terms of values at t and $t - \Delta t$. The time-stepping algorithm can be started from rest, the sources turned on, and the integration through time carried out until a dynamic steady-state has been reached.

The above finite element time-domain method requires either **E** or $\frac{\partial \mathbf{H}}{\partial t}$ be known over the boundary enclosing the domain of interest similarly to its frequency-domain counterpart, and suffers the same additional complexities when boundaries at infinity occur. A variety of approximate strategies have been posed to remedy this situation and they are briefly discussed in the next section. Hybrid schemes are also possible where time-domain finite elements are coupled to time-domain boundary elements in order to alleviate the need of applying boundary conditions at the terminations of the finite grid, but no such time-domain hybrid strategies have appeared in the hyperthermia context to date.

Note that the goal of avoiding matrix storage and inversion has been achieved due to the explicit nature of the time-domain approach; however, this typically translates into increased run times resulting from the repetitive time-stepping. In a sample two-dimensional power deposition calculation where a patient CT scan was discretized into a finite element grid, the computer storage requirements were effectively reduced to zero, but the CPU time increased by a factor of three [75]. Further study is needed to quantify the relative merits of time and frequency-domain numerical approaches for problems of interest in clinical hyperthermia. Certainly, when matrix storage reaches the limits of the computer power readily available to the user, time-domain techniques may provide an approach for obtaining solutions to problems that would otherwise go unsolved.

To summarize, the basic strength of the finite element method lies in its differential equation starting point. This allows the weighted residual reduction of the functional equation into an algebraic one to result in expressions which only have localized influence. By choosing standardized basis and weighting functions, which vary only at the element level, not only is the matrix algebra sparse, but the matrix construction, itself, is simple, consisting of differentiation and integration of elementary functions. Common direct banded matrix solvers are effective methods for solving most two-dimensional problems on readily available computer workstations. While the banded finite element system of equations is sparse, its inverse is full, and in three dimensions the sparseness can better be exploited by iteration techniques where only nonzero coefficients are of concern. Irregular boundaries and region heterogeneity can be easily accommodated with the method. Further, interfacial boundary conditions where electrical properties change abruptly are explicitly satisfied and exact energy conservation preserved as a direct consequence of the formulation. Thus, when **E** is specified on the boundary, the $\hat{\mathbf{n}} \times \mathbf{H}$ needed to sustain the imposed electric field distribution in the presence of the body can be calculated reflecting the loading of the body on the source. Both time and frequency-domain solutions are possible and their implementations involve comparable degrees of complexity.

While the major advantages of the finite element method are a result of its differential equation beginnings, its major drawback is also a consequence of such. The finite element method alone lacks a definitive boundary condition that can be applied at finite boundaries, but which represents the effects of a boundary at infinity. Further, the price paid for the capability of computing on irregular, heterogeneous geometries is in the complexity of generating the input data needed to describe such a complicated domain. Automatic finite element grid generation is reasonably sophisticated for most problems in two dimensions, including the automatic mesh construction of two-dimensional problem domains based on detailed CT scans of cancer patients. In three dimensions, however, grid generation is still problematical for other than regular shapes (spheres, rectangles, cylinders, etc.) or domains that can be considered as a combination of such regular shapes.

In terms of calculating power deposition patterns for hyperthermia applications, the advantages of finite elements suggest that they are particularly well suited for the problem. This is especially true in two-dimensional bounded problems such as the simulation of an annular array of applicators which completely surround the patient. In this case complex geometries can be automatically generated from CT scans, thus simplifying the burden of data input, and reasonable boundary conditions can be specified around the enclosing boundaries. Frequency-domain solutions are well within the computing capabilities of today's readily available and modestly priced workstations. For unbounded problems, however, conventional finite elements cannot be applied and must be supplemented with additional equations or assumptions. Exact satisfaction of infinite boundary conditions is only possible with integral equations and one strategy is to couple finite elements with such equations. This scheme has been successfully implemented for hyperthermia problems in two and three dimensions in the frequency-domain [74, 91] and is discussed in more detail in Sect. 4.5. The exact approach can significantly increase algebraic operations and storage count over pure finite elements as well as complicate matrix construction; however, in two-dimensions, unbounded problems containing realistic models of body geometry have been successfully solved with moderate computing power. Boundary conditions based on localized approximations are an alternative which preserve the computational attractiveness of finite elements, but potentially at the expense of solution integrity. Care must be exercised in implementing such approximations because of the close proximity of the source to the body (i.e., the region where accurate solutions are desired).

In theory, at least for bounded problems, the same strong arguments which favor finite element methods for use in two-dimensional hyperthermia problems are also applicable in three-dimensional hyperthermia problems. In terms of sparseness of equations and ability to account naturally for irregular geometries and inhomogeneous boundaries, this is certainly true;

however, several caveats must be mentioned. First, direct banded matrix solvers are no longer practical in three dimensions and iterative solutions strategies which more fully exploit the sparse matrix structure are needed. Further, time-domain solutions become attractive, but they have not been widely used in hyperthermia contexts and their advantages and disadvantages for hyperthermia problems need further study. Second and, more significantly, automatic finite element grid generation with the flexibility to construct the highly irregular shapes and geometries contained within the body is not presently available. The lack of such sophisticated tools for the complicated data input required to take full advantage of the power of the finite element method will limit its utility in routine hyperthermia treatment simulation in the near future. Use of finite elements in unbounded three-dimensional problems suffers from the same shortcomings as in two dimensions. While its formulation has been numerically implemented in three dimensions, the practicallity of coupling integral equations to the finite element system for three-dimensional hyperthermia problems has yet to be demonstrated and this approach calls for further study.

2.4.3 Finite Differences

In contrast to finite elements where the differential operations prescribed by L are carried out exactly on the basis function expansions, the strategy in finite differences is to approximate the differential operator, L, itself. Thus, a method is needed for differentiating functions which utilizes only algebraic operations and this technique is known as finite difference calculus [54]. The basic concept is to find these algebraic approximations by Taylor series expanding analytical functions and then truncating this series depending on the degree of accuracy desired.
As an illustrative example, consider the function f(x) shown in Fig. 2.30. If f(x) is analytical in some region,

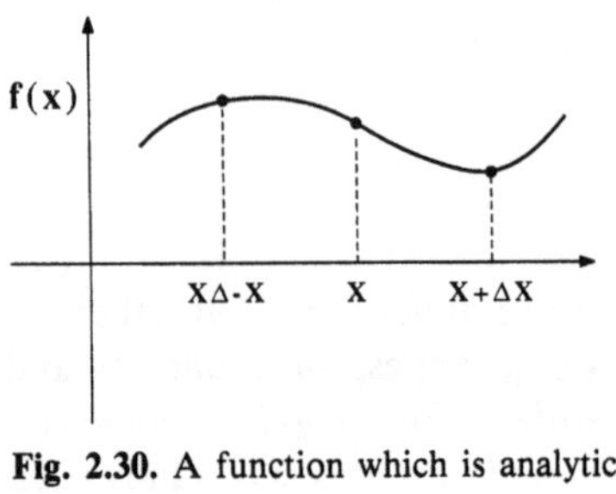

Fig. 2.30. A function which is analytical about some point x

then it can be Taylor series expanded about the point x such that f at $x+\Delta x$ can be found from the infinite series

$$f(x+\Delta x) = f(x)+\Delta x f'(x)+\frac{\Delta x^2}{2!} f''(x)+\ldots \qquad (2.60)$$

where the prime indicates differentiation with respect to x. Equation 2.60 can be rearranged to give an expression for $f'(x)$:

$$f'(x) = \frac{f(x+\Delta x)-f(x)}{\Delta x}-\frac{\Delta x}{2} f''(x)-\ldots \qquad (2.61)$$

If all terms of order Δx and higher are neglected, then Eq. 2.61 becomes an approximation of $f'(x)$

$$f'(x) \approx \frac{f(x+\Delta x)-f(x)}{\Delta x} \qquad (2.62)$$

which has an error of the order Δx. Algebraic expression 2.62 for $f'(x)$ is referred to as a forward difference approximation in that only values of the function at points greater than or equal to x are involved.
A backward difference approximation can be obtained by using the Taylor series to find f and $x-\Delta x$

$$f(x-\Delta x) = f(x)-\Delta x f'(x)+\frac{\Delta x^2}{2!} f''(x)-\ldots \qquad (2.63)$$

and rearranging terms in a similar manner to that of Eq. 2.61. The backward difference approximation with accuracy of order Δx then can be written as

$$f'(x) \approx \frac{f(x)-f(x-\Delta x)}{\Delta x} . \qquad (2.64)$$

In this case only values of the function at points less than or equal to x are needed.
A central difference approximation is possible by subtracting Eq. 2.63 from Eq. 2.60 and collecting the appropriate terms

$$f'(x) = \frac{f(x+\Delta x)-f(x-\Delta x)}{2\Delta x}-\frac{\Delta x^2}{6} f'''(x)+\ldots \qquad (2.65)$$

Note that if all terms containing higher than first derivatives are ignored, the approximation to $f'(x)$ becomes of order Δx^2 in accuracy – an important improvement over the forward and backward difference expressions 2.62 and 2.64. Now values of the function (Δx away) on either side of x are needed, but the value of f at x, itself, is not involved. A central difference approximation to the second derivative can be found by adding Eqs. 2.60 and 2.63, solving for $f''(x)$, and neglecting terms of order Δx^2 and higher

$$f''(x) \approx \frac{f(x-\Delta x)-2f(x)+f(x+\Delta x)}{\Delta x^2} . \qquad (2.66)$$

Second derivative approximations using forward or backward difference expressions can also be derived by combining two Taylor series in either the forward or backward directions (e.g., at $x+\Delta x$ and $x+2\Delta x$ for a forward difference expression) and solving for $f''(x)$. However, these approximations, like their first derivative counterparts, contain errors of order Δx. To obtain expressions having order Δx^2 errors with forward and backward differences, the first error term of order Δx can be replaced by its order Δx approximation. This maneuver results in an extra term appearing in the final expression used to approximate a given derivative. Thus, central difference approximations are to be preferred since they provide increased accuracy over forward and backward difference expressions involving the same number of terms. The increased accuracy with central difference is not surprising since it is not limited to one-sided sampling of the function as are forward and backward approximations. However, in some situations (e.g., at boundaries) central differences may not be applicable and the appropriate forward or backward difference expression will be needed.

The approximation of derivatives by finite difference calculus as described above forms the basis of the finite difference method. The algebraic expressions contained in Eqs. 2.64 and 2.66 provide one of the method's most attractive features – simplicity. In the above derivations of difference expressions, it has been implied that the sampling of the function occurs at uniform intervals. Hence the simplicity of finite differences is tied to maintaining a uniform sampling of the problem domain (i.e., a uniform mesh) and this simplicity is somewhat diminished in the presence of unequal spacing between nodes.

As an example of utilizing finite difference calculus in terms of the finite difference method for calculating power deposition patterns, consider the scalar Helmholtz equation in the z-directed electric field given in Eq. 2.10. In a two-dimensional x–y plane analysis, the finite difference approximation to Eq. 2.10 using central differences becomes

$$\frac{E_{i-1,j}-2E_{i,j}+E_{i+1,j}}{\Delta x^2}+\frac{E_{i,j-1}-2E_{i,j}+E_{i,j+1}}{\Delta y^2}+k^2E_{i,j}=0 \tag{2.67}$$

at node (ij). The subscripts in Eq. 2.67 indicate node location and Fig. 2.31 shows the relative position of the nodes involved in the equation. As indicated in Fig. 2.31, all nodes are Δx apart in the x direction and Δy apart in the y direction. Only a maximum of five unknowns are involved at any point within the mesh; thus the matrix of algebraic equations generated by enforcing Eq. 2.67 at each node in the grid lends itself to efficient matrix solution techniques which exploit its sparseness [1].

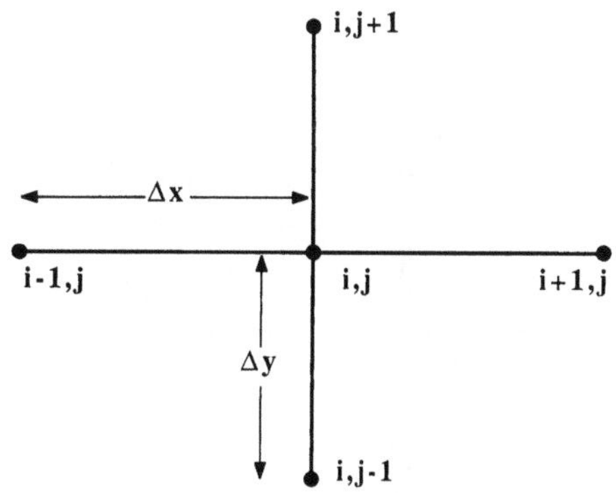

Fig. 2.31. Nodes involved in a finite difference approximation to a scalar Helmholtz equation

To close the algebraic system of equations either E_z or $\nabla E_z \cdot \hat{\mathbf{n}}$ must be specified at each boundary node. When E_z is known, Eq. 2.67 is not enforced at the boundary in favor of the specified boundary condition. Further, whenever Eq. 2.67 is centered at non-boundary nodes, but a boundary node is explicitly involved within the expression, the boundary node can be moved to the right-hand side since its value is known. If the gradient condition is given, then the finite difference equation is enforced at the boundary node. This, however, causes the involvement of nodes which are outside of the problem domain. Fortunately, the boundary condition provides the necessary additional equation to remove the extraneous node. The finite difference form of the boundary condition can be solved for the node outside of the problem domain in terms of only nodes within, thereby removing the extra node from the system. For example, assume that Eq. 2.67 is written at a boundary node (ij) as shown in Fig. 2.32, then node (i+1, j) is needed, but is outside the problem domain. If the gradient boundary condition, $\frac{\partial E_z}{\partial x}=c$ is specified at (ij), its finite difference form can be written as

$$\frac{E_{i+1,j}-E_{i-i,j}}{2\Delta x}=c \tag{2.68}$$

thus providing an expression for the outside node in terms of interior nodes. Solving Eq. 2.68 for $E_{i+1,j}$ and substituting it into 2.67 produces

$$\frac{2E_{i-1,j}-2E_{i,j}}{\Delta x^2}+\frac{E_{i,j-1}-2E_{i,j}+E_{i,j+1}}{\Delta y^2}+k^2E_{i,j}=-\frac{2c}{\Delta x} \tag{2.69}$$

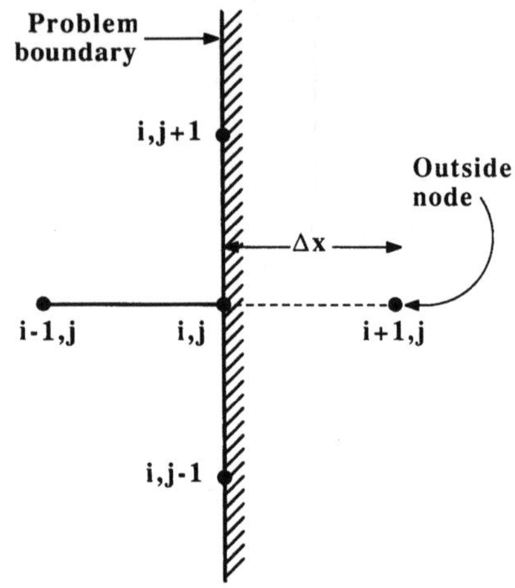

Fig. 2.32. Nodes involved in a finite difference approximation centered at a boundary point

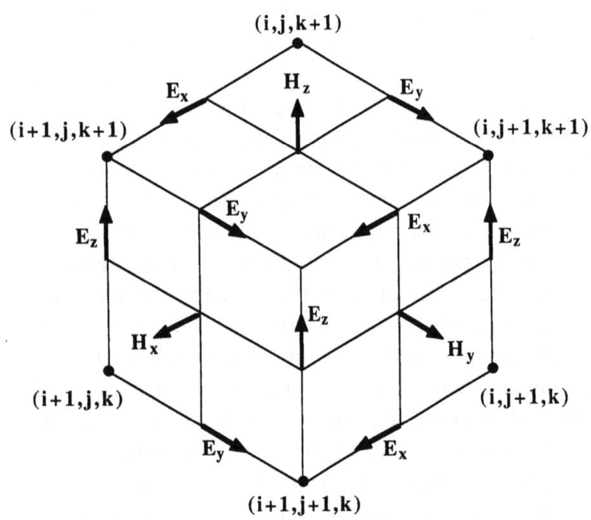

Fig. 2.33. Locations of the field components on a cube in the FDTD method

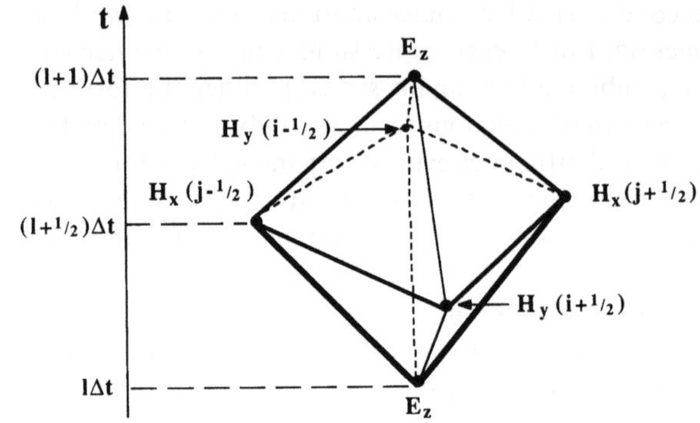

Fig. 2.34. Temporal discretization in the FDTD illustrating the computation of **E** and **H** at alternate half-time steps

which can be assembled in the usual manner since it contains only nodes within the problem domain. Note that by enforcing the boundary condition a right-hand-side term appears and closes the algebraic system of equations. The finite difference method as described above would not appear to fall under the category of a weighted residual method and typically it is not discussed as such. However, any method which reduces a functional equation into a matrix equation can be interpreted within the framework of the method of weighted residuals. The weighted residual interpretation of the finite difference expression given in Eq. 2.67 is one where point-matching has been used (i.e., delta functions have been used as weights), that is, the residual is set to zero at each node within the finite difference mesh.

The promising use of finite differences in calculating power deposition patterns for hyperthermia seems to be in the time-domain. In this case, spatial and temporal finite difference approximations have typically been implemented using the time-dependent Maxwell curl equations in their first-order partial differential form. The original appearance of this approach in electromagnetic problems is usually attributed to [141], but the method has been developed and expanded by [124, 125], and is now being used in hyperthermia contexts [121, 65]. By positioning the components of the electric and magnetic fields around a simple cube with dimensions ($\Delta x, \Delta y, \Delta z$) and by alternating the calculation of these fields as time progresses, centered difference approximations to both the space and time derivatives can be used. When the problem domain is discretized into a grid of cubes, and time is segmented into periods of length Δt, the space and time increments can be indexed such that a space-time point within the grid can be conveniently labeled by the indices (i, j, k, l). For example, under this notation a location Δx away and Δt latter than the point (i, j, k, l) can be assigned the position (i+1, j, k, l+1). Figure 2.33 shows the locations of the electric and magnetic field components on a cube where several spatial points have been labeled with this indexing notation which will be used in subsequent equations. The temporal discretization, where the electric and magnetic fields are computed alternately at half-time steps, is illustrated in Fig. 2.34. Using this scheme (Figs. 2.33, 2.34), the progression through time can be carried out explicitly with second-order accurate difference expressions in both space and time, but without the need of simultaneous equations to compute the fields at the latest time step. The time-dependent Maxwell curl equations are the starting points for the finite difference time-domain (FDTD) method

$$\nabla \times \mathbf{E} = -\mu \frac{\partial \mathbf{H}}{\partial t} \qquad (2.70a)$$

$$\nabla \times \mathbf{H} = \varepsilon \frac{\partial \mathbf{E}}{\partial t} + \sigma \mathbf{E} \ . \qquad (2.70b)$$

An explicit expression for the magnetic field can be obtained by writing the finite difference calculus equivalent of Eq. 2.70a. As an example of this procedure, consider the x component of Eq. 2.70a which provides the formula for calculating H_x at time level $l+1/2$. Referring to the index notation of Figs. 2.33 and 2.34, one can obtain

$$\mu_0 \frac{H_x(l+1/2)-H_x(l-1/2)}{\Delta t} = \frac{E_z(j)-E_z(j+1)}{\Delta y} + \frac{E_y(k+1)-E_y(k)}{\Delta z} \qquad (2.71)$$

at the spatial location $(i+1, j+1/2, k+1/2)$. Note that the arguments of the field variables only include the indices that change [i.e., if the index is missing then it is taken to be at the space-time point $(i+1, j+1/2, k+1/2, l)$, where Eq. 2.70a is centered]. Equation 2.71 can be solved for H_x at the $l+1/2$ time level in terms of **E** at the l and H_x at the $l-1/2$ time levels. Assuming that **E** and **H** are known at all time levels less than or equal to l (i.e., the time-stepping procedure has been started and the method is in the process of progressing from time level l to time level $l+1$), this equation provides a simple algebraic expression for H_x at the half-time step. Similar expressions can be obtained and solved for H_y and H_z. Thus, **H** can be explicitly computed at the $l+1/2$ level throughout the problem domain. Equation 2.70b supplies the relationship for computing **E** at the $l+1$ time level based on **E** at the l and **H** at the $l+1/2$ time levels. As an example, the z component of Eq. 2.70b is written in its finite-difference form at location $(i+1, j, k+1/2)$ as

$$\varepsilon \frac{E_z(l+1)-E_z(l)}{\Delta t} + \frac{\sigma}{2}[E_z(l+1)+E_z(l)] = \frac{H_y(i+3/2)-H_y(i+1/2)}{\Delta x} - \frac{H_x(j+1/2)-H_x(j-1/2)}{\Delta y} \qquad (2.72)$$

where ε and σ are evaluated at $(i+1, j, k+1/2)$. Again the same convention concerning the indices has been adopted in Eq. 2.72 – if they are missing then they are assumed to be at the space-time point $(i+1, j, k+1/2, l+1/2)$, where Eq. 2.70b is centered. Equation 2.72 is solved for E_z at time level $l+1$ in terms of completely known quantities. Since similar expressions can be obtained for E_x and E_y, Eq. 2.70b provides the information necessary to calculate **E** at the $l+1$ time level. Once this has been done, the procedure is carried out again to find **E** at the $l+2$ level by first calculating **H** at the $l+3/2$ level based on **E** at $l+1$ (which was just computed), and then computing **E** at $l+2$ from **H** at $l+3/2$. Note that for the second term on the right-side of Eq. 2.70b where no time derivative is involved **E** at the $l+1/2$ time level is needed, and can be found as the average of **E** at the beginning (i.e., at l) and the end (i.e., at $l+1$) of the time-step. A word of caution is in order here. If $1-\frac{\sigma \Delta t}{2\varepsilon} = 0$, then **E** at $l+1$ becomes independent of **E** at l, which can cause some stability problems and it may be safer to evaluate this term at the $l+1$ time level [69]. Hence, Eqs. 2.71 and 2.72 along with their companions for the other components of the electric and magnetic field provide a simple mechanism for marching on in time given some initial startup conditions. The procedure is fully explicit and requires no matrix storage, thus making it attractive for large-scale three-dimensional problems in hyperthermia.

While the strength of the FDTD method lies in its simplicity as suggested by expressions 2.71–2.72, and its explicit integration through time which requires no large matrices (or their inversion), this formulation has several practical problems. To maintain accuracy in the approximate spatial derivatives, the grid discretization must be sufficiently small compared with a wavelength. However, to ensure the stability of the explicit time-stepping scheme the Courant stability criterion must also be satisfied

$$c \frac{\Delta t}{\Delta R} \leq 1 \qquad (2.73)$$

where c is the velocity of wave propagation, $\Delta R = (\Delta x^2 + \Delta y^2 + \Delta z^2)^{1/2}$ is a measure of the mesh spacing, and Δt is the time-step size. Thus computer run times can become practical constraints since the time-step must get proportionately smaller as the grid spacing is reduced. These run times may counter-balance the savings in storage requirements over frequency-domain approaches. At the moment, it appears that, at least in three dimensions, this counter-balancing is not an issue because the matrices of frequency-domain approaches are often too large for available computing power.

As in the frequency-domain, boundary conditions must be applied at the outer boundaries of the grid in order to determine the solution to the interior problem. In cases where the electromagnetic fields are unbounded, this requirement can be problematical and its ramifications will be discussed below. Further, interfacial boundary conditions need to be satisfied for electrically heterogeneous problems. The interface boundary condition which requires continuity in **E** between tissues where the electrical properties change abruptly appears to be automatically satisfied by positioning the components of the electric field such that they are only tangential to adjacent cube boundaries. Closer inspection, however, reveals that a contradiction exists at an element boundary which divides two electrically distinct regions. The dichotomy is clearly illustrated in Fig. 2.35 where the equation for E_y at the boundary results in different values just to the left and just to the right of the interface due to the discontinuity in ε. These different values for E_y as the boundary is approached from opposite sides implies that E_y is discontinuous – a nonphysical result since E_y is tangential to the interface. This violation of the boundary condition is not very satisfying for problems containing severe heterogeneity where interfaces can have pronounced effects. By avoiding the involvement of the normal component of **E** at these boundaries its jump discontinuity is not satisfied either. The full implications of this for calculating the detailed power deposition patterns needed in hyperthermia are presently unknown. The type of error that can potentially be introduced is shown in Fig. 2.36 where the jump discontinuity in the normal component of the electric field at a muscle/fat interface has not been adequately accounted for as a result of the normal component boundary condition not being directly enforced. In this figure, the solid line represents the analytical solution while the circles show a corresponding FDTD calculation. For unbounded problems, the FDTD suffers from the shortcoming that only a finite mesh can be constructed, but exact boundary conditions can only be applied at infinity. Further, the field components that are required at the terminating boundaries of the grid cannot be determined directly from the differential curl equations (or their finite difference approximations). Thus, the differential equations must be supplemented with some additional equations or conditions that will allow the mesh to be truncated at a finite point in space. The exact boundary condition comes in the form of an integral equation over the entire boundary. In the frequency-domain, this expression has been used in conjunction with finite elements in order to provide a formal solution to this problem of having a finite boundary, but unbounded fields. This method has been referred to in the present chapter as the hybrid element method and it is discussed in Sect. 4.5. In the time-domain, however, this boundary condition has been formulated as an integral over time and space. The nature of this integral is such that a point on the boundary is influenced by all other boundary points (similarly to the frequency-domain representation), not at the present time, but at various times in the past (depending on their distance apart and the propagation velocity) which are a consequence of the finite speed of electromagnetic signals. Since the Courant condition must be satisfied, and the time for a signal to travel a certain distance is that distance divided by the propagation velocity, the number of time-steps over which the solution must be remembered is roughly equal to the number of grid spacing increments across the largest dimension of the mesh (i.e., the number of

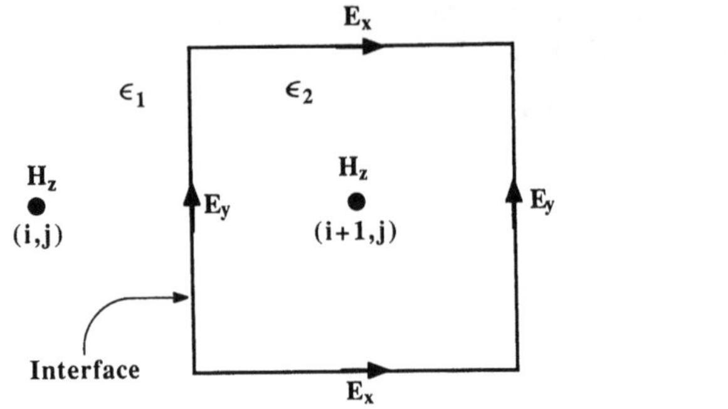

at $(i+{}^1/_2,\ j,\ l+{}^1/_2)$:

$$\epsilon\frac{\partial E_y}{\partial t} = -\frac{\partial H_z}{\partial X} \rightarrow E_y(l+1) = E_y(l) + \frac{\Delta t}{\epsilon \Delta X}\left(H_z(i) - H_z(i+1)\right)$$

Fig. 2.35. Illustration of the contradiction in calculating E_y at a dielectric interface arising from the discontinuity in ε

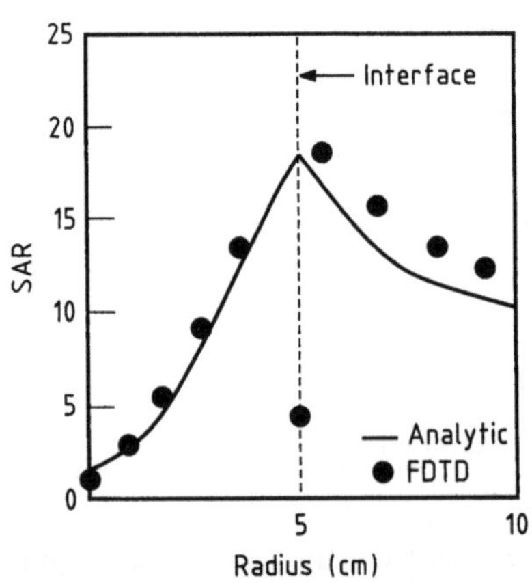

Fig. 2.36. Error in **E** at an interface resulting from not satisfying the normal component boundary condition. Redrawn from [121]

periods into the past that must be stored is determined by the number of wavelengths across the problem domain). Thus, in practical applications, the storage requirements associated with saving past values of the solution needed for future use can get large enough to nullify the advantages of the small memory requirements that were originally afforded by the time-domain approach. While a global lookback scheme has been successfully implemented for general electromagnetic applications and it formally resolves the mesh truncation issue for unbounded problems, it has been considered to be of limited practical use as presently formulated [145].

Proper termination of the mesh for unbounded electromagnetic problems requires that the outward traveling waves not be reflected back into the problem domain by the artificial boundaries imposed by the finite-sized grid. If improperly treated, the truncation of the mesh can introduce erroneous numerical reflections that will infect the interior solution as these reflected waves return from the outer boundary. Since the exact formulation as briefly described above has not yet been made a practical solution to grid termination, a number of approximate truncation schemes which lead to simplified boundary conditions have been suggested. Typically the strategies have been of three types:

1. large-volume simulations,
2. absorbing boundaries, or
3. field-matching techniques.

In large-volume simulations, the idea is to use a volume which is large enough that the reflections due to the outer boundaries do not contaminate the interior solution until after the solution times of interest have already past. Absorptive boundary conditions generally introduce an artificial layer of absorbing medium in the exterior region which continually dissipates the reflected waves as they reverberate within the lossy space, thus attempting to minimize the reflections at mesh terminations. Field-matching schemes involve the extrapolation of boundary values from interior values adjacent to the boundary using approximate formulas. Such strategies typically assume that the fields locally look like outward-traveling plane waves or that far from any sources they behave like spherical waves. Examples of these approximate grid termination schemes for finite difference meshes when unbounded problems are to be solved can be found in [31, 70, 82, 92, 124].

Each of the above types of approximate boundary conditions is not without flaws which are of some concern. Clearly, large-volume schemes require increasing amounts of storage and computation time in order to achieve accurate solutions later in time and are not readily applicable to hyperthermia problems where the dynamic steady-state is of interest. Absorptive boundary conditions based on lossy external medium only reduce the numerical boundary reflections and do not completely remove the outgoing waves from the system. Further the introduction of the lossy medium, itself, is completely artificial. Field-matching schemes based on plane-wave approximations require highly discretized meshes since only a small portion of the wave front can be locally approximated as a plane wave. In view of the Courant criterion, this leads to a reduced time-step size and concomitant increases in computational time per increment of real solution time. Spherical wave approximations also require large computational grids, since the behavior of electromagnetic fields is accurately approximated by such waves only very far from the source. This is particularly true for hyperthermia applications where the body is generally located in the near-field of the sources. Further, the implementation of this boundary condition can be complicated by the need to relate spherical waves to the Cartesian geometry of the mesh.

In summary, many of the characteristics of the finite difference method are similar to those of finite elements in that both begin with differential operators; thus the strengths and weaknesses discussed in the previous section that are intrinsic to differential equation formulations apply in general to finite differences as well. Specifically, the advantages of finite differences center around

1. the simplicity and local nature of the finite difference representation of the space (and time) derivatives contained in the Maxwell equations and
2. the calculation in the time-domain via an explicit time-stepping scheme which removes any need for matrix storage and inversion and which only involves historical values of the solution at one or two of the previous time instants.

These economies make the finite difference method a leading candidate for large-scale, three-dimensional calculations. Further, the method is most naturally applied on a uniform mesh of cubes or squares. In such cases a simple indexing system can be used to account for the nodal points comprising the mesh which approximates the problem domain. This simplicity in the data input is significant given that three-dimensional mesh generation consisting of nonuniform element sizes and shapes resolving complex geometries is a difficult problem that has not yet been adequately solved.

The numerically attractive features of the finite difference method are compromised by

1. the potential increased computational time in time-domain analysis for highly resolved geometries due to the Courant stability criterion and the need for discretizing the space exterior to the body (this limitation is a concern in time-domain analysis with finite elements as well),
2. the lack of any definitive boundary condition at the grid terminations when unbounded fields are being computed (also a problem with finite elements),
3. the inability to satisfy interface boundary conditions as a natural consequence of the method, and
4. the difficulty in adapting the method to a nonuniform irregular mesh.

Rather than only reiterate the strengths and weaknesses of finite differences relevant to hyperthermia problems, it is instructive to take as given the intrinsic advantages/disadvantages of differential equation formulations and to concentrate on the relative merits of finite difference and finite element methods for this particular application. Because the ability of finite elements to accommodate irregular boundaries and tissue heterogeneities is a natural consequence of the method, finite elements represent a more powerful approach than finite differences for calculating power deposition patterns in hyperthermia. This is a significant advantage in the hyperthermia problem on three fronts:

1. numerical boundaries can be readily constructed to conform to physical boundaries,
2. boundary conditions at tissue interfaces can be exactly satisfied, and
3. grid detail can be deployed selectively throughout the problem domain.

Advantages 1. and 2. can be especially important in hyperthermia because of the high-contrast boundaries such as muscle/fat interfaces that traditionally have caused excessive hot spots. Finite differences suffer from additional complexities when nonuniform meshes are used, and when uniform meshes are employed numerical boundaries do not readily conform to physical ones (unless excessive grid detail is used which then exists throughout the problem domain) and exact tissue boundary conditions cannot be satisfied.

This advantage of finite elements that it is intrinsically better suited for domains containing severe geometric irregularity and tissue heterogeneity, is in theory independent of problem dimensions; however, there are some practical implications that cannot be ignored. In two dimensions, finite element grid generation is only now attaining the level of automation and sophistication needed to produce meshes of CT-scan cross-sections with little user input and interaction. As these data input tools continue to improve, the advantage of finite element methods over finite differences will become more evident. In three dimensions finite differences, at the moment, may have a stronger appeal for hyperthermia power deposition calculations. Both methods can be implemented in the time-domain as completely explicit time-stepping algorithms; hence, the computer resource issue does not seem greatly to favor one method over the other (in the frequency-domain finite differences may have some computer resource advantages due to the tridiagonal structures resulting from the second-order derivative terms found in wave equations). However, it is the power of the finite element method that is also its curse in three dimensions. Three-dimensional mesh generation is considerably more demanding for irregular meshes than for uniform grids. The simplicity of uniform meshes alleviates the burdens involved in three-dimensional data input, allowing three-dimensional problems to be easily solved on the approximate geometry. Since finite differences are naturally suited for uniform grids they become the method of choice on such a mesh (finite elements can, of course, also be implemented on uniform meshes; however, assembly of an individual equation is not particularly simplified nor is the matrix structure altered, and in fact the use of a uniform grid defeats the very rationale for implementing finite elements in the first place). Currently, there are no automatic meshing programs which can assimilate the complex three-dimensional shapes associated with the clinical problem. If these data input tools become available to the level of sophistication found in two dimensions, three-dimensional finite element formulations will exert the same advantages over their finite difference counterparts that they do presently in two dimensions.

2.4.4 Boundary Element Method

The boundary element (or boundary integral) method described herein is based on the vector equivalent of Green's second identity which can be stated as

$$\int_V (\mathbf{Q}\cdot\nabla\times\nabla\times\mathbf{P}-\mathbf{P}\cdot\nabla\times\nabla\times\mathbf{Q})\,dV = \oint_S (\mathbf{P}\times\nabla\times\mathbf{Q}-\mathbf{Q}\times\nabla\times\mathbf{P})\cdot\hat{\mathbf{n}}\,da \qquad (2.74)$$

where **P** and **Q** are vector functions with continuous first and second derivatives throughout V and on S [114]. To derive the boundary element expression for the electric field, let $\mathbf{P} = \mathbf{E}$ and $\mathbf{Q} = G\hat{\mathbf{a}}$ where $\hat{\mathbf{a}}$ is an arbitrary unit vector, and G is the unbounded-space Green's function satisfying the Helmholtz equation with singularity at $\mathbf{x} = \mathbf{x}'$:

$$\nabla^2 G + k^2 G = -\delta(\mathbf{x}-\mathbf{x}') \ . \tag{2.75}$$

In two and three dimensions the Green's function is, respectively

$$G(\mathbf{x},\mathbf{x}') = \frac{i}{4}\mathbf{H}_0(k\,|\mathbf{x}-\mathbf{x}'|) \tag{2.76a}$$

$$G(\mathbf{x},\mathbf{x}') = \frac{e^{ik\,|\mathbf{x}-\mathbf{x}'|}}{4\pi\,|\mathbf{x}-\mathbf{x}'|} \tag{2.76b}$$

where $\mathbf{H}_0$ is the Hankel function of the first kind order zero. After some vector manipulations, it can be shown that the boundary expression for node i located at $\mathbf{x}'$ on S is

$$\alpha_i \mathbf{E}_i = -\oint_S \{i\omega\mu(\hat{\mathbf{n}}\times\mathbf{H})G_i + (\hat{\mathbf{n}}\times\mathbf{E})\times\nabla G_i + (\hat{\mathbf{n}}\cdot\mathbf{E})\nabla G_i\}da \tag{2.77a}$$

where $\alpha_i = \int_V \delta(\mathbf{x}-\mathbf{x}_i)dV$ and G_i is centered at node i.

The dual expression for the magnetic field can be derived using the same approach and can be shown to be

$$\alpha_i \mathbf{H}_i = \oint_S \{i\omega\varepsilon^*(\hat{\mathbf{n}}\times\mathbf{E})G_i - (\hat{\mathbf{n}}\times\mathbf{H})\times\nabla G_i - (\hat{\mathbf{n}}\cdot\mathbf{H})\nabla G_i\}da \ . \tag{2.77b}$$

Equations 2.77 are valid provided that the region contained by the surface, S, is homogeneous and source free. Formally, boundary integral Eqs. 2.77 can also involve the boundary at infinity, but under radiation condition assumptions these integrals can be shown to vanish there [58, 114]; thus integrations need only occur over finite boundaries.

Expression 2.77a can also be derived by combining the weighted residual form of Eq. 2.8a (see Eq. 2.44a) with ϕ_i replaced by G_i and the form of Eq. 2.75 weighted with $\mathbf{E}_i$

$$\langle(\nabla\times\mathbf{E})\times\nabla G_i\rangle - \langle k^2\mathbf{E}G_i\rangle = -i\omega\mu\oint \hat{\mathbf{n}}\times\mathbf{H}\,G_i\,ds \tag{2.78a}$$

$$\langle -\nabla G\cdot\nabla\mathbf{E}_i\rangle + \langle k^2 G\mathbf{E}_i\rangle = -\langle\delta(\mathbf{x}-\mathbf{x}')\mathbf{E}_i\rangle - \oint \mathbf{E}_i(\nabla G\cdot\hat{\mathbf{n}})ds \ . \tag{2.78b}$$

Using some vector identities on the leftmost terms of Eqs. 2.78, and then adding these equations produces Eq. 2.77a. A series of corresponding steps beginning with Eq. 2.8b will also generate Eq. 2.77b. Thus, the boundary element method discussed in this section can be interpreted in the vein of the weighted residual method by considering G_i as the weighting function. Relative to the variety of integral forms of the Maxwell equations that are available, Eqs. 2.77 are computationally attractive in that only a scalar Green's function is involved, the variables in the integrands are in terms of the natural boundary conditions for the electric and magnetic fields, only boundary integration is required, and sources are represented through equivalent surface fields.

As in the finite element formulation, the field variables are expressed in terms of the basis expansions given in Eq. 2.45 with the understanding that ϕ is only active on the boundary. With the variables discretized Eq. 2.77a becomes

$$\begin{aligned}\alpha_i \mathbf{E}_i = &-\sum_{j=1}^{N}\oint_S i\omega\mu\mathbf{F}_j\phi_j G(\mathbf{x}-\mathbf{x}_i)da \\ &-\sum_{j=1}^{N}\oint_S (\hat{\mathbf{n}}_j\times\mathbf{E}_j\phi_j)\times\nabla G(\mathbf{x}-\mathbf{x}_i)da \\ &-\sum_{j=1}^{N}\oint_S (\hat{\mathbf{n}}_j\cdot\mathbf{E}_j\phi_j)\nabla G(\mathbf{x}-\mathbf{x}_i)da\end{aligned} \tag{2.79}$$

where $\mathbf{F} = \hat{\mathbf{n}}\times\mathbf{H}$. By enforcing N versions of Eq. 2.79 (where N is the number of boundary nodes) using the set of Green's functions such that the ith Green's function is singular at the ith node the boundary element matrix equation can be assembled. This matrix equation provides a mechanism for calculating **E** on some boundary given that $\hat{\mathbf{n}}\times\mathbf{H}$ is known on that boundary, or, conversely, for calculating $\hat{\mathbf{n}}\times\mathbf{H}$ given **E**. Once both $\hat{\mathbf{n}}\times\mathbf{H}$ and **E** are known over some boundary, then **E** can be calculated in the homogeneous region either inside or outside this boundary via Eq. 2.79 with α equal to unity. The dual matrix formulation involving field variables, **H** and $\hat{\mathbf{n}}\times\mathbf{E}$, is reached using the same procedure on Eq. 2.77b; and, thus, provides a method for obtaining these quantities over some boundary given that one of the two variables can be specified there.

In two dimensions where the limiting TM and TE cases are considered, Eq. 2.77a and Eq. 2.77b reduce to

$$\alpha_i E_{z_i} = \oint_S (\hat{\mathbf{n}}\cdot\nabla E_z)G_i da - \oint_S E_z(\hat{\mathbf{n}}\cdot\nabla G_i)da \tag{2.80a}$$

$$\alpha_i H_{z_i} = \oint_S (\hat{\mathbf{n}}\cdot\nabla H_z)G_i da - \oint_S H_z(\hat{\mathbf{n}}\cdot\nabla G_i)da \tag{2.80b}$$

where the z subscript indicates the direction perpendicular to the analysis plane. Equations 2.80 are readily recognized as boundary integrals of the Helmholtz equation.

The interface conditions for multiple-region domains are accounted for during the assembly of Eq. 2.79 with the same strategy outlined in Sect. 4.2 where the unknowns on one side of the interface are eliminated as they arise in Eq. 2.79 in terms of their counterparts on the other side of the interface via Eqs. 2.49. These conditions, as well as Eq. 2.79 itself, require the definition of a nodal normal. In three dimensions, a nodal normal based on surface elements can be written as $\hat{\mathbf{n}}_i = (n_{x_i}, n_{y_i}, n_{z_i})$ where

$$n_{x_i} = \frac{1}{n} \oint_S n_x \phi_i \, da \ , \quad n_{y_i} = \frac{1}{n} \oint_S n_y \phi_i \, da \ ,$$

$$n_{z_i} = \oint_S n_z \phi_i \, da \tag{2.81}$$

and

$$n = \left[\left(\oint_S n_x \phi_i \, da \right)^2 + \left(\oint_S n_y \phi_i \, da \right)^2 + \left(\oint_S n_z \phi_i \, da \right)^2 \right]^{1/2} .$$

This is actually the definition of the nodal normal posed in [37], and the expression in Eq. 2.50 was derived from Eq. 2.81 via the divergence theorem.

Since the equation for the ith node utilizes the Green's function, G_i, which is singular at node i, special care must be exercised in the integrations over all elements containing this singularity. As a result of the increasing popularity of boundary element techniques as engineering analysis tools, a significant amount of research has been devoted to improving the accuracy and speed of computing singular integrals of the type that routinely appear in boundary element formulations (e.g., see [63, 67, 126, 127]). Typical strategies have included analytical integrations, semi-analytical integrations (e.g., a truncated series expansion integrated analytically term by term), and special quadratures such as those that concentrate the Gauss points near the singularity. The availability of such an array of techniques and the body of knowledge that has been accumulated about boundary element singular integrals has facilitated the acceptance of boundary-element-based analysis. Generally, all integrations over elements not containing the node where the Green's function is singular are computed with standard numerical integration schemes.

Many of the considerations surrounding the domain integral equation approach (discussed in Sect. 4.1) also apply to boundary integral formulations; however, there are some significant differences. Since only boundary integration is involved in the technique, there is a reduction of one dimensionality in the integrations that need to be performed relative to those in the domain integration problem. This not only leads to simpler integrations and consequently matrix building, but also to fewer unknowns in the algebraic system because only the boundaries need to be discretized. Note, however, that the advantage of the reduction in problem dimensionality in terms of requiring fewer unknowns tends to be diminished as the dimensions of the problem are increased due to the growing surface to volume ratio of many geometries (e.g., consider the change in this ratio as the problem domain increases in dimension from a line to a circle to a sphere). Nonetheless, algebraically speaking, the boundary element method can be viewed as superior to the domain integral equation approach on both counts described above

1. fewer unknowns and
2. easier integrations for building individual elements within the matrix.

However, one must remember that only boundary values result from the matrix solution and interior values require a set of subsequent computations, which is not the case with the domain integral equation formulation.

Further, complications begin to arise in the boundary element method as the heterogeneity within the problem domain increases. While only the boundaries need to be discretized, such boundaries also include interior ones which enclose homogeneous subdomains since the governing equations (i.e., Eq. 2.77) are only valid in homogeneous source-free regions. Part of the complication comes from the fact that, on the interior boundaries, Eq. 2.79 not only involves the unknown $\mathbf{E}$, but also the unknown $\hat{\mathbf{n}} \times \mathbf{H}$. The correct number of equations to close the algebraic system is ensured because two vector equations exist at an interior interface node – one for each region on either side of the boundary. One can, of course, carry along the unknown interior values of $\hat{\mathbf{n}} \times \mathbf{H}$ within one system of matrix algebra and solve for these quantities as part of the solution for $\mathbf{E}$. Clearly, this approach increases the number of degrees of freedom at each node and likewise increases the size of the overall system for a given number of nodes. An alternative is to perform a series of smaller matrix inversions which eliminate $\hat{\mathbf{n}} \times \mathbf{H}$ from the overall matrix algebra for $\mathbf{E}$ by expressing $\hat{\mathbf{n}} \times \mathbf{H}$ in terms of $\mathbf{E}$ for each homogeneous subregion. While this approach will accomplish the goal of reducing the size of the largest matrix that must be stored, algebraic complications begin to occur as the number of intermediate matrix manipulations increases with an increasing number of internal boundaries. A positive side effect of having two vector equations at the same boundary is that the exact interface boundary conditions can easily be applied, and are needed to provide the interconnection between the two equations. The satisfaction of these boundary conditions appears to be critical in hyperthermia because the body is in the near-field of the source, and because the body contains a number of high-contrast interfaces (e.g., muscle/fat) both of which have pronounced effects on heating patterns.

As with the frequency-domain discussions above, the time-domain also presents some of the same problems that occur in domain integral equation formulations. The space-time integral for boundary elements has the same features that the spatial integration (although only over the boundaries) is global, and the time integral requires historical values of the solution at many different time instants in order to project into the future. Time-dependent boundary element solutions for a general scalar wave equation have been successfully implemented in two and three dimensions [76, 77]. It has also been coupled in hybrid fashion with finite-difference algorithms to provide a formal outer boundary condition for unbounded problems containing regions of localized heterogeneity. This has been accomplished in both scalar [103] and vector forms [145]. To date, a time-dependent boundary element formulation has not appeared in the hyperthermia arena.

In summary, the boundary element method has the same attractive feature afforded by integral equations in general – it provides a formal treatment of problems with boundaries at infinity. Further, relative to some integral equation formulations it possesses several other advantages:

1. only boundary integration is required leading to fewer unknowns and simpler matrix assembly,
2. only a scalar Green's function is needed,
3. the quantities within the integral equation are in terms of the natural boundary conditions for **E** and **H**,
4. sources are represented through equivalent surface fields, and
5. exact interfacial boundary conditions can readily be enforced at interfaces where electrical properties change abruptly.

The negative aspects of the boundary element method center around:

1. the global nature of the integrations which lead to dense matrices,
2. the singular Green's function which requires special attention during integrations near its singularity,
3. the complicated matrix algebra when domains containing severe heterogeneity are considered (this evolves from the appearance of $\hat{\mathbf{n}} \times \mathbf{H}$ on interior boundaries when solution of **E** is sought), and
4. the lack, at least presently, of an numerically efficient time-domain equivalent, thus limiting its use to the frequency-domain.

In terms of calculating power deposition patterns in hyperthermia, the strength and weaknesses of the boundary element method suggest its use in hybrid fashion coupled to differential formulations or in three-dimensional applications. In two-dimensional hyperthermia problems, the boundary element method alone cannot be recommended for either bounded or unbounded problems. This stems from the method's inability to treat highly heterogeneous domains, such as CT scans, in a numerically efficient manner. Thus, in bounded problems differential equation methods should be favored because of their intrinsic ability to accommodate complicated domains. For unbounded two-dimensional hyperthermia problems, the boundary element method should not be considered for the body interior part of the problem for the same reasons cited above; however, it does show promise in hybrid schemes. Since boundary elements are ideal for unbounded homogeneous regions, they become leading candidates for coupling with finite elements or finite differences in many hyperthermia problems where the source is external, and the body is modeled as existing in homogeneous unbounded space. Further, these integral equations are expressed in terms of the natural boundary conditions for **E** and **H**, which facilitates the coupling procedure. Thus, two-dimensional boundary elements are best suited numerically as a means of providing the exact outer boundary condition needed for differential equation methods in unbounded hyperthermia problems. This contribution is significant given the limitations of differential equations in providing this information, the near-field positioning of the body in electromagnetic hyperthermia, and the need for solutions which account for as much of the underlying physics as possible.

In three dimensions, the same general conclusions can be reached when considering boundary element formulations – they should be avoided in bounded severely heterogeneous problems and exploited in hybrid fashion for unbounded situations with high degrees of localized heterogeneity – except for one caveat. Three-dimensional surface element grid generation is substantially simpler than its domain element counterpart. Further, no special consideration for grid uniformity is needed; thus very complex shapes and geometries can be accurately described with boundary elements. Boundary element grid construction is naturally suited for the clinical situation where planar CT scans are the usual source of anatomical information. Three-dimensional surface descriptions (of tissues and organs) can be obtained by outlining the boundaries of interest in serial CT scans and linearly connecting them in the third dimension to form the three-dimensional object. This relative ease of boundary grid construction, which readily conforms to the physical boundaries of the problem, makes the boundary element method an appealing possibility in three-dimensional simulations, despite some of its numerically less attractive features.

2.4.5 Hybrid Element Formulation

In this section a hybrid numerical method which couples the finite and boundary element methods will be discussed [74, 91]. The idea behind the hybrid approach is to exploit the strengths of differential and integral equation methods while avoiding their inherent weaknesses when each method is used alone. This technique provides a formal approach to the problem of a source which emits radiation into an infinite medium while delivering energy to a highly inhomogeneous body. The hybrid element method to be discussed below employs finite elements inside the heterogeneous body and boundary elements on the body surface and detached electromagnetic source. The coupling of these methods is realized through a single quantity which is continuous at source-free boundaries and which occurs naturally in both the finite and boundary element formulations.

Recall from Sect. 4.2 that the Galerkin-weighted residual statements of Eqs. 2.8, assuming μ constant, can be written as

$$\langle(\nabla\times\mathbf{E})\times\nabla\phi_i\rangle-\langle k^2\mathbf{E}\phi_i\rangle = -i\omega\mu \oint \hat{\mathbf{n}}\times\mathbf{H}\phi_i ds \tag{2.82a}$$

$$\left\langle\left(\frac{1}{k^2}\nabla\times\mathbf{H}\right)\times\nabla\phi_i\right\rangle-\langle\mathbf{H}\phi_i\rangle = -\frac{1}{i\omega\mu}\oint \hat{\mathbf{n}}\times\mathbf{E}\phi_i ds\ . \tag{2.82b}$$

Solution of Eq. 2.82a via finite elements requires knowledge of $\hat{\mathbf{n}}\times\mathbf{H}$ or $\mathbf{E}$ over the entire boundary of the domain of interest. Similarly, Eq. 2.82b requires that either $\hat{\mathbf{n}}\times\mathbf{E}$ or $\mathbf{H}$ be known on the boundary. In some two-dimensional models of clinical situations, these quantities can be conveniently specified over a boundary which completely encloses the patient; hence the finite element method can be used directly, and is the method of choice. However, many two-dimensional and most three-dimensional problems are fundamentally unbounded, and these quantities can only be specified over the EM source, which in general does not completely enclose the patient.

Rearranging the boundary element equations from Sect. 4.4 gives

$$-\oint_S i\omega\mu(\hat{\mathbf{n}}\times\mathbf{H})G_i da = \alpha_i\mathbf{E}_i+\oint_S(\hat{\mathbf{n}}\times\mathbf{E})\times\nabla G_i da + \oint_S(\hat{\mathbf{n}}\cdot\mathbf{E})\nabla G_i da \tag{2.83a}$$

$$\oint_S i\omega\varepsilon^*(\hat{\mathbf{n}}\times\mathbf{E})G_i da = \alpha_i\mathbf{H}_i+\oint_S(\hat{\mathbf{n}}\times\mathbf{H})\times\nabla G_i da + \oint_S(\hat{\mathbf{n}}\cdot\mathbf{H})\nabla G_i da \tag{2.83b}$$

which provide a relationship between boundary values of $\hat{\mathbf{n}}\times\mathbf{H}$ and $\mathbf{E}$ or $\hat{\mathbf{n}}\times\mathbf{E}$ and $\mathbf{H}$. These equations are applied in the homogeneous space, exterior to the patient, but containing the EM source. The boundary of this region also includes infinity, but kernels of the type found in Eq. 2.83 can be shown to vanish there; hence the only contributions to Eqs. 2.83 occur from the boundary of the patient and source. Figure 2.37 shows a typical integral path over the patient surface and a detached electromagnetic source. By integrating along such a path, unknown patient surface quantities are related to known source quantities which

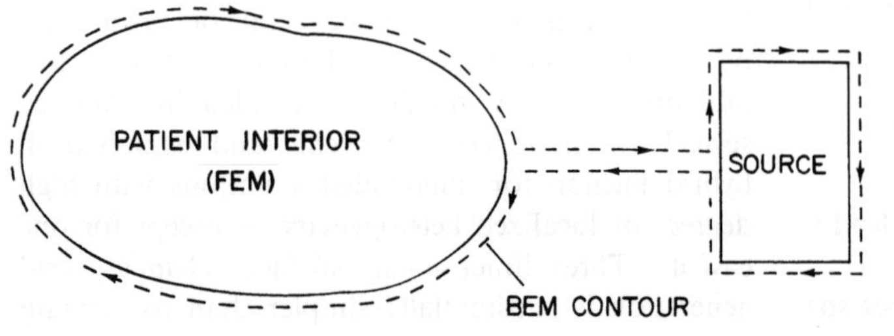

Fig. 2.37. Integration contour over the body surface and detached EM source

provide the information necessary to close the finite element matrix problem algebraically.

In matrix form, the hybrid element method for electric field solution proceeds as follows. Boundary expression Eq. 2.83a provides the algebraic statements

$$[C]\{F\}=[D]\{E\} \tag{2.84}$$

where the field variables $\hat{\mathbf{n}}\times\mathbf{H}$ and $\mathbf{E}$ are represented by the column vectors F and E, respectively. The finite element method produces matrix algebra

$$[A]\{E\}=[B]\{F\}\ . \tag{2.85}$$

Thus, the hybrid problem is handled by eliminating F between Eqs. 2.84 and 2.85:

$$[A]\{E\}=[B]\,[C]^{-1}\,[D]\{E\} \tag{2.86}$$

with direct inversion of [C] and LU decomposition of $[A-BC^{-1}D]$ subject to the boundary conditions on the source.

In the case where **E** is known on the detached source, the hybrid element method begins with the finite element formulation which provides N+m equations (for the N nodes comprising the patient interior and the m nodes constituting the patient surface) for each nodal degree of freedom:

$$\begin{bmatrix} A_{11} & A_{12} \\ A_{21} & A_{22} \end{bmatrix}\begin{Bmatrix} E_p \\ E_1 \end{Bmatrix}=\begin{bmatrix} 0 & 0 \\ 0 & B \end{bmatrix}\begin{Bmatrix} 0 \\ F_1 \end{Bmatrix} \tag{2.87}$$

where B is defined in Eq. 2.85, E_p are the unknowns on the patient interior, and E_1 and F_1 are the unknown **E** and $\hat{\mathbf{n}}\times\mathbf{H}$ on the patient surface. The boundary element method (BEM) contour shown in Fig. 2.37 provides m+n equations (for the m nodes on the patient surface and the n nodes on the source) for each nodal degree of freedom:

$$\begin{bmatrix} C_{11} & C_{12} \\ C_{21} & C_{22} \end{bmatrix}\begin{Bmatrix} F_1 \\ F_2 \end{Bmatrix}=\begin{bmatrix} D_{11} & D_{12} \\ D_{21} & D_{22} \end{bmatrix}\begin{Bmatrix} E_1 \\ E_2 \end{Bmatrix} \tag{2.88}$$

where E_2 represents the known **E** and F_2 the unknown $\hat{\mathbf{n}}\times\mathbf{H}$ on the source. Carrying out the inversion of C and denoting the partitions of this inverted matrix with a tilde results in

$$\begin{Bmatrix} F_1 \\ F_2 \end{Bmatrix}=\begin{bmatrix} \tilde{C}_{11} & \tilde{C}_{12} \\ \tilde{C}_{21} & \tilde{C}_{22} \end{bmatrix}\begin{bmatrix} D_{11} & D_{12} \\ D_{21} & D_{22} \end{bmatrix}\begin{Bmatrix} E_1 \\ E_2 \end{Bmatrix}\ . \tag{2.89}$$

By taking the top m equations of 2.89, F_1 is eliminated in Eq. 2.87; thus

$$\begin{bmatrix} A_{11} & A_{12} \\ A_{21} & A_{22}-B[\tilde{C}_{11}D_{11}+\tilde{C}_{12}D_{21}] \end{bmatrix}\begin{Bmatrix} E_p \\ E_1 \end{Bmatrix}=\begin{Bmatrix} 0 \\ B[\tilde{C}_{11}D_{12}+\tilde{C}_{12}D_{22}]\{E_2\} \end{Bmatrix}\ . \tag{2.90}$$

Note that the bottom set of Eqs. in 2.89 are not explicitly required for solution of Eq. 2.90; however, if F_2 is needed either to calculate the loading on the source or the electric field exterior to the body, F_2 can be computed from the bottom half of Eq. 2.89 once Eq. 2.90 is solved.

When $\hat{\mathbf{n}}\times\mathbf{H}$ is specified on the source boundary, the matrix algebra is similar to the above except that the bottom set of equations in 2.89 are needed. In this case, Eq. 2.90 becomes

$$\begin{bmatrix} A_{11} & A_{12} & 0 \\ A_{21} & A_{22}-B[\tilde{C}_{11}D_{11}+\tilde{C}_{12}D_{21}] & -B[\tilde{C}_{11}D_{12}+\tilde{C}_{12}D_{22}] \\ 0 & \tilde{C}_{21}D_{11}+\tilde{C}_{22}D_{21} & \tilde{C}_{21}D_{12}+\tilde{C}_{22}D_{22} \end{bmatrix}\begin{Bmatrix} E_p \\ E_1 \\ E_2 \end{Bmatrix}=\begin{Bmatrix} 0 \\ 0 \\ F_2 \end{Bmatrix}\ . \tag{2.91}$$

An alternate approach, which removes the need for the lower set of equations in 2.89, is to interchange F_2 and E_2 in Eq. 2.88 such that

$$\begin{bmatrix} C_{11} & -D_{12} \\ C_{21} & -D_{22} \end{bmatrix}\begin{Bmatrix} F_1 \\ E_2 \end{Bmatrix}=\begin{bmatrix} D_{11} & -C_{12} \\ D_{21} & -C_{22} \end{bmatrix}\begin{Bmatrix} E_1 \\ F_2 \end{Bmatrix} \tag{2.92}$$

Then, the inversion of the left side of Eq. 2.92 gives

$$\begin{Bmatrix} F_1 \\ E_2 \end{Bmatrix}=\begin{bmatrix} \tilde{C}_{11} & \tilde{D}_{12} \\ \tilde{C}_{21} & \tilde{D}_{22} \end{bmatrix}\begin{bmatrix} D_{11} & -C_{12} \\ D_{21} & -D_{22} \end{bmatrix}\begin{Bmatrix} E_1 \\ F_2 \end{Bmatrix} \tag{2.93}$$

where the tilde notation is again used to represent a partition of this inverse. Equation 2.93 can be used to eliminate F_1 in Eq. 2.87; hence,

$$\begin{bmatrix} A_{11} & A_{12} \\ A_{21} & A_{22}-B[\tilde{C}_{11}D_{11}+\tilde{D}_{12}D_{21}] \end{bmatrix}\begin{Bmatrix} E_p \\ E_1 \end{Bmatrix}=\begin{Bmatrix} 0 \\ -B[\tilde{C}_{11}C_{12}+\tilde{D}_{12}C_{22}]\{F_2\} \end{Bmatrix}\ . \tag{2.94}$$

Similarly to Eq. 2.90, the bottom set of equations in 2.93 are now not explicitly needed for the solution of Eq. 2.94. The price paid for removing the n set of equations is in terms of the inversion of the left side of Eq. 2.92. While the first approach (Eq. 2.91) contains the extra n equations, inversion of C is assured because it is effectively equivalent to a finite element mass matrix which is well conditioned. The inversion of the left side of Eq. 2.92 in theory should present no problems; however, its conditioning in terms of diagonal dominance it not as readily apparent.

The strengths and weaknesses of the hybrid element method have, in effect, already been addressed since this approach represents the coupling of finite and boundary elements and the discussions in Sects. 4.2 and 4.4, respectively, apply. Clearly, the potential contribution of the hybrid element technique is in hyperthermia problems where the quantities to be calculated are essentially unbounded. Since integral expressions cannot be avoided in rigorously treating the open boundary problem, the issue becomes the choice of method for the inhomogeneous patient interior and the competitiveness of the hybrid scheme with alternate numerical approaches must be evaluated. Recently, the algebraic requirements for the finite, boundary, and hybrid element methods as applied to two-dimensional EM field problems in hyperthermia were studied [74]. It was concluded in [74] that the advantages of the boundary element method alone, which center around reduction of the problem dimension, are lost for typical two-dimensional hyperthermia applications because of the severe degree of heterogeneity inside the patient and the concomitant multiple interior boundaries required. For many three-dimensional geometries the surface to volume ratio may actually become larger (e.g., circle vs. sphere), which further nullifies the "reduction of problem dimension" argument. In addition, the direct solution of a full boundary element matrix as compared with a banded solution of the finite element system of equations with the comparable degrees of freedom requires higher storage and more algebraic operations. However, the reduction of problem dimension with the boundary element method cannot be ignored, especially in three dimensions, where it may make some problems solvable which would otherwise be impossible because of lack of resources on present computers. Further, three-dimensional mesh generation and inspection is considerably more demanding for finite elements than for boundary elements, and may, at least presently, place some practical limitations on the use of the numerically more attractive finite element method in three-dimensional EM simulations of hyperthermia.

The competitiveness of the hybrid formulation with the FDTD method has yet to be established for three-dimensional unbounded problems. Studies are beginning to appear where detailed three-dimensional energy deposition patterns are being calculated inside inhomogeneous three-dimensional models of the body with the FDTD [121]. Certainly, the computational grids that have been used with the three-dimensional hybrid formulation (≈ 300 nodes) [91] are small relative to those achieved in [121] ($\approx 10^5$ cells). However, while the hybrid approach given above will always result in a matrix equation (as opposed to the FDTD where matrices are avoided through explicit time-stepping), iterative solution schemes should significantly reduce the storage requirements of the hybrid system of equations, thereby allowing for greater grid resolutions. Further, the hybrid technique should require considerably fewer unknowns than the FDTD for two reasons:

1. no discretization is needed in the background medium containing the source and the heterogeneous object and
2. the inherent flexibility of finite and boundary elements is such that irregular grid spacing can readily be accommodated which makes possible efficient meshing of irregular geometries, regions of little or great interest, and regions of large- or small-field gradients.

Finally, the hybrid element method does provide the formal resolution to the exact outer boundary condition where grids are terminated in unbounded problems – an issue which plagues the FDTD approach in hyperthermia where the body is in the near-field of the source. Further, exact interfacial boundary conditions are enforced in the hybrid scheme since they are satisfied naturally with the finite element method which is used in the heterogeneous patient interior. Such internal boundary conditions have also been problematical for the FDTD as used to date. More work will be required to quantify the advantages and disadvantages of the hybrid method compared with those of other numerical approaches for three-dimensional problems of interest in clinical hyperthermia.

2.4.6 Final Remarks

Each of the methods discussed above has inherent strengths and weaknesses and the purpose of Sect. 4 has been to illustrate some of these advantages and disadvantages in the context of the hyperthermia electromagnetic problem. One might expect a ranking of the numerical techniques in terms of their preferred use in hyperthermia simulation studies to follow. Unfortunately, it is difficult, if not impossible, to rank one of these methods as generally superior to the others because of the many trade-offs that exist.

Before summarizing the factors which impact the selection of one numerical technique over another, it is important to distinguish between the numerical methods (i.e., how the governing equations are solved) and the formulation of the problem itself (i.e., what the governing equations look like), since choosing one problem formulation over another has certain implications for the implementation of the numerical method. Typical problem formulation choices include time versus frequency-domain, differential versus integral equations, and total fields versus incident and scattered components. The difference between the methods and the formulation can be appreciated by realizing that it is, for example, the time-domain formulation that allows one to avoid matrix storage and inversion, not whether finite difference or finite element or domain integral equation methods are used. In some senses though, the problem formulation and the numerical method cannot be separated. Obviously, integral equations form the basis of the problem formulation in domain integral and boundary element methods. However, it is important to understand that the integral equations, themselves, have certain ramifications which are independent of whether domain integral methods or boundary element techniques are implemented.

The choice of one numerical method over another can be made by weighing a number of factors such as

1. type of calculation that needs to be made,
2. degree of accuracy required,
3. computer resources available,
4. and accessibility of relevant software and/or areas of numerical expertise of the analyst.

For example, if the problem to be solved contains numerous boundaries which play a significant role in dictating the field distribution and a high degree of detail (in the solution) is needed around these boundaries, then the finite element method would have to be considered the best choice. If, on the other hand, the boundaries must be accounted for but only approximate solutions are required, then the spatial averaging that occurs with uniform grids may be acceptable and methods such as finite differences or domain integral equations, which effectively exploit uniform grids in terms of computer resource economies, would be favored.

The degree to which the details of the problem (e.g., geometry, heterogeneity, boundary conditions) can be most accurately described is one basis for ranking the numerical methods discussed herein. Such a criterion would favor the hybrid element method because it represents the most formal solution to the typical electromagnetic problem occurring in hyperthermia treatment simulation. However, while the hybrid element method appears tractable on a moderate-sized computer in two dimensions, it has severe computer resource demands, which have yet to be overcome, thus limiting its use in three dimensions. A more approximate approach, such as FDTD, would be preferred in this situation. In many respects, this kind of trade-off between solution accuracy and numerical efficiency (and in some cases feasibility!) is the fundamental issue which surrounds the selection of one numerical method over another.

Clearly, a numerical method, which is computationally efficient, but which is based on such extensive approximations that computed results are questionable, is of little use in hyperthermia modeling. Likewise, a numerical technique which is mathematically rigorous, yet so complex (or computationally demanding) that a solution cannot even be computed, is of little value to hyperthermia research. This section has attempted to illuminate the relevant trade-offs with the hope that recognition of such will lead to the selection of numerical methods which best suit the problem at hand.

References

1. Ames WF (1977) Numerical methods for partial differential equations, 2nd edn. Academic. New York
2. Andersen JB (1985) Theoretical limitations on radiation into muscle tissue. Int J Hyperthermia 1:45–55
3. Andersen JB (1987) Electromagnetic power deposition: inhomogeneous media, applicators, and phased arrays. In: Field SB, Franconi C (eds) Physics and technology of hyperthermia. Nijhoff, Dordrecht, pp 159–210
4. Armitage DW, LeVeen HH, Pethig R (1983) Radiofrequency-induced hyperthermia: computer simulation of specific absorption rate distributions using realistic anatomical models. Phys Med Biol 28:31–42
5. Barber FE, Griffice CP (1982) Power deposition for ultrasound hyperthermia. In: Nussbaum GH (ed) Physical aspects of hyperthermia. American Institute of Physics, New York, pp 209–230
6. Bardati F (1982) Transient electromagnetic field in a lossy dielectric slab. Appl Sci Res 39:105–113
7. Bardati F (1986) Models of electromagnetic heating and radiometric microwave sensing. In: Hand JW, James JR (eds) Physical techniques in clinical hyperthermia. Research Studies, Letchworth, pp 327–382
8. Beer G, Meek JL (1981) Infinite domain elements. Int J Numer Methods Eng 17:43–52
9. Bettess P (1977) Infinite elements. Int J Numer Methods Eng 11:53–64
10. Bojarksi NN (1971) K-space formulation of the electromagnetic scattering problem. Technical Report Air Force Avionics Laboratory-TR-71-5, March, Wright-Patterson Air Force Base, Ohio, 45433
11. Bolomey JC, Durix CH, Lesselier D (1978) Time-domain integral equation approach for inhomogeneous and dispersive slab problems. IEEE Trans Antennas Propag 26: 658–667

12. Borup DT, Gandhi OP (1984) Fast-Fourier-transform method for the calculation of SAR distributions in finely discretized models of biological tissues. IEEE Trans Microwave Theory Tech 32:355–360
13. Borup DT, Sullivan DM, Gandhi OP (1987) Comparison of the FFT conjugate gradient method and the finite-difference time-domain method for the 2-D absorption problem. IEEE Trans Microwave Theory Tech 35:383–395
14. Bottomley PA, Andrew ER (1978) RF magnetic field penetration, phase shift and power dissipation in biological tissue: implications for NMR imaging. Phys Med Biol 23:630–643
15. Brebbia CA (1978) The boundary element method for engineers. Wiley, New York
16. Brebbia CA, Telles JF, Wrobel LC (1984) Boundary element techniques: theory and applications in engineering. Springer, Berlin Heidelberg New York
17. Brezovich IA, Young JH, Atkinson WJ, Wang MT (1982) Hyperthermia considerations for a conducting cylinder heated by an oscillating electric field applied parallel to the cylinder axis. Med Phys 9:746–748
18. Brezovich IA, Young JH, Wang MT (1983) Temperature distributions in hyperthermia by electromagnetic induction: a theoretical model for the thorax. Med Phys 10:57–65
19. Brezovich IA, Atkinson WJ, Chakraborty DP (1984) Temperature distributions in tumor models heated by self-regulating nickel-copper alloy thermoseeds. Med Phys 11:145–152
20. Burden RI, Douglas JD, Reynolds AC (1981) Numerical analysis, 2nd edn. Prindle, Weber and Schmidt, Boston
21. Cain CA, Umemura SI (1986) Concentric-ring and sector-vortex phased-array applicators for ultrasound hyperthermia. IEEE Trans Microwave Theory Tech 34:542–551
22. Cangellaris AC, Lin CC, Mai KK (1987) Pointed-matched time domain finite element methods for electromagnetic radiation and scattering. IEEE Trans Antennas Propag 35:1160–1173
23. Chari MK, Silvester P (eds) (1979) Finite elements in electric and magnetic field problems. Wiley, New York
24. Chen KM (1980) Interaction of electromagnetic fields with biological bodies. In: Kong JA (ed) Research topics in electromagnetic theory. Wiley, New York
25. Chen ZP, Roemer RB, Miller W, Cetas TC (1988) Three-dimensional hyperthermia patient treatment planning program. Int J Hyperthermia (to be published)
26. Collins RJ (1973) Bandwidth reduction by automatic renumbering. Int J Numer Methods Eng 6:345–356
27. DeWagter C (1986) Optimization of simulated two-dimensional temperature distributions induced by multiple electromagnetic applicators. IEEE Trans Microwave Theory Tech 34:589–596
28. Dudley DG (1986) Error minimization and convergence in numerical methods. Electromagnetics 5:89–97
29. Elliott RS, Harrison WA, Storm FK (1982) Hyperthermia: electromagnetic heating of deep-seated tumors. IEEE Trans Biomed Eng 29:61–64
30. Engleman MS, Sani RL, Gresho PM (1982) The implementation of normal and/or tangential boundary conditions in finite element codes for incompressible fluid flow. Int J Numer Methods Fluids 2:225–238
31. Engquist B, Majda A (1979) Radiation boundary conditions for acoustic and elastic wave calculations. Commun Pure Appl Math 32:313–357
32. Finlayson BA (1972) Method of weighted residuals and variational principles. Academic, New York
33. Gandhi OP, Deford JF, Kanai H (1984) Impedance method for calculation of power deposition patterns in magnetically-induced hyperthermia. IEEE Trans Biomed Eng 31:644–651
34. Gee W, Lee SW, Bong NK, Cain CA, Mittra R, Magin RL (1984) Focused array hyperthermia: theory and experiment. IEEE Trans Biomed Eng 31:38–46
35. Gex-Fabry M, Landry J, Marceau N, Gayne S (1983) Prediction of temperature profiles in tumors and surrounding normal tissues during magnetic induction heating. IEEE Trans Biomed Eng 30:271–277
36. Gibbs FA (1984) Regional hyperthermia: a clinical appraisal of noninvasive deep heating methods. Cancer Res (Suppl) 44:4765s–4770s
37. Gray WG (1984) On normal flow boundary conditions in finite element codes for two-dimensional shallow water flow. Int J Numer Methods Fluids 4:99–104
38. Grifface CP, Seydell JA (1981) A spherical wave decomposition approach to ultrasonic field calculations. J Nondestructive Eval 2:241–247
39. Guy AW, Chou CK, Luk KH (1986) 915 Mhz phased-array system for treating tumors in cylindrical structures. IEEE Trans Microwave Theory Tech 34:502–507
40. Hagmann MJ (1987) Difficulty in using two-dimensional models for calculating the energy deposition in tissues during hyperthermia. Int J Hyperthermia 3:475–476
41. Hagmann MJ, Levin RL (1986) Aberrant heating: a problem in regional hyperthermia. IEEE Trans Biomed Eng 33:405–411
42. Hagmann MJ, Gandhi OP, Durney CH (1979) Numerical calculations of electromagnetic energy deposition for a realistic model of man. IEEE Trans Microwave Theory Tech 27:804–809
43. Hagmann MJ, Massoudi H, Durney CH, Iskander MF (1985) Comments on limitations of the cubical block model of man in calculating SAR distributions. IEEE Trans Microwave Theory Tech 33:347–348
44. Hagmann MJ, Tsai CT, Massoudi H, Durney CH, Iskander MF (1987) Comments on a procedure for calculating fields inside arbitrarily shaped inhomogeneous dielectric bodies using linear basis functions with the moment method. IEEE Trans Microwave Theory Tech 35:785–786
45. Halac S, Roemer RB, Oleson JR, Cetas TC (1983) Magnetic induction heating of tissue: numerical evaluation of tumor temperature distributions. Int J Radiat Oncol Biol Phys 9:881–891
46. Hand JW, Cheetham JL, Hind AJ (1986) Absorbed power distributions from coherent microwave arrays for localized hyperthermia. IEEE Trans Microwave Theory Tech 34:484–489
47. Harrington RF (1986) Field computation by moment methods. Macmillian, New York
48. Hayes LJ, Diller KR, Pierce JA, Schick MR, Colvin DP (1985) Prediction of transient temperature fields and cumulative tissue destruction for radiofrequency heating of a tumor. Med Phys 12:684–692
49. Herman GC (1981) Scattering of transient acoustic waves by an inhomogeneous obstacle. J Acoust Soc Am 69:909–915
50. Hessary MK, Chen KM (1984) EM local heating with HF electric fields. IEEE Trans Microwave Theory Tech 32:569–576
51. Hill SC, Christensen DA, Durney CH (1983) Power deposition patterns in magnetically-induced hyperthermia: a two-dimensional low-frequency numerical analysis. Int J Radiat Oncol Biol Phys 9:893–904

52. Hill SC, Durney CH, Christensen DA (1983) Numerical calculations of low-frequency TE fields in arbitrarily shaped inhomogeneous lossy dielectric cylinders. Radio Science 18:328–336
53. Hood P (1976) Frontal solution program for unsymmetrical matrices. Int J Numer Methods Eng 10:379–399
54. Hornbeck RW (1975) Numerical methods. Quantum, New York
55. Irons BM (1970) A frontal solution program for finite element analysis. Int J Numer Methods Eng 2:5–32
56. Iskander MF (1982) Physical aspects and methods of hyperthermia production by RF currents and microwaves. In: Nussbaum GH (ed) Physical aspects of hyperthermia. American Institute of Physics, New York, pp 151–191
57. Iskander MF, Turner PF, DuBow JB, Kao J (1982) Two-dimensional technique to calculate the EM power deposition pattern in the human body. J Microwave Power 17:175–185
58. Jackson JD (1975) Classical electrodynamics, 2nd edn. Wiley, New York
59. Johnk, CTA (1988) Engineering electromagnetic fields and waves, 2nd edn. Wiley, New York
60. Kagawa Y, Takeuchi K, Yamabuchi T (1986) A simulation of ultrasonic hyperthermia using a finite element model. IEEE trans Ultrason Ferroelectrics and Frequency Control 33:765–777
61. Kantorovich LV, Krylov VI (1959) Approximate methods of higher analysis, 4th edn. (translated by Bester CD). Wiley, New York
62. Kastner R, Mittra R (1983) A new stacked two-dimensional spectral iteration technique (SIT) for analyzing microwave power deposition in biological media. IEEE Trans Microwave Theory Tech 31:898–904
63. Lachat JC, Watson JO (1976) Effective numerical treatment of boundary integrals: a formulation for three-dimensional elastostatics. Int J Numer Methods Eng 10:273–289
64. Lagendijk JJW (1983) A new coaxial TEM radiofrequency/microwave applicator for noninvasive deep-body hyperthermia. J Microwave Power 18:367–375
65. Lau RWM, Sheppard RJ (1986) The modeling of biological systems in three dimensions using the time-domain finite-difference method. I. The implementation of the model. Phys Med Biol 31:1247–1256
66. Lau RWM, Sheppard RJ, Howard G, Bleehen NM (1986) The modeling of biological systems in three dimensions using the time-domain finite-difference method: II. The application and experimental evaluation of the method in hyperthermia applicator design. Phys Med Biol 31: 1257–1266
67. Lean MH, Wexler A (1985) Accurate numerical integration of singular boundary element kernels over boundaries with curvature. Int J Numer Methods Eng 21:211–228
68. Lesselier D (1983) P waves transient scattering by 2-D penetrable targets: a direct solution. J Acoust Soc Am 74:1274–1278
69. Lin CC (1985) Numerical modeling of two-dimensional time-domain electromagnetic scattering by underground inhomogeneities. PhD thesis, University of California, Berkeley
70. Lindman EL (1975) Free-space boundary conditions for the time-dependent wave equation. J Comput Phys 18:66–78
71. Livesay DE, Chen KM (1974) Electromagnetic fields induced inside arbitrarily shaped biological bodies. IEEE Trans Biomed Eng 22:1273–1280
72. Lynch DR, Gray WG (1979) A wave equation model for finite element tidal computations. Comput Fluids 7:207–229
73. Lynch DR, Paulsen KP, Strohbehn JW (1985) Finite element solution of Maxwell's equations for hyperthermia treatment planning. J Comput Phys 58:246–269
74. Lynch DR, Paulsen KD, Strohbehn JW (1986) Hybrid element method for unbounded electromagnetic problems in hyperthermia. Int J Numer Methods Eng 23:1915–1937
75. Lynch DR, Paulsen KD, Sullivan J, Strohbehn JW (1988) Hyperthermia analysis on finite elements. Proceedings of the ninth annual conference of the IEEE Engineering in Medicine and Biology Society, pp 1293–1295
76. Mansur WJ, Brebbia CA (1982) Numerical implementation of the boundary element method for two-dimensional transient scalar wave propagation problems. Appl Math Modelling 6:299–306
77. Mansur WJ, Brebbia CA (1982) Formulation of the boundary element method for transient problems governed by the scalar wave equation. Appl Math Modelling 6:307–311
78. Matloubieh AY, Roemer RB, Cetas TC (1984) Numerical simulation of magnetic induction heating of tumors with ferromagnetic seed implants. IEEE Trans Biomed Eng 31:227–234
79. Mittra R (ed) (1973) Computer techniques for electromagnetics. Pergamon, Oxford
80. Mittra R (ed) (1975) Numerical and asymptotic techniques in electromagnetics. Springer, Berlin Heidelberg New York (Topics in applied physics, vol 3)
81. Moore J, Pizer R (eds) (1984) Moment methods in electromagnetics. Research Studies, Letchworth
82. Mur G (1981) Absorbing boundary conditions for finite-difference approximation of the time-domain electromagnetic field equations. IEEE Trans Electromagn Compat 23:1073–1077
83. Nath B (1980) The w-plane finite element method for the solution of scalar field problems is two-dimensions. Int J Numer Methods Eng 15:361–379
84. Nisson P, Larsson T, Persson B (1985) Absorbed power distributions from two tilted waveguide applicators. Int J Hyperthermia 1:29–44
85. Oleson JR (1982) Hyperthermia by magnetic induction: I. Physical characteristics of the technique. Int J Radiat Oncol Biol Phys 8:1747–1756
86. Oleson JR (1987) What is regional hyperthermia? Int J Hyperthermia 3:281–282
87. Oleson JR, Heusinkveld RS, Manning MR (1983) Hyperthermia by magnetic induction. II. Clinical experience with concentric electrodes. Int J Radiat Oncol Biol Phys 9:549–556
88. Paulsen KD, Strohbehn JW, Hill SC, Lynch DR, Kennedy FE (1984) Theoretical temperature profiles for concentric coil induction heating devices in a two-dimensional axi-asymmetric inhomogeneous patient model. Int J Radiat Oncol Biol Phys 10:1095–1107
89. Paulsen KD, Strohbehn JW, Lynch DR (1985) Comparative theoretical performance of two types of regional hyperthermia systems. Int J Radiat Oncol Biol Phys 11:1659–1671
90. Paulsen KD, Strohbehn JW, Lynch DR (1988) Theoretical electric field distributions produced by three types of regional hyperthermia devices in a three-dimensional homogeneous model of man. IEEE Trans Biomed Eng 35:36–45
91. Paulsen KD, Lynch DR, Strohbehn JW (1988) Three-dimensional finite boundary and hybrid element solutions of the

of the Maxwell equations for lossy dielectric media. IEEE Trans Microwave Theory Tech 36:682–693
92. Reynolds AC (1978) Boundary conditions for the numerical solution of wave propagation problems. Geophys 43:1099–1110
93. Richmond JH (1965) Scattering by a dielectric cylinder of arbitrary cross-section shape. IEEE Trans Antennas Propag 13:334–341
94. Rine G, Dewhirst MW, Samulski TV, Wallen A (1987) Modelling of SAR values in tissue due to slab loaded waveguide applicators. Proceedings of the ninth annual conference of the IEEE Engineering in Medicine and Biology Society, pp 1000–1001
95. Roemer RB, Cetas TC (1984) Applications of bioheat transfer simulations in hyperthermia. Cancer Res 44:4788s–4798s
96. Roemer RB, Cetas TC, Oleson JR, Halac S, Matloubieh AY (1984) Comparative evaluation of hyperthermia heating modalities. I. Numerical analysis of thermal dosimetry bracketing cases. Radiat Res 100:450–472
97. Roemer RB, Cetas CT, Oleson JR, Halac S, Matloubieh AY (1984) Comparative evaluation of hyperthermia heating modalities. II. Application of the acceptable power range technique. Radiat Res 100:473–486
98. Roemer RB, Swindell W, Clegg ST, Kress RL (1984) Simulation of focused scanned ultrasonic heating of deep-seated tumors: effects of blood perfusion. IEEE Trans Sonics Ultrason 31:457–466
99. Sapozink MD, Gibbs FA, Gates KS, Stewart JR (1984) Regional hyperthermia in the treatment of clinically advanced deep-seated malignancy: results of a pilot study employing an annular array applicator. Int J Radiat Oncol Biol Phys 10:775–786
100. Sapozink MD, Gibbs FA, Thomson JW, Eltringham JR, Stewart JR (1985) A comparison of deep regional hyperthermia from an annular array and a concentric coil in the same patients. Int J Radiat Oncol Biol Phys 11:179–190
101. Schaubert DH, Wilton DR, Glisson AW (1984) A tetrahedral modeling method for electromagnetic scattering by arbitrarily shaped inhomogeneous dielectric bodies. IEEE Trans Antennas Propag 32:77–85
102. Schwan HP, Foster KR (1980) RF-field interactions with biological systems: electrical properties and biophysical mechanism. Proc IEEE 68:104–113
103. Shaw RP (1975) An outer boundary integral equation applied to transient wave scattering in an inhomogeneous medium. J Appl Mech 42:147–152
104. Shen LC, Kong JA (1987) Applied electromagnetism, 2nd edn. Prindle, Weber, and Schmidt, Boston
105. Shen SF (1975) An aerodynamist looks at the finite element method. In: Gallagher RH et al. (eds) Finite elements in fluids, vol 2. Wiley, New York
106. Silvester PP, Ferrari RL (1983) Finite elements for electrical engineers. Cambridge University Press, Cambridge
107. Silvester PP, Lowther DA, Carptenter CJ, Wyatt EA (1977) Exterior finite elements for 2D field problems with open boundaries. Proc IEEE 124:1267–1270
108. Sloan SW, Randolph MF (1983) Automatic element reordering for finite element analysis with frontal solution schemes. Int J Numer Methods Eng 19:1153–1181
109. Storm FK, Harrison WH, Elliott RS, Hatzitheofilous C, Morton DL (1979) Human hyperthermia therapy: relation between tumor type and capacity to induce hyperthermia by radiofrequency. Am J Surg 138:170–174
110. Storm FK, Elliott RS, Harrison WH, Morton DL (1982) Clinical RF hyperthermia by magnetic-loop induction: a new approach to human cancer therapy. IEEE Trans Microwave Theory Tech 30:1149–1158
111. Storm FK, Harrison WH, Elliott RS, Silberman AW, Morton DL (1982) Thermal distribution of magnetic-loop induction hyperthermia in phantoms and animals: effect of the living state and velocity of heating. Int J Radiat Oncol Biol Phys 8:865–871
112. Storm FK et al. (1985) Magnetic induction hyperthermia: results of a 5 year multi-institutional national cooperative trial in advanced cancer patients. Cancer 55:2677–2687
113. Strang WG, Fix GJ (1973) An analysis of the finite element method. Prentice-Hall, Englewood Cliffs, NJ
114. Stratton JA (1941) Electromagnetic theory. McGraw-Hill, London
115. Strohbehn JW (1982) Theoretical temperature distributions for solenodial-type hyperthermia systems. Med Phys 9:673–682
116. Strohbehn JW (1983) Temperature distributions from interstitial RF electrode hyperthermia systems: theoretical predictions. Int J Radiat Oncol Biol Phys 9:1655–1667
117. Strohbehn JW, Douple EB (1984) Hyperthermia and cancer therapy: a review of biomedical engineering contributions and challenges. IEEE Trans Biomed Eng 31:779–787
118. Strohbehn JW, Roemer RB (1984) A survey of computer simulations of hyperthermia treatments. IEEE Trans Biomed Eng 31:136–149
119. Strohbehn JW, Mechling JA (1986) Interstitial techniques for clinical hyperthermia. In: Hand JW, James JR (eds) Physical techniques in clinical hyperthermia. Research Studies, Letchworth, pp 210–287
120. Strohbehn JW, Paulsen KD, Lynch DR (1986) Use of finite element methods in computerized thermal dosimetry. In: Hand JW, James JR (eds) Physical techniques in clinical hyperthermia. Research Studies, Letchworth, pp 383–451
121. Sullivan DM, Borup DT, Gandhi OP (1987) Use of the finite-difference time-domain method in calculating EM absorption in human tissues. IEEE Trans Biomed Eng 34:148–157
122. Sultran MF, Mittra R (1985) An iterative moment method for analyzing the electromagnetic field distribution inside homogeneous lossy dielectric objects. IEEE Trans Microwave Theory Tech 33:163–168
123. Swindell W (1986) Ultrasonic hyperthermia. In: Hand JW, James JR (eds) Physical techniques in clinical hyperthermia. Research Studies, Letchworth, pp 288–326
124. Taflove A (1980) Application of the finite difference time-domain method to sinusoidal steady-state electromagnetic penetration problems. IEEE Trans Electromagn Compat 22:191–202
125. Taflove A, Brodwin ME (1975) Numerical solution to steady-state electromagnetic scattering problems using the time-dependent Maxwell's equations. IEEE Trans Microwave Theory Tech 23:623–630
126. Telles JCF (1987) A self-adaptive coordinate transformation for efficient numerical evaluation of general boundary element integrals. Int J Numer Methods Eng 24:959–973
127. Theocaris PS, Ioakimidis NI, Kazantzakis JG (1980) On numerical evaluation of two-dimensional principle value integrals. Int J Numer Methods Eng 15:629–634
128. Tijhius AG (1984) Toward a stable marching-on-in-time method for two-dimensional transient electromagnetic scattering problems. Radio Science 19:1311–1317
129. Trembly BS (1985) The effects of driving frequency and antenna length on power deposition within a microwave

array used for hyperthermia. IEEE Trans Biomed Eng 32:152–157
130. Trembly BS, Wilson AH, Sullivan MJ, Stein AD, Wong TZ, Strohbehn JW (1986) Control of SAR patterns with an interstitial microwave array through variation of antenna driving phase. IEEE Trans Microwave Theory Tech 34:568–571
131. Tsai CT, Massoudi H, Durney CH, Iskander MF (1986) A procedure for calculating fields inside arbitrary shaped inhomogeneous dielectric bodies using linear basis functions with the moment method. IEEE Trans Microwave Theory Tech 34:1131–1139
132. Turner PF (1984) Hyperthermia and inhomogeneous tissue effects using an annular phased array. IEEE Trans Microwave Theory Tech 32:874–882
133. Turner PF (1984) Regional hyperthermia with an annular phased array. IEEE Trans Biomed Eng 31:106–114
134. Turner PF (1986) Interstitial equal-phased arrays for EM hyperthermia. IEEE Trans Microwave Theory Tech 34:572–578
135. Turner PF, Kumar L (1982) Computer solution for applicator heating patterns. Natl Cancer Inst Monogr 61: 521–523
136. Van Den Berg PM, DeHoop AT, Segal A, Praagman N (1983) A computational model of electromagnetic heating of biological tissue with application to hyperthermic cancer therapy. IEEE Trans Biomed Eng 30:797–805
137. Visser AG, Van Rhoon GV, Van Den Berg PM, Reinhold HS (1987) Evaluation of calculated temperature distributions for a 27 MHz ridged waveguide used in localized deep hyperthermia. Int J Hyperthermia 3:245–256
138. Wait JR (1985) Focused heating in cylindrical targets. Part I. IEEE Trans Microwave Theory Tech 33:647–654
139. Wait JR, Lumori M (1986) Focused heating in cylindrical targets. Part II. IEEE Trans Microwave Theory Tech 34:357–359
140. Wong TZ, Strohbehn JW, Jones KM, Mechling JA, Trembly BS (1986) SAR patterns from an interstitial microwave antenna array hyperthermia system. IEEE Trans Microwave Theory Tech 34:560–567
141. Yee KS (1966) Numerical solutions of initial boundary value problems involving Maxwell's equations in isotropic media. IEEE Trans Antennas Propag 14:302–307
142. Young JH, Wang MT, Brezovich IA (1980) Frequency/depth-penetration considerations in hyperthermia by magnetically induced currents. Electron Lett 16:358–359
143. Zienkiewicz OC (1977) The finite element method. McGraw-Hill, London
144. Zienkiewicz OC, Emson C, Bettess P (1983) A novel boundary infinite element. Int J Numer Methods Eng 19:393–404
145. Ziolkowski RW, Madsen NK, Carpenter RC (1983) Three-dimensional computer modeling of electromagnetic fields: a global lookback lattice truncation scheme. J Comput Phys 50:360–408

3 Thermal Dosimetry

R. B. ROEMER

3.1 Introduction

If hyperthermia becomes a common clinical treatment modality, then it is inevitable that sophisticated, computerized treatment planning procedures will be utilized, just as has historically occurred with radiation treatments. This task will be more difficult and complex than for radiation, primarily because hyperthermia planning requires knowledge of both the anatomical and physiological characteristics of the patient, whereas current radiation planning does not utilized any physiological information. That is, during radiation planning, one needs to know only the energy deposition pattern, a calculation which involves taking into account the relatively well known tissue anatomy and energy absorption characteristics. In hyperthermia, however, one must not only know the energy deposition pattern (which again depends on the tissue anatomy and energy absorption characteristics) but also the energy removal pattern. It is the difference between these deposition and removal terms which results in the final tissue temperatures in hyperthermia, while deposition is the only important variable in radiation treatments. Thus, in hyperthermia one has an additional problem to solve, and a difficult one at that. In particular, the energy removal pattern depends on both

1. the distribution and magnitude of the tissue blood perfusion and
2. the temperatures produced during the treatment

two factors which interact and can significantly affect one another. Thus one must not only know, a priori, the tissue blood perfusion characteristics to be present during the treatment, characteristics which are dynamic with time, but one must also be able to solve a relatively complex partial differential equation in order to calculate the temperature distributions. However, while the problem is indeed more difficult than for radiation, it does appear tractable. The need for such treatment planning is rapidly increasing as hyperthermia heating systems become more complex and flexible, and as improved treatments are sought for more deeply situated tumors.

Just as radiation therapy has evolved from simple treatments with relatively crude and inflexible equipment, so is hyperthermia heating equipment evolving – and at a relatively rapid rate. The first generation of equipment with inflexible, fixed power deposition patterns is being replaced by a second generation that can deposit power in much more variable patterns, patterns which can be tailored to the region one wants to heat, thus potentially giving significantly improved temperature distributions. However, to utilize these improved systems, one must be able to understand their performance and to plan and control their application in an optimal manner. This will require the utilization of complex, computer-based patient treatment-planning programs, programs which are in their infancy at present and whose use is restricted to a few research centers. This lack of program development can be directly related to the relatively youthful age of hyperthermia. That is, such programs have not been needed since the equipment in use to date has generally been inflexible, with a fixed power deposition pattern and only one type of control – the power amplitude could be increased or decreased, primarily dependent upon verbal feedback from the patient. As a result of these limited capabilities, there was very little to plan for – the patient was positioned in the heating field of the equipment and the power was increased until the patient's tolerance level was reached or, in some cases, until the thermometry indicated that therapeutic temperatures had been reached at the tumor temperature measurement locations.

This situation is changing because of the never-ending impetus to improve the temperature distributions in treatments and the more frequent attempts to treat deeper-seated tumors (with their neighboring critical organs and tissues), two taskmasters which are pushing the development and use of more sophisticated equipment. As this maturation of hyperthermia occurs, the use of mathematical models of hyperthermia treatments will become commonplace.

Indeed, such simulations are already beginning to demonstrate their value in clinical situations. This is occurring in all of the traditional manners in which mathematical models are known to be useful:

1. invoking mathematical rigor and precision in the formulation and evaluation of problems;
2. providing a theoretical framework which can be used to substantiate, evaluate, and interpret experimental results;
3. allowing extensive parametric studies to be performed quickly and inexpensively so that sensitive (and insensitive) parameters can be determined, different heating systems and configurations can be evaluated, and critical experiments can be identified;
4. giving the ability to predict, a priori, the outcome of proposed experiments or treatments (in terms of temperature distributions for hyperthermia applications); and
5. extending the capabilities of available instrumentation by predicting the values of quantities which are difficult or impossible to measure.

The applications of hyperthermia simulations can be divided under four main headings [106, 110], which can be thought of as progressing in time through a patient treatment: comparative, prospective, concurrent, and retrospective thermal dosimetry.

The goal of comparative thermal dosimetry is to compare the abilities of different heating modalities and configurations to heat general classes of patients and tumors properly. Such calculations can be done using standardized patient models which contain only the most significant anatomical and physiological features of "typical" patients and the major characteristics of the power deposition patterns.

Conversely, in prospective thermal dosimetry (individual patient treatment planning) more detailed information is needed regarding the particular patient's anatomy and expected blood perfusion responses so that detailed power deposition patterns can be calculated and used to determine the complete temperature distribution for that patient. The goal of such simulations is to optimize the proposed thermal treatment by maximizing the therapeutic effects of the tumor temperature distribution while minimizing normal tissue damage and patient stress.

Concurrent thermal dosimetry (feedback control during a treatment) involves calculating complete temperature fields during a treatment and adjusting power deposition parameters (and other variable quantities) to optimize the actual treatments. In present applications, measured temperatures at discrete locations are controlled, while the eventual goal is to evaluate and control the complete temperature field.

Retrospective thermal dosimetry (post-treatment evaluation of a complemented therapy) has as its goal the calculation of the complete temperature field (and thermal dose) that was attained during the treatment, based on knowledge of temperatures at the measurement locations. Such data are needed for determining the efficacy of the hyperthermia treatments, as well as for meaningful clinical evaluations of the equipment's performance and of the heating protocol utilized during the treatment. If this task can be performed in real time, it will be equivalent to noninvasive thermometry and could then be used not only for treatment evaluation but also for real-time feedback control.

Each of these four areas will be discussed in detail – after a general discussion of the application of the basic principles of heat transfer to typical hyperthermia situations has been provided. In all cases, mathematical results will be presented for the interested reader, but derivations will not be provided in the interest of brevity. The discussion will be structured so that the results can be understood without reference to the mathematics. The present chapter does not cover the subject of temperature measurement, which is discussed in depth in other volumes of this series, but rather the need for and applications of modeling principles in treatment planning, control, and evaluation. Likewise, many practical clinical techniques presently used in these areas are also discussed in the companion volumes of this series and by T.C. Cetas (1982), and thus will not be covered in depth here.

3.2 Applications of Basic Heat Transfer Modeling Principles to Hyperthermia

This section applies the basic heat transfer principles described in Chap. 1 to the many practical problems that arise in hyperthermia treatments. Several situations and problems are common for all heating modalities, and they than thus be analyzed generically. For example: What constitutes an ideal, or optimal, treatment, including the effects of blood flow and blood vessels? What spatial distributions are present and, in particular, what are the distances through which thermal conduction effects can be felt (an important problem for skin or surface cooling in regional and local external hyperthermia, for forced convection cooling and/or heating by various interstitial techniques, and for blood vessel cooling effects)? What are the time scales involved in the heating and cooling of tissue? What are the relative roles of thermal conduction and blood perfusion in cooling the tissue?

3.2.1 The "Ideal" Hyperthermia Temperature Distribution

Two fundamental, unanswered questions within the hyperthermia community are: "What is an ideal, or optimal, hyperthermia treatment?" and "What are the equipment characteristics that are needed to attain that goal?" In concrete terms, this latter question often arises between engineers, who ask clinicians, "What are the temperature distribution performance characteristics we should use to design our equipment?", and the clinicians, who often give different, and sometimes ambiguous, responses. These imprecise answers are partly caused by our lack of complete knowledge of the basic biothermal processes and clinical responses associated with hyperthermia treatments, and partly by the clinicians knowing that, even if such goals were specified closely, they could probably not be reached because of today's inflexible equipment and software and, thus, one should just do the best one can to heat tumors selectively. The same basic question is also raised when the tables are turned and the physician asks, "What machine should I buy?" or "How good is your machine?" To which general, vague responses can, at best, be given by the engineering and physics community, which has never had a clear, well-articulated, common goal. This leaves us in an unsettled state, without even an imperfect target to shoot at and discuss to see what we could learn from that debate. This section attempts to move along that path by providing a description of several possible goals, starting from the "perfectly ideal", in which no practical constraints are considered, through a set of other ideal, but "less ideal", goals which take into account the various equipment and clinical constraints that are present. This exercise will perhaps:

1. make us explicitly aware of some of the decisions we are making, and the rationale behind those decisions;
2. illustrate the interrelationships between several phenomena; and
3. help clarify and unify the hyperthermia nomenclature and terminology.

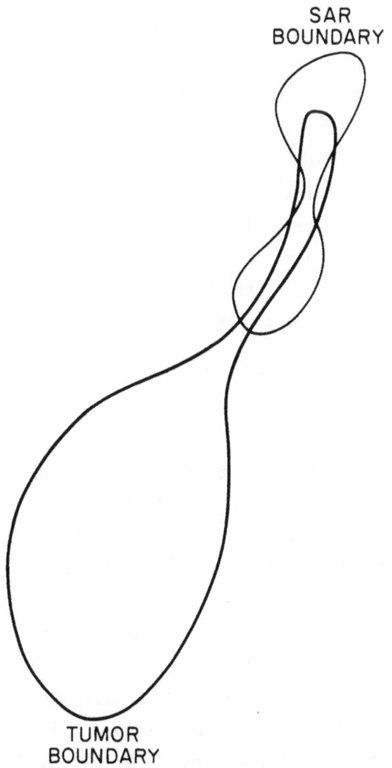

Fig. 3.1. The conformability problem: For all practical hyperthermia equipment, the size of the region in which significant power deposition occurs (the SAR boundary) is so large and has such a shape that the temperature cannot be selectively elevated to desired values in all the malignant cells alone (the tumor boundary)

Clearly, in a perfectly ideal clinical setting one would selectively raise the temperature of every cancerous cell to provide it with a therapeutic thermal dose. Technically this is impossible due to both the lack of methods for identifying all malignant cells and because of the supracellular sizes of the power deposition fields available at present. One could try to decrease the number of cells to be treated by attempting to selectively raise the temperature of only the malignant cells that will not be necrosed by a complementary modality (e.g., radiation, drugs), but, again, the same two problems are present. One must thus move up the anatomical scale to practical geometrical sizes, where we can see what it is we want to treat (the identifiability problem) and are able effectively to treat that volume. The identifiability problem will be placed aside temporarily to let us concentrate on the problem of the size and shape of the power deposition fields produced by existing hyperthermia equipment and, in particular, on the inability of that equipment to have its SAR pattern conform exactly to the necessary boundaries, i.e., the fundamental problem of conformability (Fig. 3.1):

Conformability: A Fundamental Limitation of All Hyperthermia Heating Equipment

No hyperthermia heating equipment exists which has an SAR distribution which can be configured such that all malignant cells are treated to a therapeutic thermal dose while no normal tissue cells are treated to a necrotic thermal dose. That is, the boundary outlining the volume of tissue at or above the necrotic or therapeutic thermal dose cannot be made to conform exactly to the boundary of the tumor.

It follows directly from this fundamental limitation that a compromise needs to be made during any practical treatment – if we treat the complete tumor volume to a therapeutic thermal dose, we will perforce give some tissue a necrotic thermal dose, whereas if we avoid giving any normal tissue a necrotic thermal dose, we will not be able to treat all of the tumor volume to therapeutic thermal dose. Here, a therapeutic thermal dose for tumor cells is one that either directly kills the tumor cells or will result in the death of tumor cells when used in conjuction with another treatment modality. The therapeutic thermal dose will then be different for different treatment combinations. Similarly, the necrotic thermal dose for normal cells will also be different for different treatment combinations. The treatment volume is defined here to include all normal and tumor cells that have been given the desired thermal treatment dose. Mathematically, we define the treatment volume (V_{tr}), i.e., that volume of tissue treated to the thermal treatment dose, as the sum of the volume of tumor tissue treated to that dose, $V_{tu}(T_{tr})$, plus the volume of normal tissue treated to that dose, $V_{no}(T_{tr})$, i.e.,

$$V_{tr} = V_{tu}(T_{tr}) + V_{no}(T_{tr}) \ . \tag{3.1}$$

It should be noted here that we have temporarily framed the above discussion in terms of a thermal dose rather than a therapeutic temperature because of the more all-encompassing nature of the concept of a dose. However, because the concept of a thermal dose is not adequately defined at present (see *International Journal of Hyperthermia*, Vol. 3, No. 4, July-August 1987, for several articles covering a recent workshop on this subject), we will frame our future discussions in terms of the physically measurable quantity temperature. In so doing, several observations are pertinent. First, the therapeutic temperature in the tumor could well be a function of position in the tumor, i.e., $T_{th} = T_{th}(\vec{r})$, since it is well known that the pH level, the blood supply, and the oxygen levels vary within the tumor and that these factors can affect the cellular energy stature and response at a given temperature (e.g. [38, 41]). Likewise, for normal tissues the type of tissue present in the treated volume is a function of position and thus so is the unacceptable level of temperature, i.e., $T_{ne} = T_{ne}(\vec{r})$. Furthermore, we must consider time, a factor which is quite important since the temperature elevation needed to produce a given amount of cell death is clearly a function of the length of time the cells are kept at that temperature (e.g. [38]). Thus, in all of our discussions, when we say that a volume of tissue has reached therapeutic temperatures, that implies that the tissue has been kept at that temperature for a sufficiently long time to produce some specified thermal dose to yield a given percentage of cell death, e.g., 99.9%. It it also pertinent to note here that, in general, there does not appear to exist a significant difference in response to hyperthermia between normal and malignant cells (e.g., [38, 96]) if their physiological conditions are the same. Thus, the small infiltrative fibers of cancerous cells, which are in the same physiological environment as the normal cells, will not respond preferentially – and to necrose them all by hyperthermia would require sacrificing their adjacent normal tissue. As a final point, it should be noted that it is generally believed that the insides of tumors often contain regions of tissue which are relatively radioresistant due to a meager vasculature structure causing regions of low oxygen content (e.g., [39]). And, for chemotherapy, this same poor vascular supply hinders the drugs from reaching all of the cancerous cells. These facts, while important clinically, interestingly do not affect our definition of a practical hyperthermia treatment goal because of the identifiability problem. This is also true when one considers the different possible biological treatment mechanisms [96], direct hyperthermia cell kill (or cell kill as a result of tumor microcirculatory collapse after hyperthermia), or radiosensitization.

Returning to the needed compromise, there are two possible directions in which to proceed, each with its own logical goal (Fig. 3.2): First, we can extend the size of the treatment volume so that all tumor cells are included in the volume of tissue which is heated to therapeutic temperatures, i.e., set $V_{tu}(T_{tr})$ equal to the complete tumor volume, $V_{tu}(T_{tr}) = V_{tumor}$. This approach could be called the complete tumor volume approach and would have the following goal:

Goal of the Ideal Complete Tumor Volume Treatment Approach

Given the constraint that the volume of tissue raised to the treatment temperature (V_{tr}) always contains the complete volume of malignant tumor cells (V_{tumor}), that treatment volume should be minimized so that the volume of normal tissues subjected to necrotic

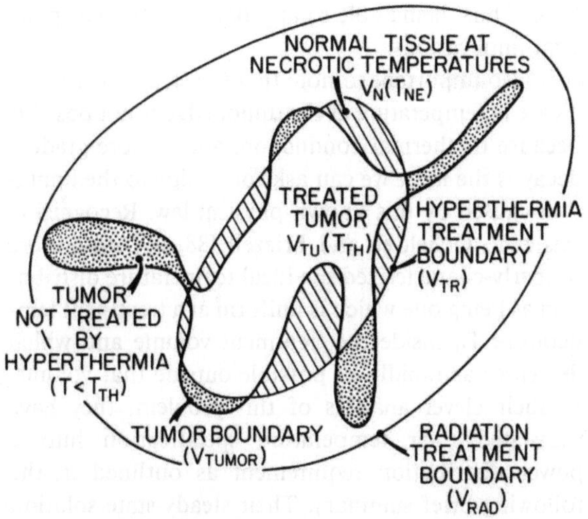

Fig. 3.2. Tissue regions involved in the practical approach to hyperthermia treatments. The hyperthermia treatment boundary can be retracted or expanded to reach either of two extremes or ideal goals. First, for an ideal partial tumor volume approach (ideal in the clinical sense of zero normal tissue damage), the treatment volume would be retracted so that $V_{no}(T_{ne}) = 0$. Second, for an ideal complete tumor volume treatment (ideal in the clinical sense of providing a therapeutic dose to all tumor cells), the hyperthermia treatment boundary would be extended to include all of the tumor volume. A large-field radiation treatment boundary has also been shown

temperatures, $V_{no}(T_{ne})$, is minimized. Mathematically: Minimize V_{tr} subject to the constraint that $V_{tumor} \in V_{tr}$.

The second logical possibility would be to go in the other direction and treat a volume which is smaller than the tumor volume, leaving the treatment of the malignant cells outside the treatment volume to another modality, or leaving it untreated. In this second approach, one pulls back the ideal hyperthermia treatment boundary so that any infiltrative threads or vague areas on the tumor boundary are not treated by hyperthermia, and only the "bulk" of the tumor is treated. Here, of course, we would not be treating the complete tumor ($V_{tumor} \notin V_{tr}$) and, hence, the name partial tumor volume treatment approach. In contrast to the complete tumor volume approach, the logical extremum of this second direction would have as its goal the maintenance of the largest treatment volume which would not destroy any normal tissue (the sense in which this treatment would be clinically ideal). This could be called the ideal partial tumor volume treatment approach:

Goal of the Ideal Partial Tumor Volume Treatment Approach
With the volume of normal tissue raised to necrotic temperatures, $V_{no}(T_{ne})$, kept at zero, the largest possible volume of malignant tumor should be treated therapeutically. Mathematically: Maximize V_{tr} subject to the constraint that $V_{no}(T_{ne}) = 0$.

Turning from the ideal to the practical, some normal tissue can generally be sacrificed in practical clinical cases, putting us somewhere between the above two "ideal" limits and giving us a good working definition for our treatment goal, a definition which we can use as a base for further discussion:

Goal of the Technically and Clinically Practical Treatment Approach
With the volume of normal tissue raised to necrotic temperatures, $V_{no}(T_{ne})$, kept below some clinically specified value $[V_{no,acc}(T_{ne})]$, the largest possible volume of malignant tumor should be treated therapeutically. Mathematically: Maximize $V_{tu}(T_{tr})$ subject to the constraint that $V_{no}(T_{ne}) < V_{no,acc}(T_{ne})$. Table 3.1 summarizes the various possible goals we have considered and, given the acceptability of the last entry, we can now begin to investigate the characteristics of the temperature distribution in the treatment volume in order to gain further insights into the possibility of refining the goal. That is, to this point we have only considered what volumes to treat, not the details of the temperature distributions in those volumes. Because of the identifiability problem, we cannot detect the physiological and cellular differences inside the tumor; thus, as a first step, we will utilize a single treatment temperature, T_{tr}, for the complete tumor. Then, an ideal treatment would have a uniform temperature T_{tr} inside the tumor and that temperature would drop off immediately outside the treatment volume to a low, nontherapeutic temperature in a step function manner (Fig. 3.3). The uniform temperature inside the treatment volume is ideal in the

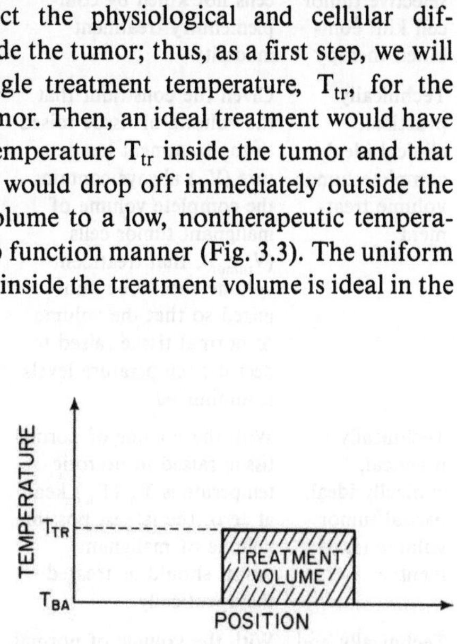

Fig. 3.3. Ideal temperature distribution: A uniform therapeutic temperature (T_{th}) inside the treatment volume and no increase in temperature outside that volume (basal temperature, T_{ba}, everywhere). If the identifiability problem did not exist (i.e., we could identify the physiological and biological status of the tumor as a function of position inside the tumor), then the ideal treatment temperature inside the tumor would not be constant, but would be a function of position

sense that it minimizes the amount of power required and it makes our accounting task simpler, while the instantaneous decrease in temperature is ideal in that it spares all of the normal tissue from damage. It should be noted that to obtain this ideal will require a perfectly conformable power deposition source with infinitely fine resolution. The power supplied by that conformable source will also be ideal in the sense that it will be the minimum power required to heat the tumor to T_{tr}. That is, no power will be wasted in heating the normal tissue, nor in heating the tumor or its blood supply, to temperatures greater than T_{tr}. This factor is important clinically since many treatments with regional and local devices are limited by the fact that excessive power is deposited in the patient. Thus, being able to approach ideality has practical implications.

It is also important to note that the step function decrease in temperature at the tumor edge is not possible because of thermal conduction, and a more gradual decay is the most we can ask for – due to the limitation caused by this known physical law. Recognizing this fact, Ocheltree and Frizzell [88, 89] have more properly characterized the ideal temperature distribution as being one which is uniform at a treatment temperature T_{tr} inside the treatment volume and which decreases as rapidly as possible outside that volume. In their clever analysis of this problem, they have translated their temperature specification into a power distribution requirement as outlined in the following brief summary. Their steady-state solution assumes that the bioheat transfer equation

$$-k\nabla^2 T + \dot{W}c(T - T_{ar}) = \dot{Q}_a(\vec{r}) \tag{3.2a}$$

is valid. They recognized that $\nabla^2 T = 0$ for the case of a uniform temperature (T_{tr}) inside the tumor and thus

$$\dot{Q}_a(\vec{r}) = \dot{W}(\vec{r})c(T_{tr} - T_{ar}) \ . \tag{3.3}$$

Thus, if T_{ar} is also fixed, then $\dot{Q}_a(\vec{r})$ is a linear function of $\dot{W}(\vec{r})$. To extend their analysis, if one uses a more general energy balance (i.e., with a general term for the removal of energy by blood flow, $\dot{Q}_b$) rather than the bioheat transfer equation, one has

$$-k\nabla^2 T + \dot{Q}_b(\vec{r}) = \dot{Q}_a(\vec{r}) \ . \tag{3.2b}$$

Again, for a uniform temperature (T_{tr}) in the tumor, we have $\nabla^2 T = \nabla^2 T_{tr} = 0$, giving

$$\dot{Q}_a(\vec{r}) = \dot{Q}_b(\vec{r}) \ ; \tag{3.4}$$

i.e., the energy added locally by the power deposition source must just compensate for the local losses due to blood perfusion. Next, they recognized that to obtain the maximum rate of decrease of temperature in the normal tissue simply implies that the power must be zero outside the treated volume. Finally, the outer surface of the treatment volume requires additional power deposition to compensate for the conduction losses into the normal tissue, a factor accounted for in their bioheat transfer equation-based analysis. Figures 3.4 and 3.5 show the blood perfusion, temperature, and applied power distributions for two different situations with $T_{tr} = T_0$. Figure 3.4 is for both a cylinder and a sphere which have a uniform perfusion inside the treated volume of radius r_0, and Fig. 3.5 is for a spherical tumor with a nonuniform internal blood perfusion.

These results clearly show the effects of thermal conduction, which causes a gradual temperature decrease

Table 3.1. Possible hyperthermia treatment goals

Approach	Hyperthermia treatment goal	Reason for discarding
Technically and clinically ideal, selective tumor cell kill: hyperthermia alone	Therapeutically and selectively treat all malignant cells	Tumor cell identifiability problem; conformability problem
Technically and clinically ideal, selective tumor cell kill: combined therapy	Therapeutically and selectively treat all malignant cells not killed by complementary treatment modality	Tumor cell identifiability problem; conformability problem
Technically practical, clinical ideal, complete tumor volume treatment	Given the constraint that the volume of tissue raised to the treatment temperature (V_{tr}) always contains the complete volume of malignant tumor cells (V_{tumor}), that treatment volume should be minimized so that the volume of normal tissue raised to necrotic temperature levels is minimized	Possible excessive normal tissue damage
Technically practical, clinically ideal, partial tumor volume treatment	With the volume of normal tissue raised to necrotic temperatues $V_{no}(T_{ne})$ kept at zero, the largest possible volume of malignant tumor should be treated therapeutically	Does not allow for some clinically acceptable normal tissue damage
Technically and clinically practical treatment	With the volume of normal tissue raised to necrotic temperatures $V_{no}(T_{ne})$ kept below some clinically specified value, the largest possible volume of malignant tumor should be treated therapeutically	None

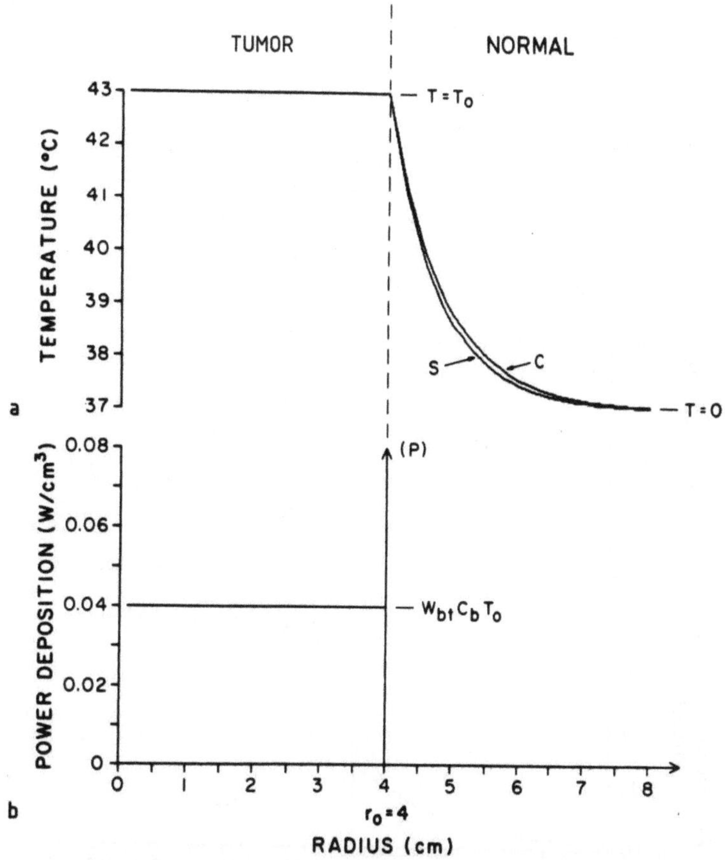

Fig. 3.4a, b. Temperature (**a**) and power deposition (**b**) distributions in cylindrical (C) and spherical (S) tumor models which have uniform perfusion of $\dot{W}_{bt}$. The blood perfusion has one value, $\dot{W}_{bt}$, inside the tumor and another, $\dot{W}_{bn}$, in the normal tissue. Note the extra power spike required to overcome conduction at the tumor boundary (r_0), as indicated by the *arrow*. k_n is the normal tissue thermal conductivity; T_0 is the treatment temperature. [88]

outside the treatment volume rather than the ideal square wave of Fig. 3.3. In this respect, it is also of interest to note that, for these ideal treatments, manipulations of the normal tissue blood perfusion using vasoactive drugs as proposed and studied by several investigators [4, 5, 86, 117] will only have the effect of limiting the amount of normal tissue subject to elevated temperatures at the expense of increased power at the tumor edge. For example, from Ocheltree and Frizzell's [88] calculations for a planar, half-space tumor, the value of $\dot{Q}(r_0)$ at the tumor edge is given by

$$\dot{Q}(r_0) = T_{tr} \sqrt{\dot{W}_{no} c_b k_{no}} \, , \tag{3.5a}$$

and the normal tissue temperature decreases away from the tumor exponentially,

$$T_{no}(x) = T_{tr} \exp\left[-(\dot{W}_{no} c_b / k_{no})^{1/2} x\right] \, . \tag{3.5b}$$

Thus, increasing the normal tissue blood flow will cause the normal tissue temperature to decay more rapidly (Eq. 3.5b) and will require more power at the tumor edge (Eq. 3.5a), but it will not affect the temperatures in the tumor itself after the additional power is added at the tumor edge (Eq. 3.5a) – in this ideal treatment. Possible decreases in the tumor perfusion would likewise only lower the overall power requirement for these ideal treatments without affecting the ideal temperature distributions.

Their model is a very useful tool, and it clearly illustrates several of the major requirements for good hyperthermia systems: the ability to deposit power in a specified volume (conformability); the need to increase power in regions of increased blood perfusion within a tumor; and the necessity for overcoming conduction losses at the tumor boundary, a goal attained in their ideal case by putting an additional spike of power on the tumor boundary. (Note that if power cannot be preferentially deposited at the tumor edge, then overcoming conduction effects into the surrounding normal tissue – so that the tumor edge is kept at the therapeutic temperature – will require that the interior of the tumor be raised to an even higher temperature, a subject we will return to later; see Fig. 3.13.) It is significant to note that these general conclusions hold regardless of their model's limitations, the major ones of which are its dependence on the bioheat transfer equation (and its inherent limitations as previously described in Chap. 1) both for the tumor and the normal tissue, and the assumption that power can be applied in an arbitrari-

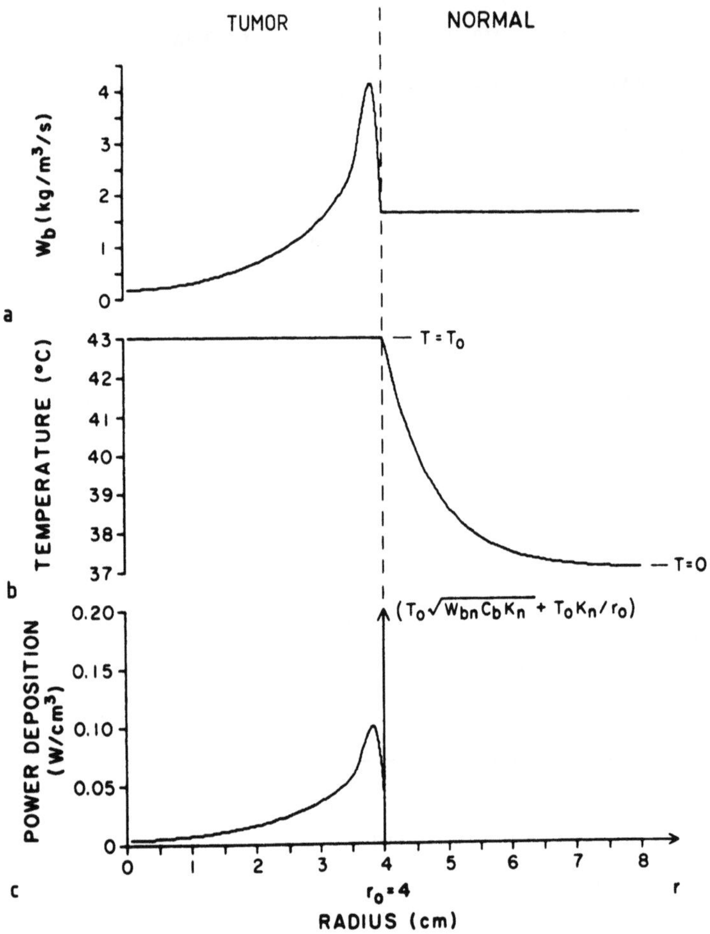

Fig. 3.5a–c. Example of variable perfusion within the tumor (**a**), associated temperature (**b**), and power deposition (**c**) distributions for a spherical tumor model. [88]

ly fine pattern – including the point source distributed around the tumor surface. In reality, clinical power sources will have spatially distributed power deposition fields with some finite, minimal spatial dimension that cannot be reduced. Also, even if the bioheat transfer equation did hold and one had an ideal power source so the conformability problem was avoided, their ideal distribution of power could only be implemented if one knew the actual distribution of blood perfusion in the tumor and normal tissue (Fig. 3.5) – something which is not known. This lack of knowledge of the tissue perfusion patterns is one of the major problems in all hyperthermia treatments, both actual and simulated.

An additional factor which needs to be addressed is the problem of large blood vessels, structures which we know do not obey the bioheat transfer equation and which need to be analyzed separately. In several previous publications [66, 68, 69, 71], Lagendijk and colleagues have emphasized the importance of preheating large vessels in hyperthermia treatments. This concern, first observed clinically and reported by Overgaard and Nielsen [95], has also been more recently analyzed by Baish et al. [7], who also show the need for preheating large blood vessels. While the general problem of the temperature distribution around and within such vessels will be analyzed later, here we can look at the simple case of a single pair of countercurrent vessels (Fig. 3.6) in order to continue our study of some "ideal cases". Since large vessels frequently occur in countercurrent pairs [153], this is the case we will analyze here.

For the ideal case of a uniform treatment temperature in a tumor (Fig. 3.7), we know that

1. if all the returning venous blood has been collected from the tumor which is at the temperature T_{tr}, the venous blood will also be at the treatment temperature when if leaves the tumor, i.e., $T_v(x = L) = T_{tr}$; and
2. for an ideal treatment, we must have the arterial blood temperature equal to the treatment temperature when the arterial blood enters the treatment volume, i.e., $T_{ar}(x = L) = T_{tr}$.

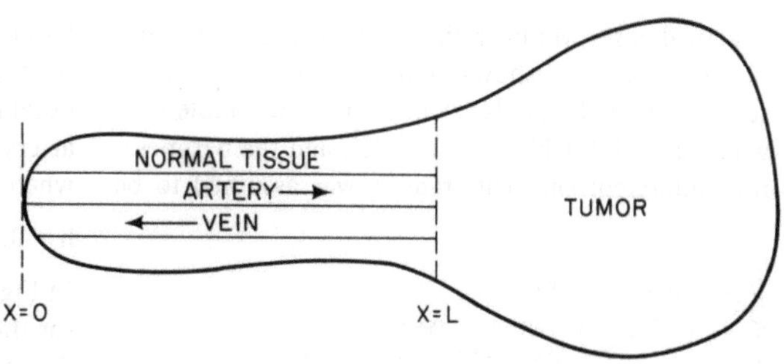

Fig. 3.6. Schematic diagram of countercurrent vessel pair and associated normal and tumor tissue

This latter requirement is essential because the tumor tissues immediately adjacent to the arteries will be at a nontherapeutic temperature if the arterial blood is indeed at a nontherapeutic temperature when it enters the treatment volume – thus giving an inadequate thermal treatment. Thus, we need to determine the power required to raise the arterial blood to the treatment temperature just as it enters the treatment volume $T_{ar}(x = L) = T_{tr}$. Let us do that in a simple, conservative way which will allow us to calculate a power that is less than that which will probably be needed. So, given the above ideal conditions, plus the assumptions that the vessels can be located, that power can be selectively deposited in them, and that their heat transfer losses to the surrounding tissue can be neglected, we can construct a model to calculate this power. (It should be noted here that if in this ideal case the surrounding normal tissue is at or close to its resting temperature, then losses from arteries and veins to the tissue would require even larger power values than those to be calculated in this analysis and, in that sense, this ideal case will give us conservative results. This analysis also neglects the fact that the venous blood will be heated above the treatment temperature; another conservative assumption that will result in an underestimation of the power density required in real cases.) The energy balance equations for the two blood vessels then become

$$-\dot{M}c\,\frac{dT_v}{dx} = (UP)(T_{ar} - T_v) + A_c\dot{Q}_a \tag{3.6}$$

and

$$+\dot{M}c\,\frac{dT_{ar}}{dx} = (UP)(T_v - T_{ar}) + A_c\dot{Q}_a\ , \tag{3.7}$$

where we have assumed

1. that the mass flow rates in the countercurrent artery and vein have the same value ($\dot{M}$);
2. that the power depositions in the artery and vein are identical ($\dot{Q}_a$); and
3. that both vessels have approximately the same cross-sectional area (A_c), overall countercurrent heat transfer coefficient (U), specific heat (c), and perimeter (P).

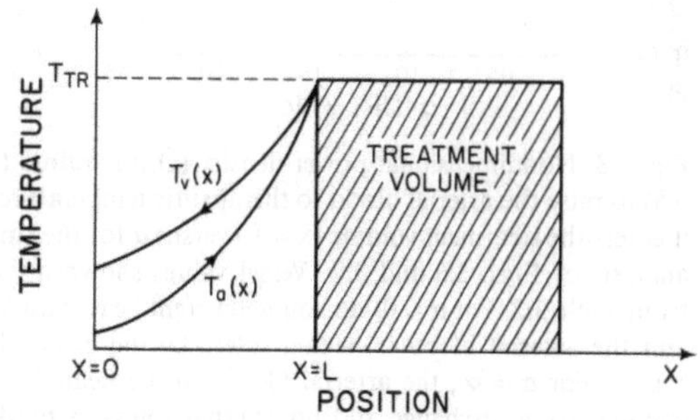

Fig. 3.7. Schematic diagram of ideal temperature distributions for tumor and countercurrent vessels of Fig. 3.6

These simplifications are not present in the more general analysis [111], but the practical trends can easily be shown for this simpler case. Solving these equations gives the uniformly applied power required to raise the arterial blood temperature to the therapeutic temperature when it reaches the tumor, x = L. In its most compact, nondimensional form, it is given by

$$\dot{Q}_N = \frac{\dot{Q}_a A_c L}{\dot{M}c\,[T_{tr} - T_{ar}(0)]} = \frac{1}{1+\alpha}\ , \tag{3.8}$$

as shown in Fig. 3.8, where $\alpha = UPL/\dot{M}c$. Here, $\dot{Q}_N$ is the ratio of the total amount of energy which has been added to the artery in the length L by the power deposition source, i.e., $\dot{Q}_a A_c L$, divided by the total amount of energy which is required to raise the flow of arterial blood from its initial temperature, $T_{ar}(0)$, to the treatment temperature, T_{tr}. At $\alpha = 0$ (i.e., no countercurrent heat exchange), all of the energy must come from the power deposition; for $\alpha = \infty$ (perfect countercurrent heat exchange), no additional power is needed since the energy transferred from the vein is just enough to raise the arterial blood to a therapeutic value. (In the traditional heat transfer literature, α is the number of transfer units for the heat exchanger.)

Practical cases will have finite values of α; for example, Fig. 3.8 also shows some typical numbers for several arterial vessels characterized in Table 3.2, where c = 3700 J/kg°C, $A_c = \pi R^2$, and the perimeter for countercurrent heat transfer was assumed to be half of the vessels perimeter, $P = \pi R$. Here, it has also been assumed that the heat transfer coefficient can be obtained from Eq. 3.9 for laminar flow and that the artery and vein represent a series circuit with U = h/2, where

$$h = 3.66\,k/D\ . \tag{3.9}$$

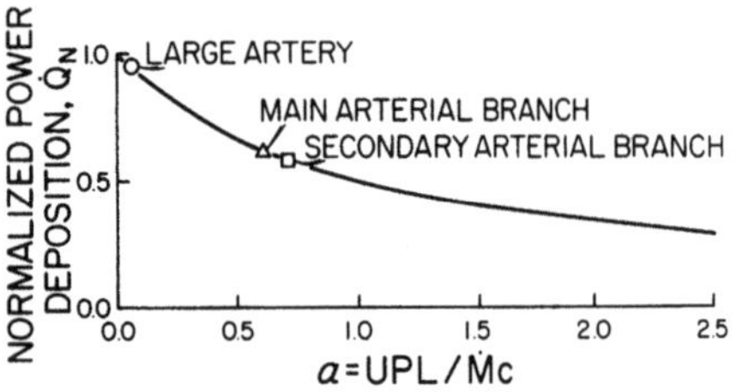

Fig. 3.8. Nondimensional power density ($\dot{Q}_N$) required (see Eq. 3.8) to raise the arterial blood to therapeutic temperature just as it enters the treatment volume (x = L) versus α for the simplified analysis of Figs. 3.6 and 3.7. Vessel values shown are derived from Table 3.2. For $\alpha = 0$, no countercurrent heat transfer exists and the arterial blood is heated solely by the external power source. For $\alpha = \infty$, the arterial blood can be heated solely by countercurrent exchange and no external source is needed

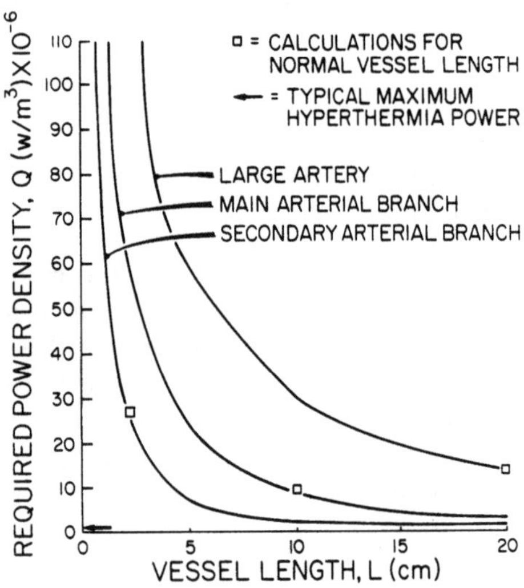

Fig. 3.9. Power density required ($\dot{Q}_a$, Eq. 3.8) to raise the arterial blood temperature of typical "large" vessels (see Table 3.2) by 5 °C as a function of heated vessel length (L). The marked lengths (□) indicate the typical lengths (L*) of these vessels. Note that typical maximum hyperthermia powers are very small (*see arrow*) compared with these required powers

In Fig. 3.8, the dominance of direct power deposition (or the weakness of countercurrent exchange, even in this case where the countercurrent exchange process has been overestimated since the venous blood has been allowed to reach temperatures greater than the treatment temperature) can be seen for the large artery (since $\dot{Q}_N \cong 1.0$), and the approximate equality of the two effects seen for the smaller vessels ($\dot{Q}_N \cong 0.5$).

Next, given these assumptions, one can ask: If different lengths of vessel are heated, what values of $\dot{Q}_a$ are needed using Eq. 3.8 to obtain a 5 °C rise in arterial temperature, i.e., $T_{tr} - T_{ar}(0) = 5\,°C$? The results are shown in Fig. 3.9 for a range of lengths spanning those typical of these large vessels (Table 3.2). It is very significant to note that these conservative estimates of the required power densities are approximately ten times typical hyperthermia values, which range from approximately 10–100 kw/m^3 (0.01–0.1 w/cm^3) for regional heating devices, up to approximately 500–1000 kw/m^3 (0.5–1 w/cm^3) for external, localized heating systems such as superficial microwave applicators. Given these low power values encountered in practice, if the above blood vessel numbers are indeed typical of tumors, then there will definitely be tumor locations adjacent to these vessels that will not be adequately treated in clinical cases where typical clinical power density values are used. This may not be true if there is a reduced blood perfusion in the tumor (thus implying a reduced flow in the larger vessels supplying and draining those tumors), which seems to be the case for many situations, although definitive human clinical data are lacking [104].

Since most clinical devices also have rather broad spatial distributions of power, these large power

Table 3.2. Approximate anatomical and physiological parameter values for large blood vessels (R, A_c, L, V, $\dot{M}$) based on Chato's [17] presentation for a 13-kg dog and the resulting heat transfer coefficients (h) and approximate values of UP/$\dot{M}$c and $\dot{M}$c/A_c needed to solve Eq. 3.8 for different length (L) values (see Figs. 3.8 and 3.9); c_p = 4000 J/kg-°C, ϱ = 1000 kg/m^3

Vessel	R (mm)	A_c (mm^2)	L* (mm)	V (mm/s)	$\dot{M}$ (kg/s)	h (W/m^2-°C)	UP/$\dot{M}$c (m^{-1})	$\dot{M}$c/A_c (W/m^2-°C)
Large artery	1.5	7	200	150	1.0×10^{-3}	600	0.33	600×10^3
Main arterial branch	0.5	0.8	100	80	0.06×10^{-3}	1800	5.6	320×10^3
Secondary arterial branch	0.25	0.2	20	60	0.01×10^{-3}	3600	29.9	240×10^3

values are likely to be deposited in the surrounding tissue. Thus, it is of interest to estimate the approximate tissue temperature rise for the above powers. If one assumes as a first estimate that the power distribution is broad enough so that the tissue somewhat away from the vessels (i.e., not significantly affected by the local vessel temperatures) is heated and that the temperature rise is approximately uniform for that tissue, then conduction can again be ignored in Eq. 3.2a, giving

$$T_{no} = T_{ar}(0) + \frac{\dot{Q}_a}{\dot{W}c} . \tag{3.10}$$

Combining Eqs. 3.10 and 3.8 gives the ratio of the normal tissue temperature (T_{no}) rise to the arterial blood temperature rise,

$$R_T = \frac{T_{no} - T_{ar}(0)}{T_{tr} - T_{ar}(0)} = \frac{\dot{M}/A_c L}{\dot{W}} \left[\frac{1}{1+\alpha}\right] \tag{3.11 a}$$

or

$$R_T = \frac{T_{no} - T_{ar}(0)}{T_{tr} - T_{ar}(0)} = \frac{R_M}{1+\alpha} , \tag{3.11 b}$$

where R_M is the ratio of mass flow rates per unit volume in the vessel and the surrounding tissue. For typical tissues, $\dot{W} \cong 1.0\ \mathrm{kg/m^3\,s}$ for resting muscle and $\dot{W} \cong 10\ \mathrm{kg/m^3\,s}$ for brain. For the vessels given in Table 3.2 and using $L = 2L^*$ in order to give a low (conservative) estimate of R_T, this gives the results shown in Fig. 3.10. Unfortunately, it is easily seen here that if the required power densities could be reached, even with the conservative vessel lengths used, then the normal tissue temperature rises would be quite large.

From the results of these simple analysis (Fig. 3.9, 3.10), two obvious conclusions can be drawn: First, we can easily recognize the need for preheating these large vessels for relatively long lengths when practical powers are applied. Second, in doing so, we will need to be careful not to overheat either the normal tissue or the venous blood. Because of the importance of these phenomena, and the crude assumptions made in this first analysis, we can also see the need for performing more detailed analyses of these phenomena to obtain better estimates of the numbers involved. This will be done later (see Fig. 3.33), but for now we have enough information to further refine our definitions of the ideal power and temperature distributions. A revised ideal tissue temperature distribution is sketched in Fig. 3.11 where the new need for pretreating the blood vessels is illustrated. This is a significant departure from the pattern required by a bioheat transfer-based equation alone, since now some power *must be* deposited outside the treatment volume in order to ensure that the blood is at a therapeutic temperature when it enters the treatment volume. If this preheating is not done, then there will be unacceptably cold spots surrounding these vessels in the tumor. Thus, the ideal power deposition pattern of Ocheltree and Frizzell [88, 89], which calls for zero power deposition outside the tumor boundary, must be modified when the directionality of blood flow in large vessels is considered. Because of the convective, directional flow in these vessels, power needs to be deposited over a finite distance in order to raise the blood temperature, and thus they must be preheated *before* reaching the tumor. This can perhaps be seen most simply by regarding only the artery in Fig. 3.6 and noting that if one only considers power deposition in the artery and neglects countercurrent exchange (U = 0), the solution of Eq. 3.7 becomes

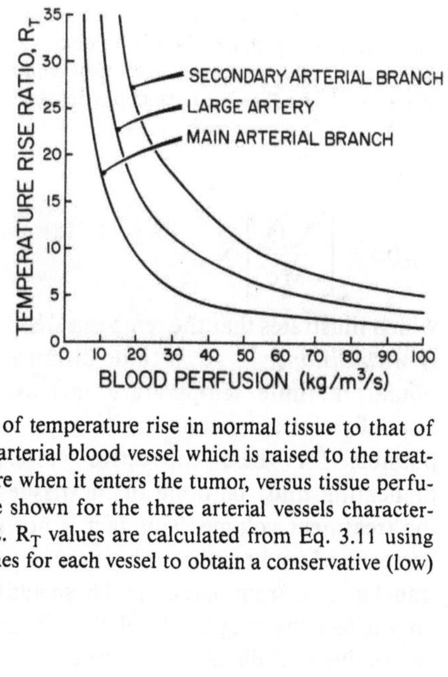

Fig. 3.10. Ratio of temperature rise in normal tissue to that of the blood in an arterial blood vessel which is raised to the treatment temperature when it enters the tumor, versus tissue perfusion. Results are shown for the three arterial vessels characterized in Table 3.2. R_T values are calculated from Eq. 3.11 using twice the L* values for each vessel to obtain a conservative (low) estimate of R_T

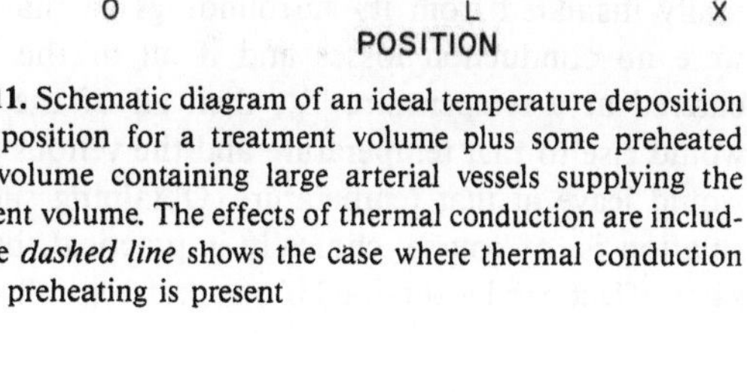

Fig. 3.11. Schematic diagram of an ideal temperature deposition versus position for a treatment volume plus some preheated tissue volume containing large arterial vessels supplying the treatment volume. The effects of thermal conduction are included. The *dashed line* shows the case where thermal conduction but no preheating is present

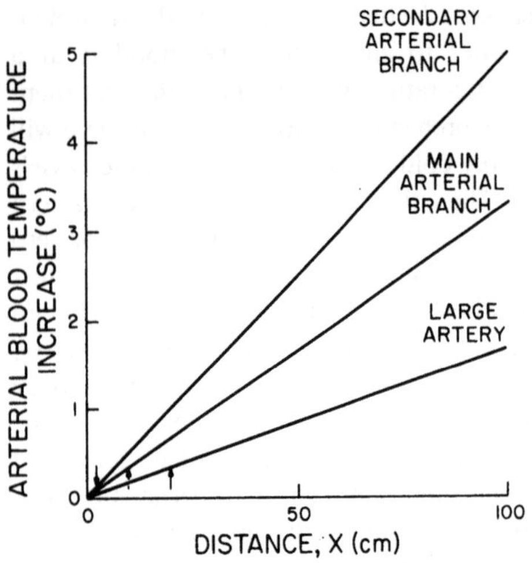

Fig. 3.12. Temperature versus distance (Eq. 3.12) for arterial blood heated uniformly by a power source of strength $\dot{Q}_a = 1000\,\text{KW/m}^3$ (1 W/cm^3); a very strong local field for a hyperthermia treatment. The three curves are for the three blood vessels of Table 3.2. The approximate normal physiological lengths (L^* of Table 3.2) are given by the *arrows*. Note that the heated lengths which are required to obtain a 5 °C temperature rise – a typical hyperthermia treatment requirement – are significantly longer than the normal physiological lengths of these vessels

$$T_{ar}(x) = \left[\frac{A_c \dot{Q}_a}{\dot{M} c}\right] x \,, \tag{3.12}$$

which illustrates that the temperature increases *linearly with distance* – i.e., a finite distance is required to obtain a finite temperature increase (Fig. 3.12). Spatially instantaneous heating is not physically possible for these convective vessels, and some preheating must be done in the tissues surrounding the treatment volume. This fact is not altered by the presence of countercurrent heat exchange and/or heat transfer to or from the tissue. These additional factors only affect the magnitude of the effect, not its basic convective and directional nature.

The presence of this preheated region to overcome convective blood flow will affect the amount of power needed inside the tumor to overcome conduction effects, and it is worthwhile here to consider these two processes together. Their interaction is illustrated in an interesting, simple way in Fig. 3.13. Figure 3.13a shows that if one had a tissue region which was thermally insulated from its surroundings so that there were no conduction losses and if all of the blood entered at a temperature T_{tr}, then all of the tissue would rise to that temperature and the venous blood would leave at that temperature. Obtaining such insulation is, of course, clinically impractical, but the same effect can be obtained if one preferentially heats the tumor boundary to overcome conduction effects, such as suggested by Ocheltree and Frizzell [88, 89] for their infinitely conformable power source. For a power source of finite size, but some selectivity, this would give a nonideal temperature pattern like the one in Fig. 3.13b. For most practical systems, however, the conformability problem prevents the power from being deposited so selectively, so even more nonideal temperature patterns such as those seen in Fig. 3.13c are generally obtained. While the blood preheating and boundary conduction phenomena are closely related, no matter what their relative magnitudes are, it will always be necessary both to preheat the arterial blood and then to add power to the tumor to overcome conduction effects at the treatment volume boundaries in order to approach or obtain an ideal treatment. Indeed, the only reasons for adding power to and around the tumor in any treatment are to achieve these two goals of overcoming boundary losses and heating the blood to the treatment temperature. Thus, the above observations can be formalized as two rules for an ideal hyperthermia treatment:

Two Rules for an Ideal Hyperthermia Treatment

1. Enough power must be deposited in the normal tissue outside the treatment volume to raise all of the arterial blood to the treatment temperature when it reaches the boundary of the treatment volume.
2. Enough power must be added to the treatment volume to overcome conduction effects so that the temperatures on the boundary of the treatment volume are maintained at the treatment value.

Given these rules, it is interesting to note that any hyperthermia modality which confines power only to the tumor will not provide an ideal hyperthermia treatment since cold spots will inevitably exist when any "large" blood vessels are present. In those cases, the cells in the cold spots will need to be treated by radiation or by another complementary modality (Fig. 3.14).

In summary, regarding the goal of a hyperthermia treatment, the basic definition given at the end of Table 3.1 for the technically and clinically practical treatment approach is still valid; i.e., although not stated explicitly, it implicitly includes the need for preheating blood vessels as part of maximizing the therapeutic volume. However, for a clearer definition of our goal, that implicit requirement should be clearly stated, as should several other previously discussed aspects of this problem. Thus, our final definition is given below:

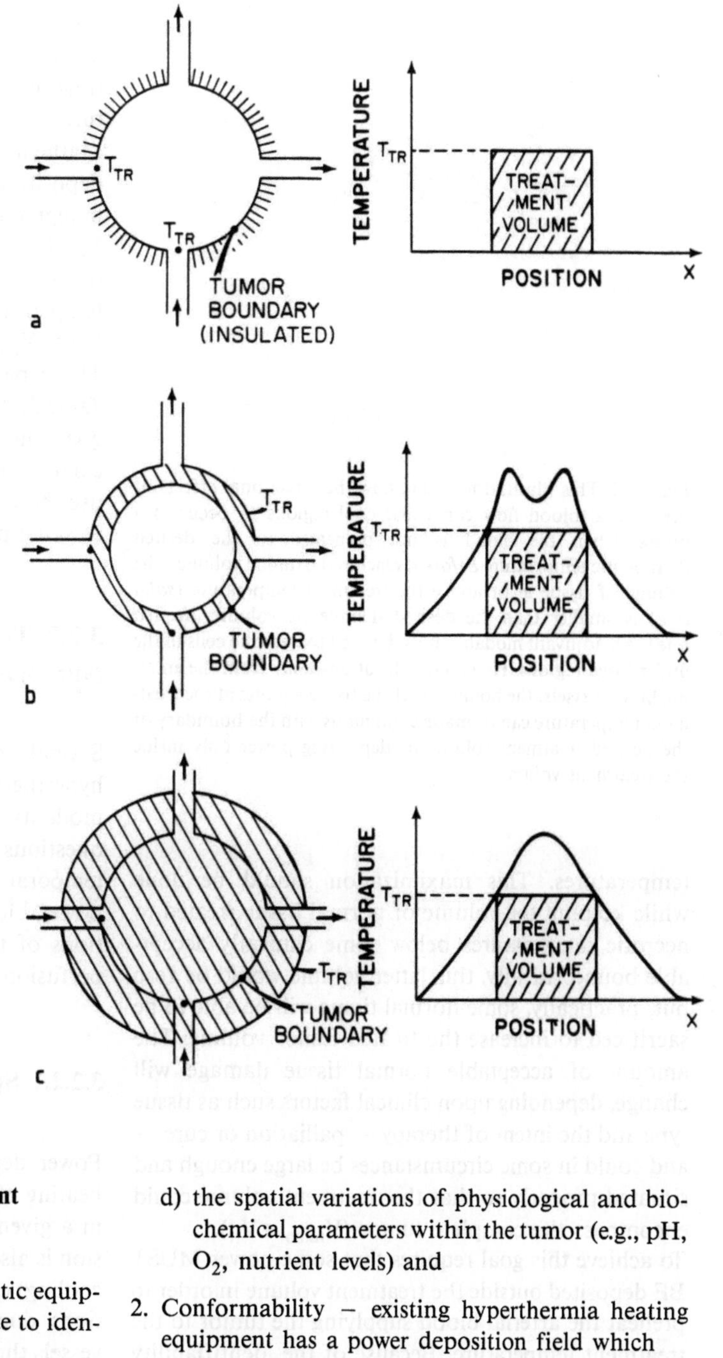

Fig. 3.13a–c. Temperature distribution: **a** in a perfectly insulated treatment volume in which all temperatures are equal to the incoming blood temperature. If that blood has been heated to the treatment temperature (T_{tr}), then all of the treatment volume will be heated to that temperature; **b** for a treatment volume which is selectively heated around the periphery (*hatched area*) to overcome conductive losses from the boundary and for which the incoming blood has been heated to the treatment temperature; and **c** for a treatment volume which has been heated by a distributed power source which cannot conform to the treatment volume boundary and for which the incoming blood has been preheated to the treatment temperature

Goal of a Practical Hyperthermia Treatment

Given the technological restrictions of:

1. Identifiability – existing clinical diagnostic equipment has a resolution which is inadequate to identify clearly:
   a) the actual boundary of the irregularly shaped tumor/normal tissue interface, both at the macroscopic level of several millimeters, or even centimeters for some cases, and always for any small infiltrative fibrils of tumor tissue extending into the normal tissue
   b) those tumor cells/locations which have been and/or will be necrosed by a complementary therapy modality
   c) the locations of the blood vessels supplying the tumor
   d) the spatial variations of physiological and biochemical parameters within the tumor (e.g., pH, O_2, nutrient levels) and
2. Conformability – existing hyperthermia heating equipment has a power deposition field which
   a) Has a resolution (minimum dimension) which is larger than the smallest characteristic dimension of the tumor and its irregularly shaped boundary
   b) Has a shape which cannot be configured such that all tumor cells are treated at a therapeutic temperature while no normal tissue cells are treated to necrotic temperatures.

Thus, the thermal goal of a technically and clinically practical hyperthermia treatment is to maximize the volume of malignant tissue subject to therapeutic

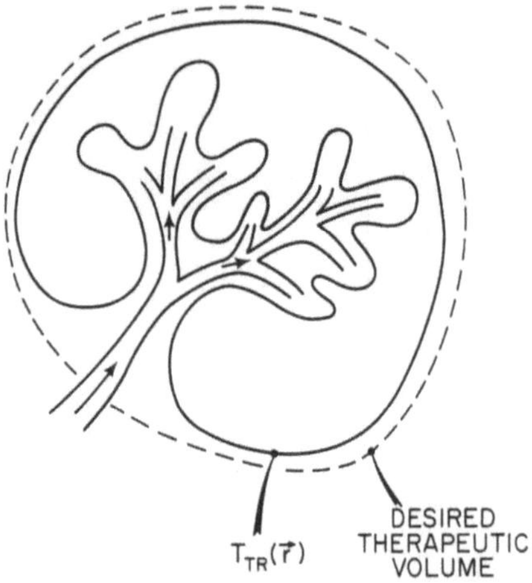

Fig. 3.14. This illustration shows how the directional effects of the arterial blood flow can cause cool regions to occur in a tumor when the blood is not preheated to the desired therapeutic temperature *before* it reaches the tumor volume. The volume of tissue at or above the treatment temperature (*solid line*) is smaller than the desired therapeutic volume (*dashed line*). An adjuvant modality must be used to treat the cells in the underdosed regions. However, at locations away from the entering blood vessels, the boundary of the tissue volume at the treatment temperature can be made contiguous with the boundary of the desired treatment volume by depositing power only inside the treatment volume

temperatures. This maximization should be done while keeping the volume of normal tissue treated to necrotic temperatures below some clinically acceptable bound. Ideally, this latter volume would be zero but, practically, some normal tissue will be able to be sacrificed to increase the treated tumor volume. The amount of acceptable normal tissue damage will change, depending upon clinical factors such as tissue type and the intent of therapy – palliation or cure – and could in some circumstances be large enough and situated properly so that the treatment volume could encompass the complete tumor ($V_{tumor} \in V_{tr}$).

To achieve this goal requires that some power MUST BE deposited outside the treatment volume in order to preheat the arterial blood supplying the tumor to the treatment temperature. Because of the identifiability problem, the treatment temperature must be chosen as that value appropriate for the least thermally sensitive malignant cell conditions, e.g., well nourished and oxygenated tumor cells at a normal pH value. The ideal power deposition pattern would be one which followed the two rules for an effective hyperthermia treatment: (a) enough power is deposited in or near the arterial blood vessels in the normal tissues surrounding the tumor such that all of the arterial blood is at the treatment temperature when it reaches the boundary of the treatment volume and (b) enough power is added inside the treatment volume to overcome conduction effects so that the boundary of the treatment volume is kept at the treatment temperature.

Mathematically, one wants to determine the power deposition pattern $\dot{Q}_a(\vec{r})$ such that the volume of malignant cells raised to therapeutic temperatures, $V_{tu}(T_{th})$, is maximized subject to the constraint that the volume of normal tissues subjected to necrotic temperature elevations is kept within an acceptable limit, $V_{no,acc}$; i.e., $V_{no}(T_{ne}) \in V_{no,acc}$.

The expanded definition just given (compared with Table 3.1) allows us to have a good definition of our goal, the rationale behind it, and the implications it carries for a good hyperthermia treatment. We will use these results at a later time, after looking closely at some practical, typical hyperthermia numbers.

3.2.2 Typical Hyperthermia Thermal Numbers

Several common, basic considerations arise in all hyperthermia applications, regardless of heating modality. These can be conveniently categoried into questions regarding the magnitudes of the spatial and temporal variations of a few important quantities – power, blood flow, and temperature – and considerations of the relative roles of conduction and blood perfusion in the energy removal process.

3.2.2.1 Spatial Variations

Power deposition is a distributed quantity, with its heating effects being felt immediately at all locations in a given heated field. Similarly, local blood perfusion is also a distributed quantity, with its heating (or cooling) effects also being felt immediately at all locations due to the ubiquitous distribution of small vessels throughout the body. On the other hand, large blood vessel effects are quite different since they have a convective nature with highly directional characteristics and the concomitant time delays. The final temperatures reached in a heated field are a result of the interaction of the above factors plus the effect of thermal conduction, which is again significantly different in that it relies on a diffusive process and thus is neither a localized distributed source or sink effect nor a highly directional convective term. Thus, the characteristics of each of the above factors must be analyzed separately.

Power Deposition – The Conformability Problem

By suitable choice of frequency and applicator(s) configuration, both electromagnetic and ultrasonic methods can either provide power deposition at depth or, alternatively, by choosing a high enough frequency, the power can be concentrated into a more superficial and smaller volume. This trade-off between increased resolution and increased penetration represents a fundamental spatial conflict when choosing a power deposition modality for a given treatment. It arises primarily out of the fact that as frequency increases and wavelengths get smaller (which allows for a finer resolution of the power), tissue absorptivity increases and thus the achievable penetration depth decreases. This is illustrated in Figs. 3.15 and 3.16 for the ideal cases of plane wave ultrasound and microwaves. While both graphs have roughly the same shape, it is significant to note that, for a given penetration depth, the wavelengths for the ultrasound are several orders of magnitude smaller than the corresponding electromagnetic values. This has the significant result that ultrasound can be focused to a much finer degree than electromagnetic waves (Fig. 3.17) at any given depth while using practical applicators. However, electromagnetic techniques can obtain some power concentration through the use of phase and amplitude control of multiple, interfering applicators. While the power concentration abilities of electromagnetics (Fig. 3.18) are not as good as ultrasound's, they will definitely be useful in situations where ultrasound cannot be used (due to air or bone barriers) and in cases where their concentrating abilities are sufficient to be useful in approaching the

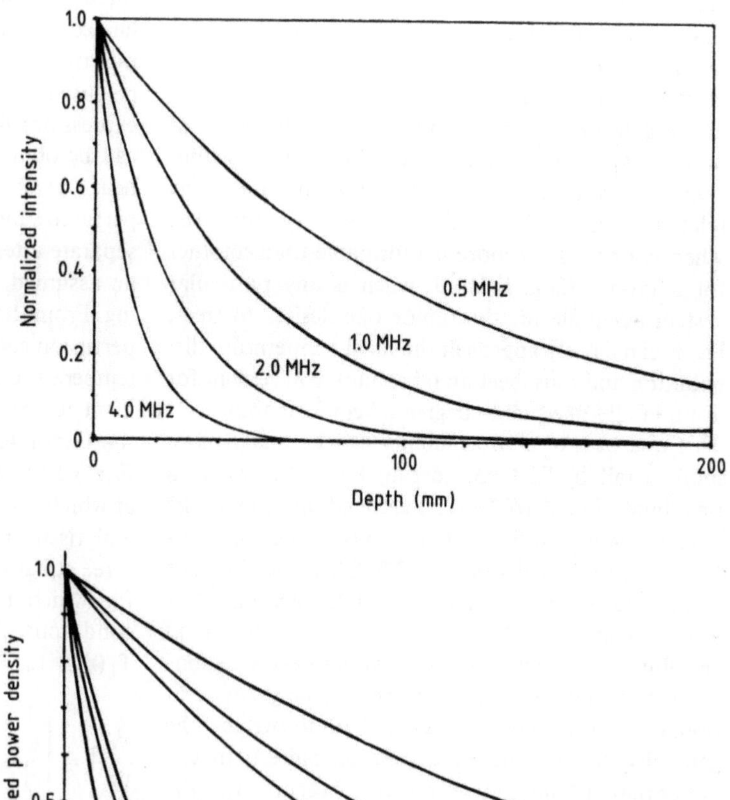

Fig. 3.15. The effect of frequency (f) on the axial intensity distribution of a plane-wave ultrasonic field in tissue (attenuation 10 Np/m/MHz). The wavelength in millimeters is calculated for muscle from $\lambda \cong 1.51$ f. [55]

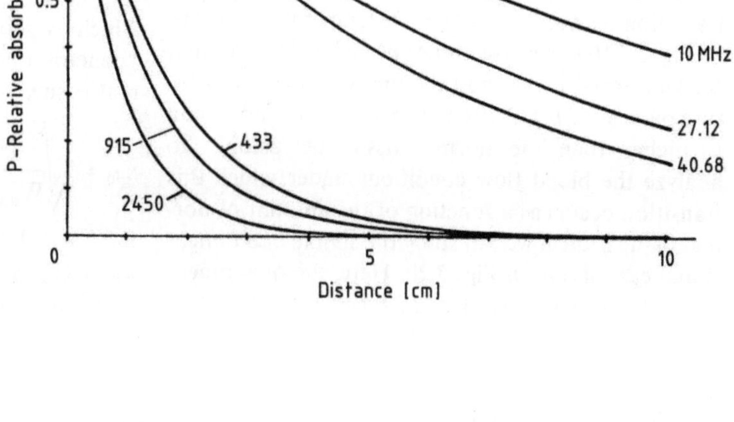

Fig. 3.16. Relative power absorbtion versus distance for an electromagnetic plane wave propagating in a dielectric halfspace $z > 0$. The dielectric has the permittivity of muscle tissue. The graphs are normalized to values at $z = 0$. At 10 MHz, the wavelength in muscle tissue is approximately 118 cm, while for 2450 MHz it is approximately 1.76 cm [34]. Note the scale change between Figs. 3.15 and 3.16

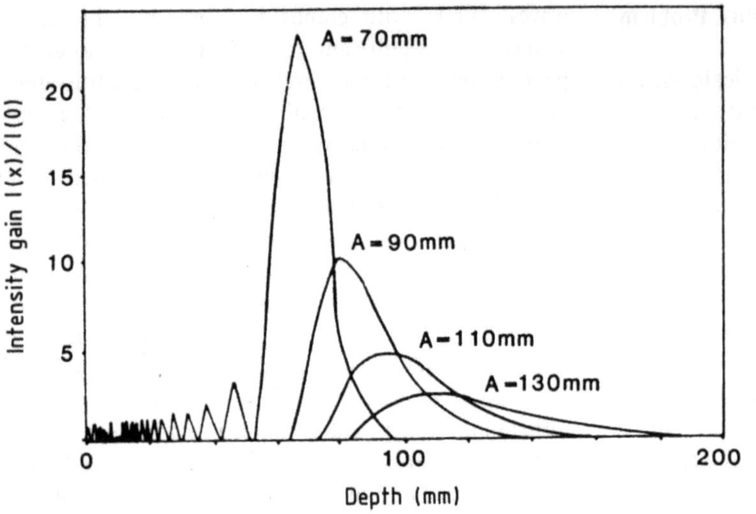

Fig. 3.17. The effect of radius of curvature (A) of a spherically curved transducer on the axial intensity distribution in tissue. [55]

ideal temperature distribution (Fig. 3.11). That is, since some preheating is required, there may be a lower limit on the amount of focusing needed for a particular situation. Indeed, the general question of how much power focusing is needed is only pertinent in relation to obtaining the ideal temperature distribution. Clinically, one faces two questions: First, the relative question of ranking different systems, i.e., when is one system more conformable than another for a given tumor. Second, when is any particular system adequate for the tumor one desires to treat, i.e., it can closely approach the ideal temperature distribution and thus meet an (absolute) requirement for a minimally acceptable degree of conformability.

This question of conformability can be analyzed in more detail by first considering Fig. 3.19, where a one-dimensional problem is illustrated. In general, the sizes of some significant dimensions of the SAR pattern (e.g., the lengths of the 50% SAR lines in three orthogonal directions; L_x, L_y, and L_z) are only important relative to the tumor dimensions, the blood vessel sizes, and the sizes and locations of any regions of high (or low) perfusion that need to be given additional (or less) power. Figure 3.19 illustrates the general case for a power deposition pattern that is larger than a tumor. Here, we are concerned with the transition between the acceptable temperature pattern of Fig. 3.19b (where the tumor perfusion is lower that of the normal tissue) and the unacceptable temperature pattern of Fig. 3.19c (where the tumor perfusion is higher than the normal tissue perfusion). To analyze the blood flow conditions under which this transition occurs as a function of the amount of normal tissue heated, we can study the simple one-dimensional case shown in Fig. 3.20. Here, the one-dimensional bioheat transfer Eq. 3.2a can be utilized for three separate regions: the uniformly perfused and heated tumor, the uniformly perfused and heated normal tissue adjacent to the tumor, and the uniformly perfused but unheated normal tissue. The analytical expressions for the temperatures in these three regions can be obtained by solving the one-dimensional bioheat transfer equation separately for each uniformly perfused and heated (or unheated) region with a separate arterial temperature in the tumor to simulate an assumed amount of preferential arterial preheating. From these solutions, we can determine the blood perfusion conditions under which it is possible for the temperature at the tumor boundary to equal the treatment temperature and for the temperature profile in the tumor to change from convex to concave (from Fig. 3.19b to Fig. 3.19c), i.e., to determine the point at which the maximum temperature occurs in the normal tissue rather than in the tumor. Solving these three equations, and then determining the conditions for which this change occurs [i.e., the blood flow conditions for which $dT_1/dx \ (x_1 = L_{tu/2}) = 0$ and $T_1(x_1 = L_{tu/2}) = T_{tr}$] gives the following expression:

$$\frac{\dot{W}_{tu}}{\dot{W}_{no}} = \left[\frac{T_{tr}}{T_{tr} - T_{aph}}\right]\left[\frac{1}{(1 - e^{-L_{hn}/x_{pn}})}\right] \tag{3.13a}$$

which is illustrated in Fig. 3.21, where x_{pn} is the "penetration depth" of the cooling effect of the normal tissue,

$$x_{pn} = \sqrt{\frac{k}{\dot{W}_{no} c_b}} \tag{3.13b}$$

L_{hn} is the length of heated normal tissue, $L_{hn} = (L_{SAR} - L_{tu})/2$, T_{tr} is the treatment temperature that is specified at the tumor/normal tissue boundary,

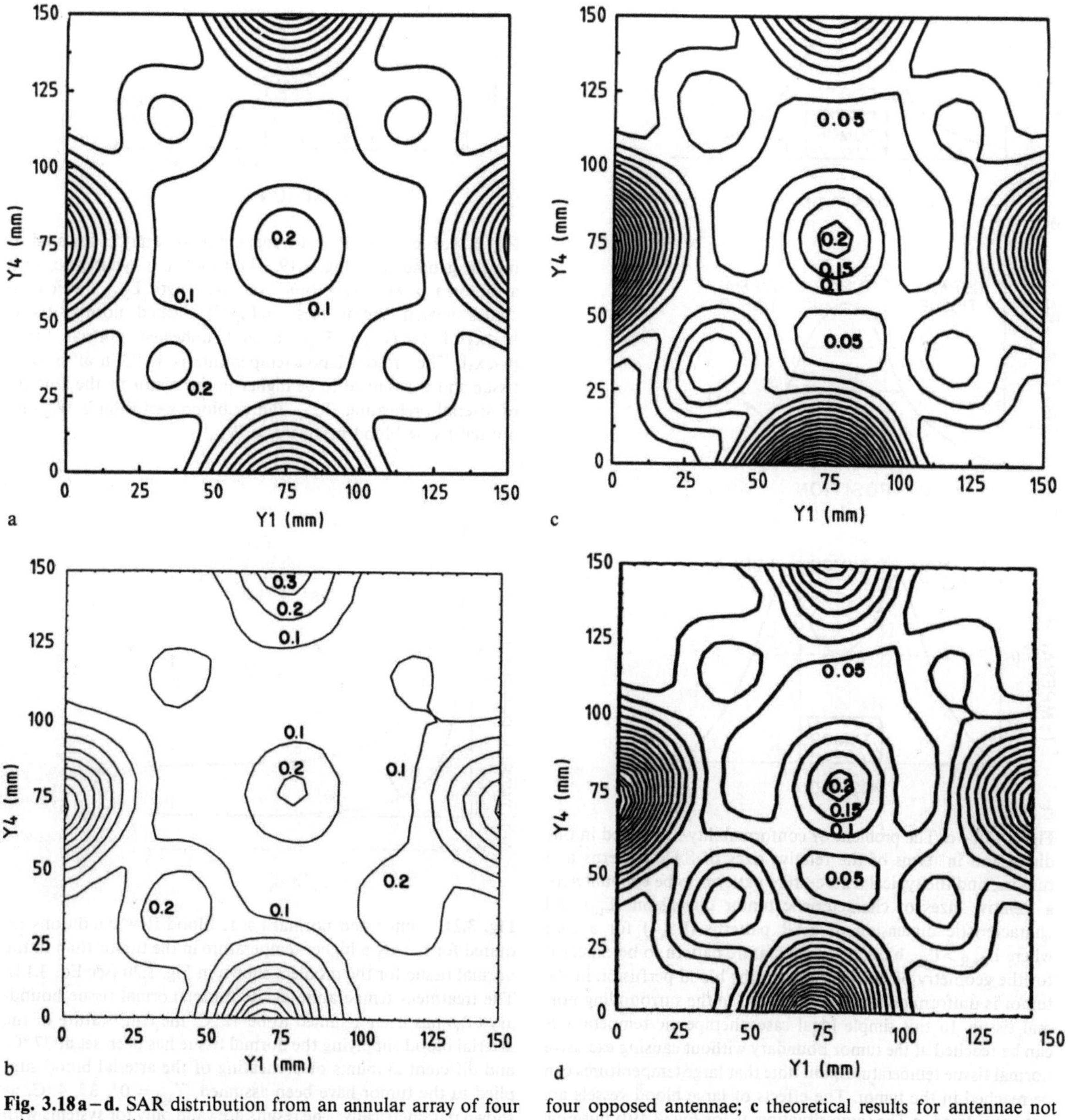

Fig. 3.18 a – d. SAR distribution from an annular array of four microwave applicators irradiating a homogeneous saline media (3.32 g/liter) at 400 MHz: **a** ideal theoretical results for four perfectly aligned antennae in phase; **b** experimental results for four opposed antennae; **c** theoretical results for antennae not perfectly aligned nor in perfect phase agreement; **d** experimental results at higher resolution [73]. The contourintervals are given as percentages of the maximum value

and T_{aph} is the amount of preferential preheating of the arterial blood supplying the tumor tissue.

With this graph, for a given heating situation and a given normal tissue perfusion (i.e., a given L_{hn}/x_{pn}, the abscissa of Fig. 3.21), and a given amount of preferential preheating of the arterial blood supplying the tumor (i.e., a given T_{aph}, the parameter shown in Fig. 3.21), one can determine the maximum allowable tumor blood perfusion that will still have the maximum temperature in the tumor rather than in the normal tissue. That is, any points above and to the right of a given preheating curve will have the maximum temperature in the normal tissue. Here, one can readily see that shorter normal tissue heating lengths (where $L_{hn} \rightarrow 0$ and the conformability problem disappears) and increased preheating of the blood supplying the tumor both push the temperature maximum into the tumor – i.e., they allow a tumor with a higher $\dot{W}_{tu}$ value to be preferentially heated. Increased normal tissue blood perfusions have the same effect. It is also interesting to note here (see Eq. 3.13) that the conditions that make this change possible are

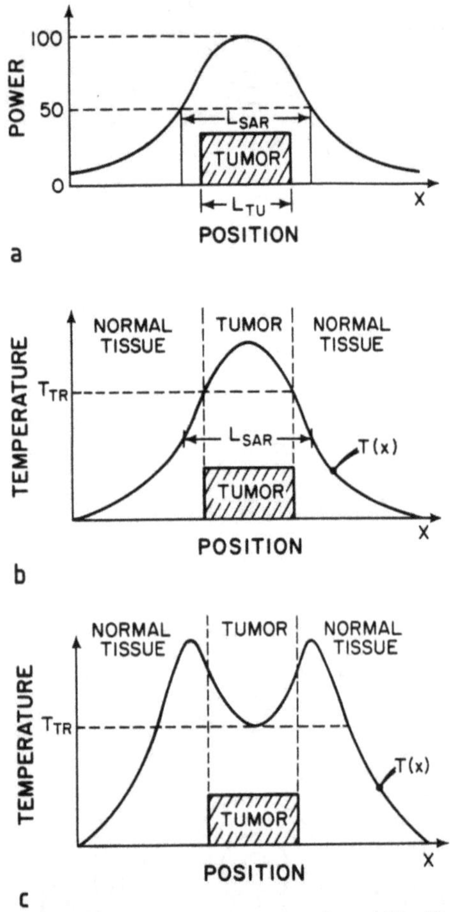

Fig. 3.19 a–c. The problem of conformability illustrated in one dimension in terms of the relative sizes of SAR patterns and tumors, and the typical temperature patterns to be encountered: **a** Relative sizes of characteristic tumor dimension (L_{tu}) and characteristic dimension of SAR patterns (L_{SAR}) for a case where $L_{SAR} > L_{tu}$. **b** General temperature pattern to be expected for the geometry of Fig. 3.19a when the blood perfusion in the tumor is uniform and smaller than that in the surrounding normal tissue. In this simple ideal case, therapeutic temperatures can be reached at the tumor boundary without causing excessive normal tissue temperatures, but note that large temperatures can be reached in the tumor. The effects of large blood vessels are not considered. **c** The same situation as for Fig. 3.19b but now the homogeneous tumor perfusion is larger than the normal tissue perfusion, causing the maximum temperature to occur in the normal tissue when the minimum tumor temperature is raised to therapeutic values. Again, large blood vessel effects are not considered

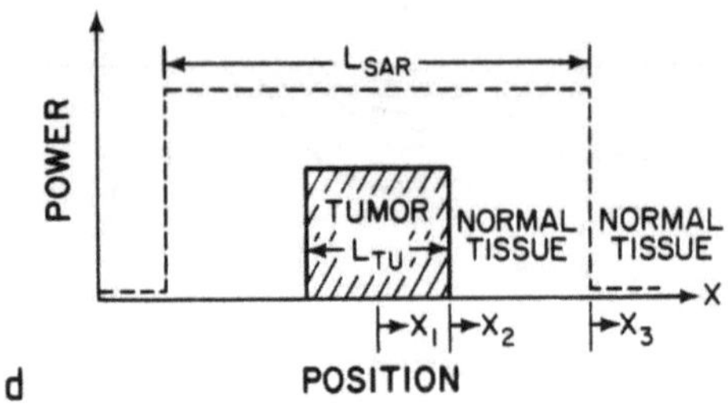

Fig. 3.20. Idealized bioheat transfer equation model for analyzing the geometry of Fig. 3.19. The problem is symmetric, with a uniform power deposition over the length L_{SAR}, which includes heated tumor $[0 \leq x_1 < L_{tu}/2]$, heated normal tissue $[0 \leq x_2 < L_{hn} = (L_{SAR} - L_{tu})/2]$, and unheated normal tissue $[0 < x_3]$. The arterial blood temperature is 37 °C in all normal tissue and is assumed to be higher in the tumor by the amount of arterial preheating, T_{aph}. Tumor blood perfusion is $\dot{W}_{tu}$ and normal tissue blood perfusion is $\dot{W}_{no}$

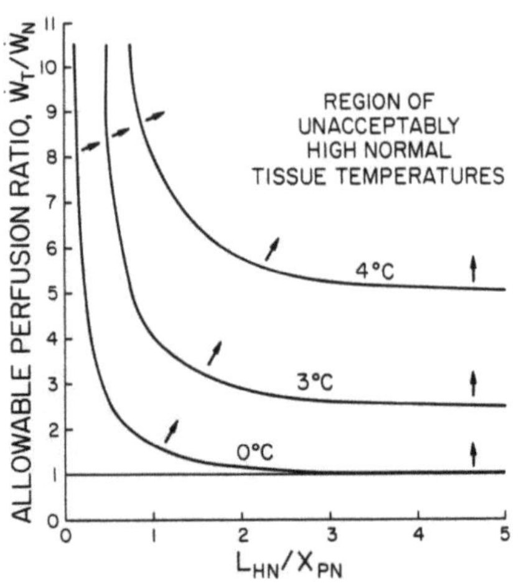

Fig. 3.21. Tumor and normal tissue blood flow conditions required for having a higher temperature in the tumor than in the normal tissue for the problem shown in Fig. 3.20 (see Eq. 3.13). The treatment temperature at the tumor/normal tissue boundary (T_{tr}) has been assumed to be 42 °C, the temperature of the arterial blood supplying the normal tissue has been set at 37 °C, and different amounts of preheating of the arterial blood supplied to the tumor have been assumed, $T_{aph} = 0°, 3°, 4°C$, as shown parametrically. The results are valid only for systems with $L_{SAR} > L_{tu}$. For a given length of heated normal tissue and a given normal tissue perfusion, i.e., a fixed L_{hn}/x_{pn}, the blood perfusion conditions above a given preheat line have the maximum temperature in the normal tissue and are thus not acceptable

not a function of the values of L_{tu}, the tumor size. Also, given practical values of the penetration depth for normal tissues (see Table 3.6 below), one can see that after L_{hn} is several centimeters at most, $\dot{W}_{tu}/\dot{W}_{no}$ has approached its lowest value, and heating more normal tissue has no effect – unless it adds to the arterial blood preheating effect, a phenomenon studied later. That is, this analysis has assumed that the arterial blood supplied to the tumor can be selectively preheated (i.e., $T_{aph} > 0$ in the tumor only), a task which is difficult to perform. This subject will be discussed in a later section where the effect of large blood vessels is investigated.

The general situation illustrated in Figs. 3.19–3.21 ($L_{SAR} > L_{tu}$) is quite common at present for many practical clinical treatments. Most certainly, all regional power deposition devices (concentric and opposed coils [91, 136], APAS [144, 145], helical coil [118], and TEM [28, 67] and many RF applicators (e.g., large plate electrodes, e.g. [87, 130] and ring electrodes [150]) fall into this category ($L_{SAR} > L_{tu}$), as do many external microwave applicator treatments used on small superficial tumors. While this simplified analysis has been for a uniform perfusion case with preferential preheating of the arterial blood supplied to the tumor (a difficult practical task), it clearly illustrates the basic problems present when there is a lack of conformability in the power source. The conclusions drawn from Fig. 3.21 remain true for the more general case – systems with $L_{SAR} \gg L_{tu}$ will have trouble in properly heating inhomogeneously perfused tissues containing either tumors with regions of high perfusion or normal tissues with regions of low perfusion – a fact borne out in the limited tumor temperature and patient pain data obtained clinically with such regional devices (e.g. [94, 122]). For these systems, adjusting the power deposition pattern (or the patient's position) offers little hope for significant gains since the basic problem of a lack of conformability will remain.

In summary, these systems are very passive and inherently rely on a preferential blood perfusion difference (i.e., tumor blood perfusion less than the normal tissue blood perfusion since $L_{hn}/x_{pn} \gg 1$ for these methods in general) to obtain good treatments. (Many of these devices do, however, have the inherent advantage of having large lengths of normal tissue being given significant power deposition, thus potentially providing large lengths for preheating the arterial blood. This is also done, however, in an uncontrolled, passive manner.) This reliance on thermal opportunism, a characteristic of all first-generation heating devices, is no longer an acceptable design philosophy, and thus newer second-generation systems are more active and provide some control over the pattern of power deposition. Also, even some of the original devices with large SAR distributions ($L_{SAR} > L_{tu}$) are now being used in an "active" mode [120] to obtain some control over the amount of blood preheating, to overcome cold tumor spots, to heat adjacent tumor masses, or to reduce excessive normal tissue heating at some locations – or a combination of some or all of these reasons. Although improved patient tolerance was attained, the initial results of these trials are not thermally optimistic [120], a not unexpected result considering the lack of conformability of the system used, even with some manipulation of the power field.

On the other hand, scanning of the SAR pattern around the tumor volume is a necessity for devices with SAR patterns typified by those illustrated in Fig. 3.22, where the significant SAR distribution falls over a distance smaller then the tumor ($L_{SAR} < L_{tu}$). If such scanning is not possible, treatment of the complete tumor will generally not be possible – although one might treat the tumor in sections. The scanning (electrical or mechanical) must be done in an intelligent fashion in order to achieve the closest approach to the ideal temperature distribution – both to overcome conduction at the tumor boundary and to preheat the arterial blood supplies. As shown in Fig. 3.23, the smaller the value of L_{SAR}, i.e., the more conformable the system is, the more control one has over the tissue temperature distribution and the closer one can approach the ideal. However, to utilize such capabilities, one must have both the knowledge of where, exactly, one wants to deposite the power and the practical ability to implement that power deposi-

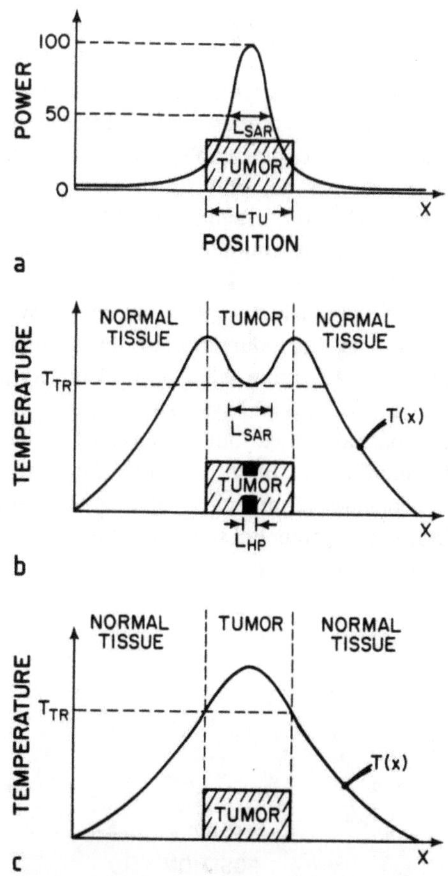

Fig. 3.22 a–c. Illustration of SAR and temperatures for a system where $L_{SAR} < L_{tu}$: **a** Relative SAR and tumor sizes; **b** temperature distribution for a system where $L_{SAR} < L_{tu}$ but a small, highly perfused region (L_{hp}) exists with dimensions smaller than L_{SAR}; **c** temperature distribution for the case where $L_{SAR} < L_{hp} < L_{tu}$ and the system is thus conformable and can compensate for the effects of the small, highly perfused region

tion pattern. This optimization problem will be considered in the section on interface cooling/heating of "large" blood vessels since it will be important to consider the effects of these vessels. In general, as systems become less conformable, the temperature distribution becomes not only much more spread out, but also much more irregular (Fig. 3.23).

In summary, to evaluate the performance of different systems, we can look at the two requirements mentioned previously: Can the system both overcome conduction at the boundary, by depositing significant power at the tumor edge, and selectively preheat the blood? For regional systems ($L_{SAR} > L_{tu}$), both goals are partially met, but because of a lack of conformability in these systems, they cannot be independently approached and solved, thus strictly limiting the potential success of such methods. On the other hand, while a system which puts power *everywhere* is not desirable, neither is one where all power, is in the tumor, i.e., for interstitial systems it is essential to note that they only preheat the blood by a small amount (since the implants are generally restricted to the interior of the tumor). Thus, they too have a serious design deficiency. To meet the above requirements properly, one needs a single highly conformable system, such as scanned, focused ultrasound,

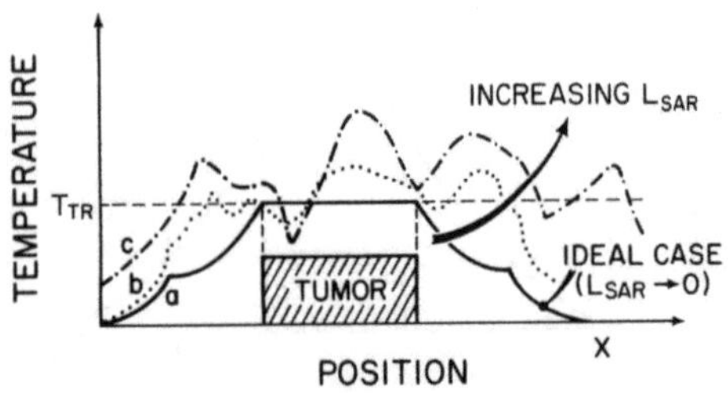

Fig. 3.23. The effect of decreasing conformability is to increase the amount of tissue heated and to increase the variability of the temperature distribution. To obtain the ideal temperature distribution not only requires that $L_{SAR} \to 0$, but also that the identifiability problem be solved – so that one knows where to put the power. Curve *a* shows the ideal case ($L_{SAR} \to 0$) while curves *b* and *c* show the effect of increasing L_{SAR}

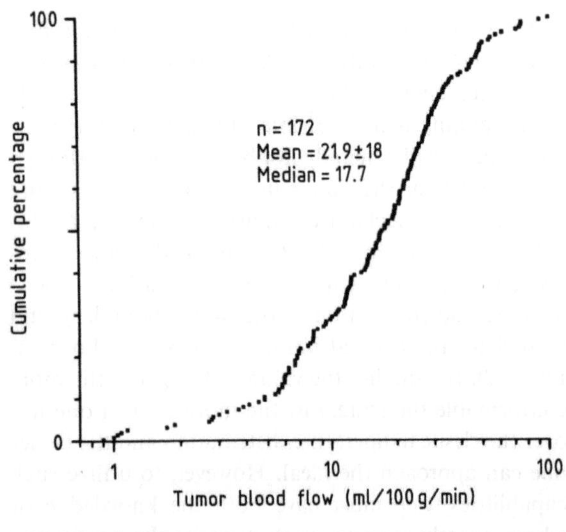

Fig. 3.24. Summary of reported perfusions of human tumors (pooled data). [103]

Table 3.3. Typical blood perfusion rates of various tissues and organs. Condensed from [124]

Tissue	Anatomical locations and qualifications	Specific flow rate (ml/min-100 g)
Skin	Foot (dorsal surface, normal resting flow)	14.3 ± 2.6 (SD)
	Calf (normal resting flow)	10.6 ± 1.3 (SD)
	Thigh (normal resting flow)	9.8 ± 2.6 (SD)
	Arms (normal resting flow)	8.39
	Hands (normal resting flow)	20.07
	Abdomen (normal resting flow)	8.65
	Thorax (normal resting flow)	6.45
	Head (normal resting flow)	42.9
	Face (normal resting flow)	70.3
	Forearm: hyperthermia (reaction to ultraviolet radiation, "fully developed redness")	55.3 ± 11.2 (SD)
	Forearm: reactive hyperthermia ("peak value, rough approximation")	280.0
Subcutaneous fat	Abdomen adipose tissue; several subjects; thickness 10 – 29 mm	3.04 ± 2.09 (SD)
	Abdomen adipose tissue; several subjects; thickness 30 – 49 mm	2.15 ± 1.22 (SD)
	Abdomen adipose tissue; several subjects; thickness > 40 mm	1.84 ± 0.71 (SD)
Muscle	Anterior calf, resting flow	2.75 ± 0.65 (SD)
	Anterior thigh, resting flow	2.6 ± 1.0 (SD)
	Forearm, resting flow	3.2 ± 1.4 (SD)
	Calf: reactive hyperthermia, peak value	54.9 ± 11.6 (SD)
	Forearm: reactive hyperthermia, peak value	50.3 ± 19.4 (SD)
	Anterior thigh: hyperthermia in response to microwave diathermy	36.0
Bone	Estimated range of flow in human humerus; flow in marrow only	0.33 – 0.67
Organ	Brain	54.0
	Heart	84.0
	Kidney	420.0
	Liver	57.7

or a combination approach with one mechanism for preheating the arterial blood and a second mechanism for overcoming conduction effects at the boundary of the treatment volume. The reliance of these conclusions on the nature of the tumor blood supplies cannot be underemphasized. If the blood supply is slow and sluggish and occurs in small vessels, then preheating will be much easier, as will obtaining a close-to-ideal temperature distribution.

Blood Flow

The effects of blood flow, both in terms of localized blood perfusion in the tissue and in terms of large blood vessels, play a central role in hyperthermia. As was discussed previously, both the tissue perfusion rate and the "large" blood vessel characteristics are important, and they will be discussed separately here.

Tissue Perfusion Variations

Tissue perfusion, measured in terms of a net flow of blood per unit volume of tissue, $\dot{W}$ (kg/m^3-s), varies from tissue to tissue, as documented in Table 3.3, and with position within an organ as the tissue function and composition change (e.g., white and gray matter in the brain). The spatial rates of change of these perfusion values are as abrupt as the tissue anatomical changes, and the perfusion magnitudes can change in time, depending on the physiological demands on the organ, as indicated by some of the data in Table 3.3. In hyperthermia, the physiological changes we are primarily interested in are the variations of local perfusion with temperature. A considerable amount of data concerning the thermal response of skin and muscle is available, primarily because of the work that has been performed for thermoregulatory studies and for physical therapy. This is also a direct result of the fact that these two tissues are quite accessible, while for deeper-seated organs the available information is almost nonexistent, as reflected in Table 3.3.

The above data are for normal tissues. For human tumors, some information on the magnitudes of tumor perfusion is available, as summarized in Figs. 3.24 and 3.25, but this knowledge is quite incomplete – as illustrated in the following quote:

A great number of investigators have, independently, shown that tumour blood flow is affected by a hyperthermic treatment to a larger extent than normal tissue blood flow. While the majority of the studies on experimental tumours show a decrease and even a lapse in blood flow within the microcirculation during or after hyperthermia, the data on human tumours are less con-

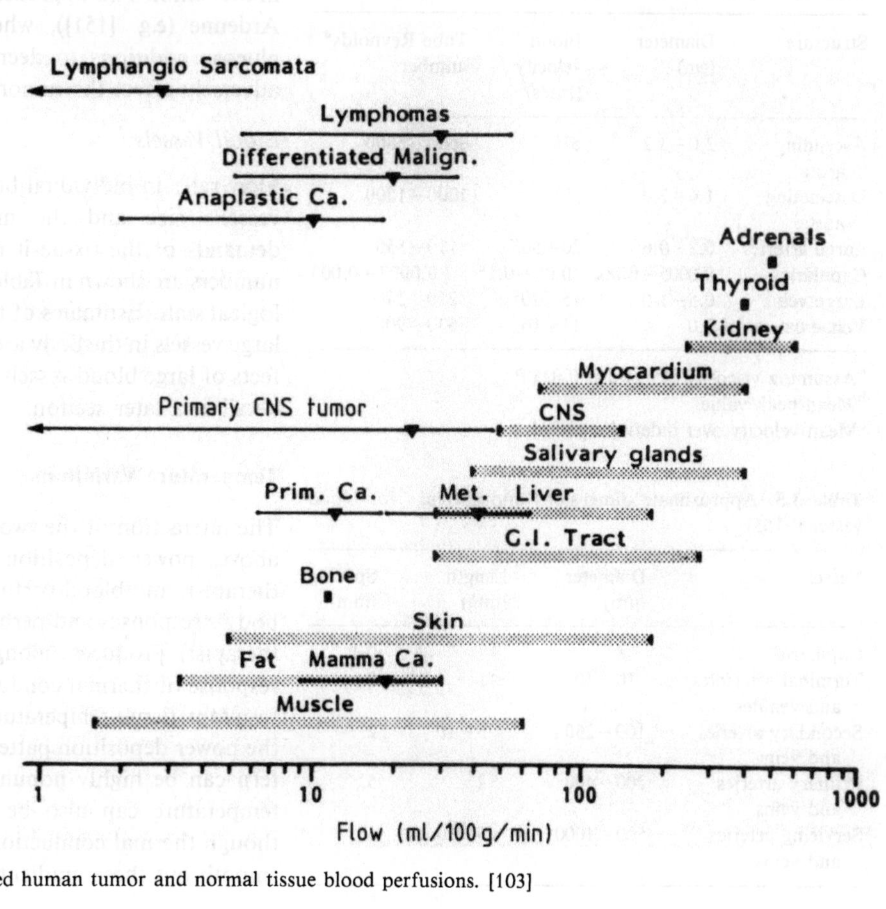

Fig. 3.25. Variations of reported human tumor and normal tissue blood perfusions. [103]

clusive. Some of the investigators do not find a decrease in circulation, while others do. Obviously, this is an important field of investigation in the clinical application of hyperthermia because a shut down of the circulation would not only facilitate tumour heating (by reducing venous outflow, thus reducing the "heat clearance" from the tumour), but would also facilitate tumour cell destruction...
With all these considerations in mind, one should be aware of the fact that effects, secondary to heat-induced vascular stasis *alone* will never be efficient enough to eliminate all tumour cells, even through a heat reservoir is created. This is so because some malignant cells will inevitably have already infiltrated normal, surrounding structures and will therefore not be affected by changes in the tumour vascular bed. On the other hand, vascular stasis, with its subsequent necrosis, will result in elimination of large numbers of tumour cells, leaving substantially fewer numbers of tumour cells to be sterilized by radiation therapy [105]. It is in this fashion that the heat sensitivity of tumour microcirculation may be exploited in the combination of radiation therapy and hyperthermia [104 p. 115].

Because of the significance of the blood perfusion in affecting the temperatures obtained clinically, there is considerable interest in manipulating the tumor and normal tissue perfusions. One such effort has been aimed at using vasoactive drugs to increase blood perfusion in normal tissues, particularly with the drug hydralazine, as previously discussed. Any such increase in normal tissue perfusion will have the effect of protecting that tissue and increasing power requirements, as previously described for an ideal treatment, or allowing one to increase tumor temperatures by increasing power levels for a given amount of normal tissue damage – a worthwhile goal for real treatments in which the ideal temperature distribution is not present. Also, these manipulations have the potential for decreasing tumor perfusion [86] through the mechanism of vascular "stealing", i.e., the increased blood perfusion in the normal tissue could steal some perfusion from the tumor (for a supply at a fixed magnitude). Again for a fixed applied power, this decreased tumor perfusion will allow increased temperatures to be reached in practical situations where low tumor temperatures are common. This same effect can be obtained by surgical or compressive obstruction of major vessels supplying a tumor – if they can be located and obstructed without also causing unacceptable normal tissue damage, an impractical task at present. Alternatively, one can attempt to augment any damage or destruction of the tumor vasculature caused by hyperthermia itself by modification of the chemical concentrations in the tumor. This approach has been espoused by von Ardenne (e.g. [151]), who uses hyperthermia plus glucose additions to decrease tumor pH and thus adversely affect the tumor vasculature.

Table 3.4. Systemic circulation of man ([154] p. 93)

Structure	Diameter (cm)	Blood velocity (cm/s)	Tube Reynolds[a] number
Ascending aorta	2.0 – 3.2	63[b]	3600 – 5800
Descending aorta	1.6 – 2.0	27[b]	1200 – 1500
Large arteries	0.2 – 0.6	20 – 50[b]	110 – 850
Capillaries	0.0005 – 0.001	0.05 – 0.1[c]	0.0007 – 0.003
Large veins	0.5 – 1.0	15 – 20[c]	210 – 570
Venae cavae	2.0	11 – 16[c]	630 – 900

[a] Assuming viscosity of bood is 0.035 P
[b] Mean peak value
[c] Mean velocity over indefinite period

Table 3.5. Approximate dimensions and spacings for blood vessels. [155]

Vessel	Diameter (μm)	Length (mm)	Spacing (mm)
Capillaries	8	1	0.1
Terminal arterioles and venules	10 – 40	≤1	2
Secondary arteries and veins	100 – 250	5 – 10	2
Primary arteries and veins	200 – 400	2	5
Servicing arteries and veins	500 – 1000	5 – 10	5

Blood Vessels

Flow rates in individual blood vessels depend on the vessel's size and the metabolic/thermoregulatory demands of the tissue it is supplying. Some typical numbers are shown in Table 3.4 for the resting physiological state. Estimates of the approximate spacing of large vessels in the body are given in Table 3.5. The effects of large blood vessels will be considered in more detail in a later section.

Temperature Variations

The interaction of the two active processes described above, power deposition (active in terms of the therapist) and blood perfusion (active in terms of the body's responses and perhaps the intervention of the therapist) produces, along with the totally passive response of thermal conduction within the tissue, the resultant tissue temperature distribution. Since both the power deposition pattern and the blood flow pattern can be highly nonuniform, the resultant tissue temperature can also be highly nonuniform, even though thermal conduction is continuously trying to smooth out these gradients.

Clinical Treatments

During practical hyperthermia treatments, temperature measurements are generally made at a few discrete points, or, when possible, at several points along a line using either multiple sensor probes or pull-back techniques. In no case is the complete temperature field measured or known – one of the fundamental problems in hyperthermia. Thus, knowledge of the magnitudes of spatial variations in temperature is quite limited, even though it is well known that these variations can be quite dramatic, up to 10 °C/cm. Figures 3.26–3.28 illustrate some typical situations. These sharp variations even occur for power deposition patterns which are known to change gradually in space (e.g., Fig. 3.26), thus implying that the rapid temperature variations are due to variations in blood perfusion.

Tissue temperature variations are also present during whole-body hyperthermia, and while the magnitudes of these variations are smaller in this application (see Fig. 3.29), they are also more critical since the temperatures in these treatments are brought as close as possible to the tolerance level of normal tissues.

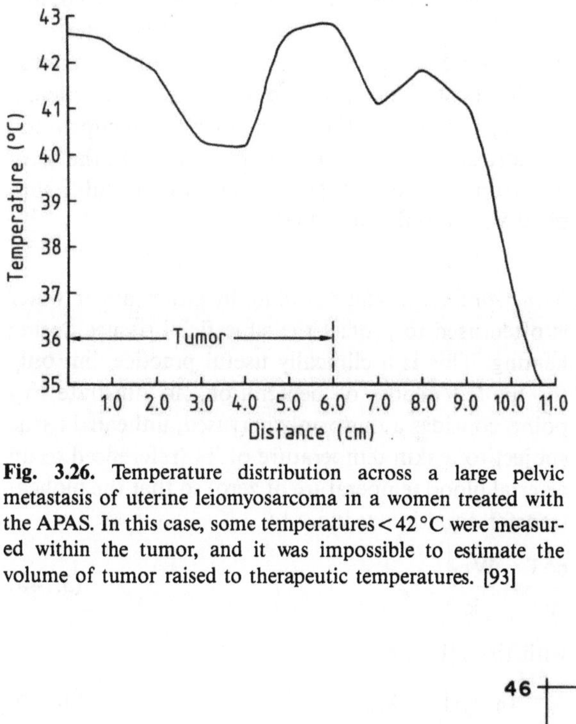

Fig. 3.26. Temperature distribution across a large pelvic metastasis of uterine leiomyosarcoma in a women treated with the APAS. In this case, some temperatures < 42 °C were measured within the tumor, and it was impossible to estimate the volume of tumor raised to therapeutic temperatures. [93]

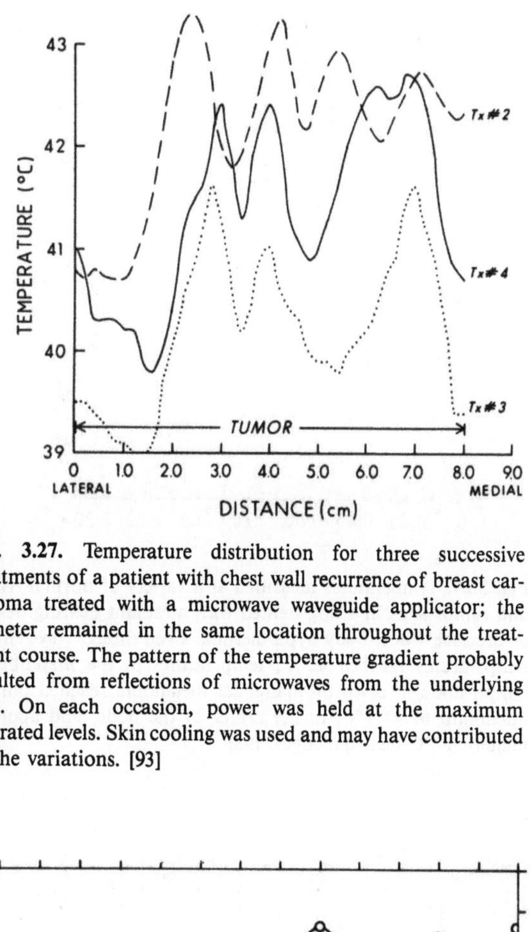

Fig. 3.27. Temperature distribution for three successive treatments of a patient with chest wall recurrence of breast carcinoma treated with a microwave waveguide applicator; the catheter remained in the same location throughout the treatment course. The pattern of the temperature gradient probably resulted from reflections of microwaves from the underlying ribs. On each occasion, power was held at the maximum tolerated levels. Skin cooling was used and may have contributed to the variations. [93]

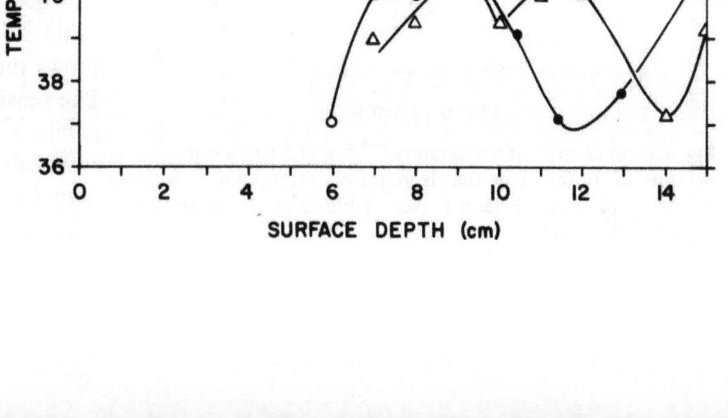

Fig. 3.28. Temperature variations with depth (for three tracks parallel to the electrodes) during an interstitial RF treatment. [14]

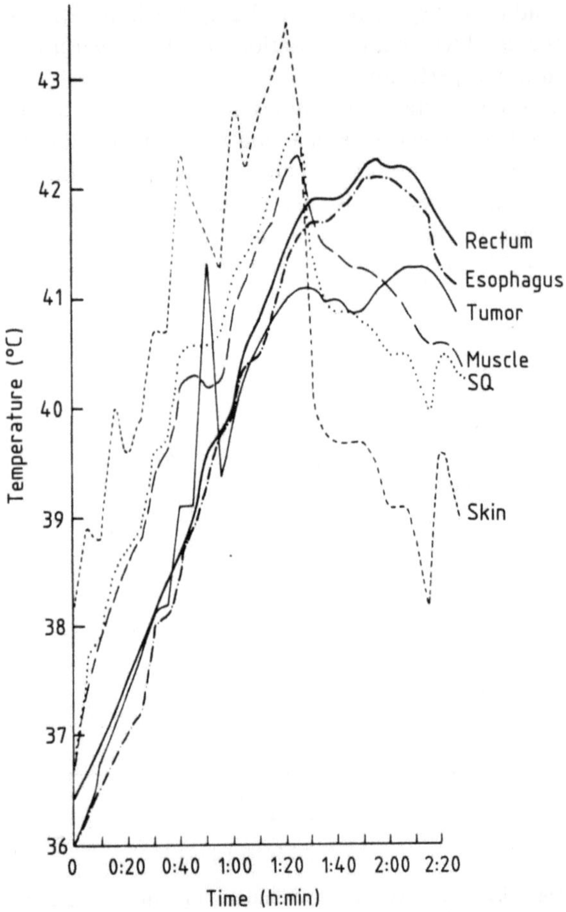

Fig. 3.29. Temperatures measured at a variety of normal tissue and tumor sites in a dog treated with a radiant heating device to produce whole-body hyperthermia. Even though "systemic" temperatures reached 42 °C, temperatures in the mandibular lymph node involved by malignant melanoma reached only a maximum of 41.3 °C, in the center of the node, and approximately 40 °C near the edges. [93]

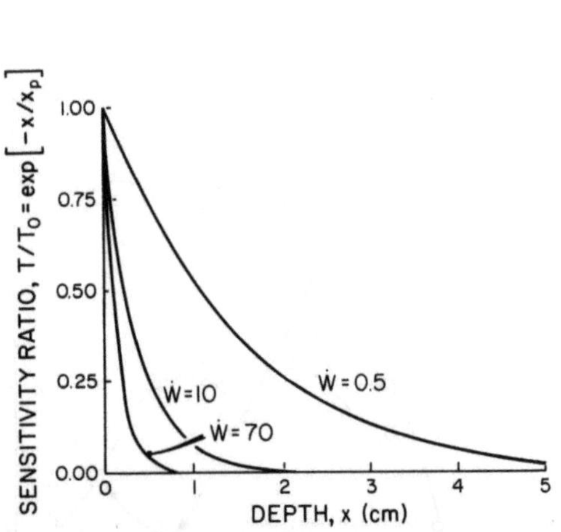

Fig. 3.30. Sensitivity of temperature (T) at depth x to a skin temperature of T_0 for tissue that is uniformly perfused at a value $\dot{W}$. The penetration depth (see Table 3.6) is given by $x_{pn} = \sqrt{k/\dot{W}c_b}$. [108]

Table 3.6. Penetration depths for skin cooling of uniformly perfused tissue

Tissue	$\dot{W}$ (kg/m³/s)	x_{pn} (cm)
Resting muscle	0.5	1.6
Resting muscle	1.0	1.1
Brain	10.0	0.35
Kidney	70.0	0.13

Interface Cooling/Heating

Surface cooling or heating can be used at all interfaces between tissue and external or interstitial applicators. The most common applications are skin cooling for use with surface applicators and skin heating for whole-body hyperthermia, while cooling of cylindrical electrodes/antenna for interstitial RF/microwave treatments is currently under intense development. Closely related to the electrode/antenna cooling problem is the use of constant-temperature cylindrical sources to heat tumors, either in the form of ferromagnetic seeds [11, 12, 132, 133] or tubes supplied with a hot liquid [53].

Skin Cooling. Surface cooling by either air or water is often used to protect the superficial tissues during heating. This is a clinically useful practice, but only for limited depths of penetration. To illustrate this point, consider a uniformly perfused, unheated tissue subject to a skin temperature of T_0 (referenced to an arterial blood temperature of zero) so that the bioheat transfer equation reduces to

$$\frac{d^2T}{dx^2} = \frac{\dot{W}c_b}{k}T \ , \qquad (3.14\text{a})$$

with the solution

$$T = T_0 \exp[-x/x_{pn}] \ , \qquad (3.14\text{b})$$

where x_{pn} is a penetration depth for the skin temperature,

$$x_{pn} = \sqrt{\frac{k}{\dot{W}c_b}} \ . \qquad (3.14\text{c})$$

For typical tissues, $k = 0.5$ w/m°C and $c_b = 4000$ J/kg°C, giving the penetration depths of Table 3.6 for a range of typical tissues. Figure 3.30 shows the T/T_0 values versus depth for these cases. The sensitivity of the tissue temperature to skin temperature changes (dT/dT_0) is quite small at depth even will small perfusions, as shown in Fig. 3.30 – note that this sensitivity is the same as T/T_0; i.e., $dT/dT_0 = \exp[-x/x_{pn}]$ as plotted. This result is independent of adding a heating modality, as can be seen by considering the case of an idealized, planar microwave heating of the above tissues. The bioheat transfer equation then becomes

$$-k\frac{d^2T}{dx^2} = \dot{Q}_0 \exp[-x/\mu] - \dot{W} c_b T \ , \qquad (3.15\,a)$$

where μ is the exponential penetration depth of the microwave heating. Again, for skin cooling so that $T_0 = T(x = 0)$ and $T(x = \infty) = T_{ar} = 0$, the solution is

$$T(x) = \left[T_0 - \frac{\dot{Q}_0}{(\dot{W} c_b - k/\mu^2)} \right] \exp[-x/x_{pn}] + \left[\frac{\dot{Q}_0}{(\dot{W} c_b - k/\mu^2)} \right] \exp[-x/\mu] \qquad (3.15\,b)$$

where, due to the linear nature of this problem, the solution contains the additive effects of skin cooling as given by the first term $[T_0 \exp(-x/x_{pn})]$, plus the effect of the distributed heating source given by the remaining terms. The sensitivity of $T(x)$ to T_0 is given by the same expression as before

$$\frac{dT}{dT_0} = \exp[-x/x_{pn}] \ . \qquad (3.16)$$

That is, at a given depth, regardless of the presence of a heating modality or its magnitude, a given change in surface temperature, dT_0, will give the same change in tissue temperature, dT – a change which decreases rapidly with depth, as shown in Fig. 3.30. These limited depth effects of skin cooling have also been noted in clinical applications.

Cylindrical Cooling/Heating Systems. Long cylindrical sources placed in tissue have an even more limited penetration depth than planar surface cooling because of the small size of the needles used and their cylindrical shape, which means that more tissue must be cooled as the distance away from the cylinder increases. Again, if one solves the one-dimensional bioheat transfer equation for a cylindrical needle (radius r_0) at temperature T_0 imbedded in a homogeneous media of tissue of perfusion $\dot{W}$ and conductivity k, the resultant temperature distribution is [49]

$$\frac{T}{T_0} = \frac{K_0(r/x_{pn})}{K_0(r_0/x_{pn})} \qquad (3.17)$$

where K_0 is the modified Bessel function of order zero and $x_{pn} = (k/\dot{W} c_b)^{1/2}$ as before. Figure 3.31 shows the temperature profile for typical tissue values. Note particularly the more rapid fall-off in temperature in this case compared with the planar case (Fig. 3.30). Again, because of the linear nature of the bioheat transfer equation, these results are independent of the presence of a source term as in the case of microwave or RF needle heating. For these situations, in which cooling is primarily supplied to prevent overheating of the electrodes/antennae and the immediately adjacent tissues where power deposition values are high, this limited penetration depth is not a problem since cooling is only desired very close to the antennae. However, for applications such as ferromagnetic seeds and tubular heating sources, the limited penetration depth means that the thermal sources must be placed relatively close together and that these methods could have difficulty in heating regions of high perfusion.

"Large" Blood Vessels

The effects of large blood vessels need to be analyzed slightly differently than the above cylindrical constant temperature sources since one is generally interested in the temperature variations in both the blood and in the tissue as a function of position along the vessel (or vessel pair), as well as in the radial distributions illustrated above. Also, the larger vessels frequently occur in countercurrent pairs, thus requiring a separate analysis. However, if one is not interested in the axial tissue/blood temperature variations and wants to know the approximate effect of a single blood vessel (of surface temperature T_0) on the surrounding tissue, then the result in Fig. 3.31 (from Eq. 3.17) is applicable. However, in general, axial effects cannot be ignored since the blood vessel surface temperature is not known at any given position and needs to be

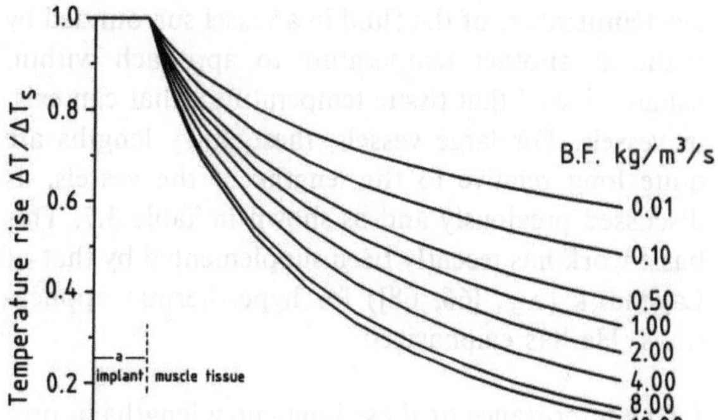

Fig. 3.31. Temperature versus radius around a cylinder of radius *"a"* at a surface temperature T_0, surrounded by muscle-like tissue with a perfusion of $\dot{W}$ (see Eq. 3.17) [49]. a = 0.5 mm. B.F. indicates the perfusion in the muscle

determined from knowledge of the interactions between the blood and the tissue, countercurrent heat transfer effects, and of any direct heating caused by power deposition into the blood. Two problems are important here, dependent on the blood vessel locations. If the vessel is outside of the treatment volume, then one wants to know how best to heat the vessel so that the blood is at a therapeutic temperature when it reaches the tumor and, second, if that has not been done and a "cold" vessel inside of a tumor is being analyzed, then one may also want to determine the extent of the temperature depression caused by the vessel. [Before going further, it is important to note that none of the field equations which are designed to predict temperature fields in tissue include the specific effect of "large" blood vessels, as expected by the nature of a field equation. This holds for the bioheat transfer equation [101], for Chen and Holmes' [18] recent formulation, and for the work by Jiji et al. [58], Weinbaum et al. [153], Weinbaum and Jiji [152], Dagan et al. [27], and Song et al. [131].

For the problem of determining the temperature of the blood prior to the tumor, several analytical solutions are possible for simple cases. On the other hand, for more realistic cases, the general problem of solving for the temperature distribution in both countercurrent vessels and in the surrounding tissue is a much more complicated one, called the fully conjugated problem in the standard heat transfer literature, which has only been solved in a semi-analytical form by Mori et al. [82] for a single tube placed in a conducting medium. For studying these large vessels, the early work of Mitchell and Myers [81] and Chato [17] on the importance of large vessels in other applications illustrated the large thermal equilibrium lengths, or entry lengths, x_{eq} (the distance required for the average temperature of the fluid in a vessel surrounded by tissue at another temperature to approach within, usually, $1/e$ of that tissue temperature), that can exist in vessels. For large vessels, these entry lengths are quite long relative to the lengths of the vessels, as discussed previously and as shown in Table 3.7. This basic work has recently been supplemented by that of Lagendijk (e.g., [66, 68]) for hyperthermia applications. He has emphasized

1. the importance of these long-entry lengths in producing cold spots (or lines) in tumors traversed by vessels with relatively large flow rates and
2. the subsequent necessity of preheating such vessels (by possibly heating the large tissue volume which the vessel passes through before it reaches the tumor, as was discussed earlier) to eliminate these cold spots.

Another detailed study of heat transfer processes in isolated and countercurrent vessels has been performed specifically for hyperthermia applications by Baish et al. [6–8]. They used the basic model of Weinbaum and Jiji, instead of the bioheat transfer equation, to describe the tissue, but relaxed the assumption that $(T_{ar}+T_v)/2 \rightarrow T_t$, and analyzed cases for two Nusselt numbers, both $Nu = \infty$, as done by Weinbaum and Jiji, and $Nu = 4$, as done by Chen and Holmes. (The Nusselt number is given by $Nu = hD/k_b$, where h is the convective heat transfer coefficient between the blood and the solid, D is the vessel diameter, and k_b is the blood thermal conductivity.) They determined new equilibration lengths for vessels and showed that

Table 3.7. Properties of vascular compartments[a] ($j = 1, \ldots, 12$). [18]

j	Vessel	% Vasculature volume	r_j (μm)	x_{ej} (m)	l_j/x_{ej}
1	Aorta	3.30	5000	190	0.002
2	Large artery	6.59	1500	4	0.05
3	Arterial branch	5.49	500	0.3	0.3
4	Terminal branch	0.55	300	0.08	0.1
5	Terminal branch	1.00	175	0.009	1
6	Arteriole	2.75	10	5E-6	400
7	Capillary	6.59	4	2E-7	6000
8	Venules	12.09	15	2E-6	800
9	Terminal veins	3.30	750	0.1	0.1
10	Venous branch	29.67	1200	0.3	0.3
11	Large veins	24.18	3000	5	0.04
12	Vena cava	5.49	6250	190	0.002

[a] Compartment fraction of total vascular volume, % vasculature volume; typical vessel radius, r_j (micrometers); equilibration length, x_{ej} (meters); ratio of typical vessel length to the equilibration length, l_j/x_{ej}

Table 3.8. Parameter values[a] for typical blood vessels ($Nu = 4$). [7]

	r_0 (μm)	$\frac{r_s}{r_0}$	$\frac{sp}{r_0}$	ū (cm/s)	$\left(\frac{\sigma_\Sigma}{\sigma_\Delta}\right)^{1/2}$	L_{cc} (cm)	L_α (cm)
Large artery	1500	40	0.5	13	0.95	300	440
Main arterial branch	500	35	0.5	8	0.96	21	29
Terminal branch	300	30	1	6	1.10	6	7
Small artery	200	20	3	2	1.35	0.8	0.8

[a] r_0 is the vessel radius; r_s is the radius of the tissue cylinder surrounding a countercurrent pair; sp is the spacing between the pair of countercurrent vessels; ū is the average blood velocity; σ_Σ and σ_Δ are conduction coupling parameters between the two vessels and between those vessels and the tissue, respectively; L_{cc} is the equilibrium length for the countercurrent pairs; and L_α is the equilibrium length for a single vessel with the same parameters

x_{eq} decreases significantly for countercurrent vessels, causing the vessels to come to equilibrium with the tissue more rapidly; e.g., compare L_{cc} and L_α in Table 3.8. Their calculations still show, however, that for some conditions expected to be found in typical treatments, e.g., if terminal branch arteries and veins ($r_0 \cong 300\ \mu$) are present in a heated field of 3 cm diameter, then very significant local cold spots can be produced around these vessels.

To further analyze the thermal interactions between vessels and tissue in a more general vein, consider the close-to-ideal case of two countercurrent heat transfer vessels imbedded in perfused normal tissue, as in Fig. 3.32. Here, it is again assumed that the edge of the tumor is at T_{tr}, that the venous blood returning from the tumor is also at T_{tr}, and that power is deposited uniformly in the blood flowing in the vessels and in the surrounding normal tissue. As a performance measure in this situation, we can attempt to determine what length of a heated region is needed surrounding the actual tumor in order adequately to preheat the arterial blood to T_{tr}. The previous simple analyses performed (Figs. 3.9, 3.10 and 3.12) have indicated that, in general, either excessive power density levels or impractical vessel heating lengths were needed to raise the arterial blood temperature to the therapeutic temperature at the tumor boundary. Thus, it is worthwhile to reinvestigate this problem using a more realistic, conservative model, i.e., to look at conditions under which the amount of external heating would be even further minimized. To do this, consider the ideal case where the venous blood remains at T_{tr} for all positions (to thus maximize the amount of countercurrent heat exchange and therefore minimize the amount of external energy deposition needed) and for which the normal tissue is also maintained at T_{tr} for the same ideal, conservative rationale. For this ideal case, we know that if the normal tissue is supplied by the arterial blood at the entry condition $T_{ar}(0) = 0$ and the normal tissue temperature is uniform at T_{tr}, then the applied power must be $\dot{W}_{no} c_b T_{tr}$ (see Eq. 3.3). In this more optimistic case (optimistic since the tissue and venous blood are assumed to be kept at the treatment temperature, thus increasing the heat transfer to the blood), the equation to be solved is now given by

$$\dot{M} c_b \frac{dT_{ar}}{dx} = (UP)_{cc}(T_{tr} - T_{ar}) + (UP)_{an}(T_{tr} - T_{ar}) + \dot{Q}_a A_c \ . \qquad (3.18)$$

If the same assumptions are made that $(UP)_{cc} \cong (UP)_{an} = UP$, then the solution is given by (here, $\dot{Q}_a$ has been replaced by the maximum allowable power $\dot{W}_{no} c_b T_{tr}$):

$$T_{ar}(x) = T_{tr}\left[1 + \frac{\dot{W}_{no} c_b A_c}{2UP}\right][1 - e^{-(2UP/\dot{M}c)x}] \qquad (3.19)$$

where one can see the separate effects of the direct heating (the linear term) and of the highly idealized countercurrent heat exchange (the exponential term). We can now solve for the heated lengths (L) needed to reach our goal of $T_{ar}(L) = 42\,°C$. The results of solving this equation are shown in Fig. 3.33, where one can see that we still require quite large lengths (L) to properly preheat the arterial blood, even under the highly idealized and conservative conditions assumed in this analysis. Also, the conformability problem has been ignored since this analysis has assumed that both the normal tissue and the venous blood are maintain-

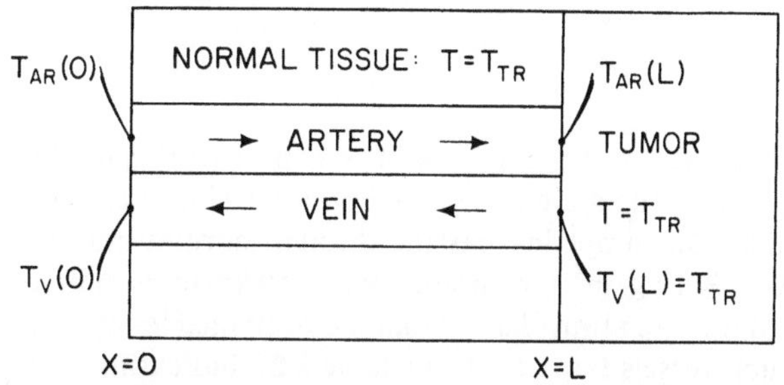

Fig. 3.32. Idealized countercurrent pair of vessels suppyling an idealized tumor at temperature T_{tr}. Power is assumed to be deposited uniformly in the homogeneously perfused normal tissue so that it is just at (or slightly below) the treatment temperature. Figure 3.33 shows the heated length (L) needed to preheat the arterial blood to T_{tr}

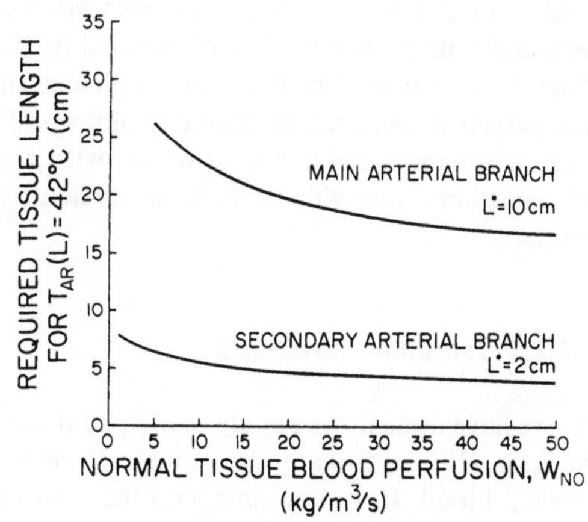

Fig. 3.33. Length of tissue that needs to be heated to therapeutic temperature (or slightly below) in order to preheat the arterial blood to T_{tr} before it enters the tumor (Fig. 3.32). The normal vessel lengths (L*) from Table 3.2 are listed. Results calculated using Eq. 3.19 and the numerical values of Table 3.2. The applied power is related to the blood perfusion as $\dot{Q}_a = \dot{W} c_b (T_{tr} - T_{ar})$. In this example, $T_{tr} - T_{ar} = 5\,°C$, $UP = h\pi R$

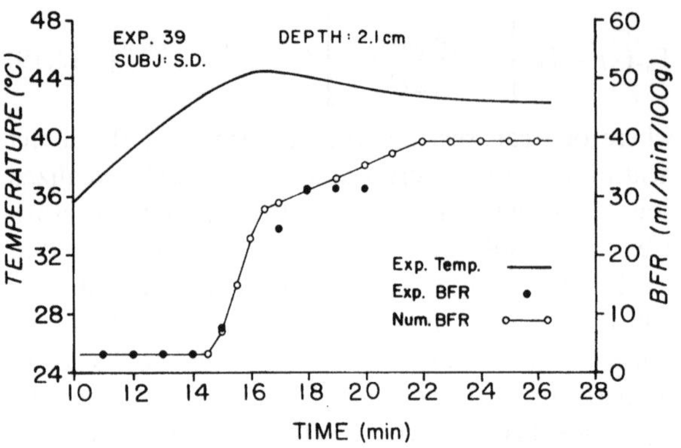

Fig. 3.34. Transient temperature and experimental and numerical blood flow response (BFR) occurring at the site of the xenon injection depot in the thigh of a subject exposed to microwave hyperthermia. Note the rapid response of blood flow, which increased an order of magnitude in a 2-min period. [124]

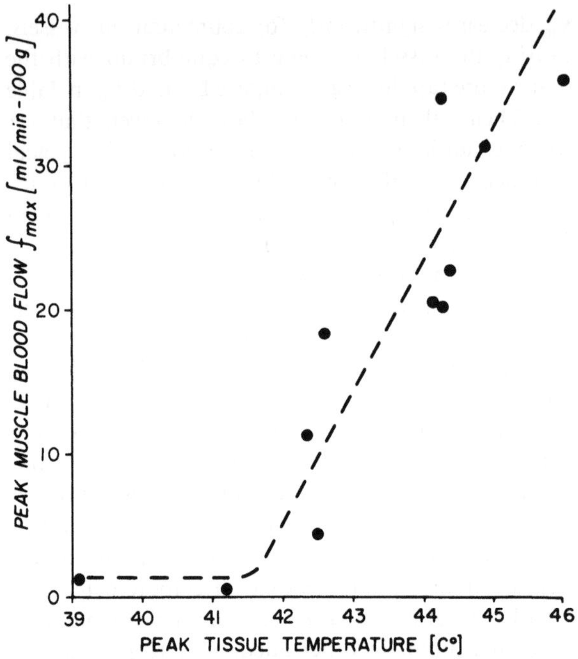

Fig. 3.35. Perfusion rates occurring in the quadricepts muscles at the time of peak temperature in response to microwave diathermy as shown in Fig. 3.34. The elevation from basal levels of blood flow to the peak values shown occurred over about 60–90 s, in most cases, beginning after the tissue temperature exceeded threshold values corresponding to the respective peak temperature values shown on the abscissa. [125]

ed at T_{tr}, a difficult task. For a practical example, consider the main and secondary arterial branches of Table 3.2 supplying/passing through normal muscle, $\dot{W}_{no} = 1$ kg/m^3-s, or brain, $\dot{W}_{no} = 10$ kg/m^3/s. These lengths are always larger than the combined lengths of such vessels ($\cong$ 12 cm from Table 3.2), indicating that even larger vessels need to be heated, a task which becomes even more difficult because of their high flow rates and long entry lengths.

In summary, considering the results from both of the idealized models (Figs. 3.9, 3.10, 3.12, and 3.33), we end up with a similar conclusion – if "large" vessels are present, one must preheat them in order to avoid cold spots or lines in a tumor, and this will not be an easy task without overheating the normal tissue. Here, "large" is a rather deceptive adjective since the thermal effects of even rather geometrically small vessels such as the main and servicing vessels with diameters of less than 1 mm will make them difficult to heat properly.

3.2.2.2 Temporal Variations

As we have done for the analysis of spatial variations, we can also investigate the temporal variations in power, blood flow, and temperature, although the power variations will not be discussed here since they are under the control of the operator or of a feedback control system (a case to be evaluated later) and are generally increased relatively slowly to avoid unexpected patient pain and/or damage. Likewise, little is known regarding the actual time rates of changes of blood perfusion, especially in tumors during (after, or between) hyperthermia treatments. For normal muscle tissue, the rate of change of blood perfusion can be quite large in response to elevated temperatures, especially after a "critical" temperature of approximately 43 °C has been reached (Figs. 3.34 and 3.35). When long times are involved, these blood perfusions can become oscillatory (Fig. 3.36). Finally, a considerable amount is known concerning the time rate of change of tissue temperatures during hyperthermia treatments, both for cooling and heating processes. This latter subject will be discussed in this section.

Tissue Heating

For tissue heating, the initial response to a sudden increase in power is a linear increase in temperature reflecting the fact that all of the absorbed power is going into increasing the local tissue temperature before any significant temperature rise (and the associated heat transfer losses) is produced. From a local energy balance (without regard to any form of the bioheat transfer equation), one knows that since metabolism is negligible for almost all regional and local hyperthermia [107]

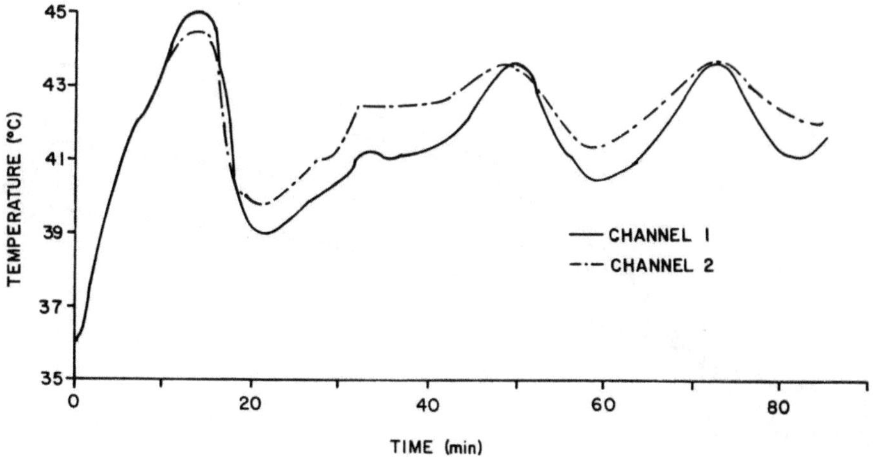

Fig. 3.36. Transient temperature oscillations in dogs' thighs subjected to external microwave hyperthermia. The rapid changes in temperature are a consequence of rapid blood perfusion changes in response to elevated temperatures. [116]

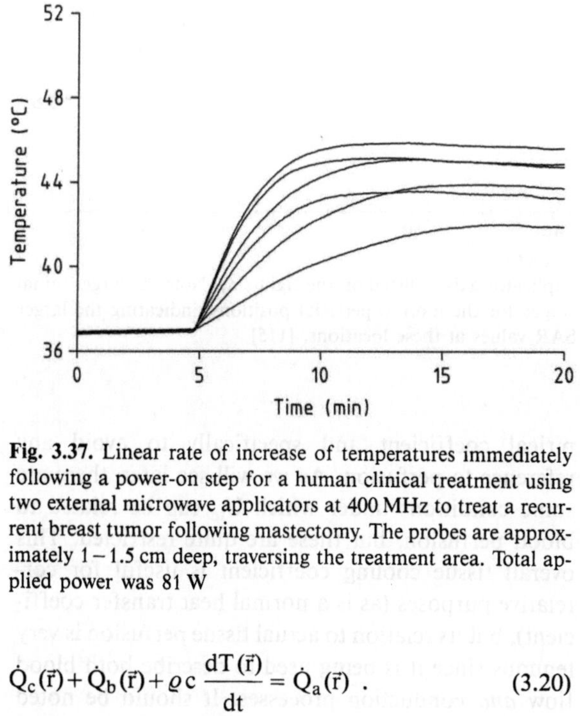

Fig. 3.37. Linear rate of increase of temperatures immediately following a power-on step for a human clinical treatment using two external microwave applicators at 400 MHz to treat a recurrent breast tumor following mastectomy. The probes are approximately 1–1.5 cm deep, traversing the treatment area. Total applied power was 81 W

$$\dot{Q}_c(\vec{r})+\dot{Q}_b(\vec{r})+\varrho c\,\frac{dT(\vec{r})}{dt}=\dot{Q}_a(\vec{r})\ . \tag{3.20}$$

If conduction ($\dot{Q}_c$) and blood flow cooling ($\dot{Q}_b$) can be neglected for the initial short times,

$$\varrho c\,\frac{dT(\vec{r})}{dt}=\dot{Q}_a(\vec{r}) \tag{3.21}$$

and thus for constant applied power

$$T(\vec{r},t)=\left(\frac{\dot{Q}_a(\vec{r})}{\varrho c}\right)t \tag{3.22}$$

which gives the resultant linear increase in temperature (Fig. 3.37). This relationship between the linear rate of increase in temperature with time and the locally applied power can be used to measure $\dot{Q}_a$ and SAR (specific absorption rate) distributions [SAR (w/kg) = $\dot{Q}_a/\varrho$] in phantoms and tissues when ϱ and c are known (as described in a later section on prospective thermal dosimetry). These initial rates of temperature increase could reach up to 15 °C/min for a superficial treatment which had a power deposition value of 1 w/cm^3. Clinically, however, this is unacceptably high and values closer to 1 °C/min are more commonly used [72] for superficial treatments; deep-seated tumors heated with regional power deposition systems, with their associated lower power densities (on the order of 0.1 w/cm^3), have practical rates of increase of less than 1 °C/min [120]. For long times, the blood flow and conduction terms become significant due to the increased tissue temperatures, and the rate of temperature increase becomes smaller (Fig. 3.38). In practical hyperthermia situations, one does not generally know which term, blood flow, or thermal conduction contributes most significantly to the tissue cooling – an issue to be discussed later. In the face of this ignorance, for simplicity one can lump both effects into a single term which is linear in the local temperature increase (above the arterial temperature), giving the following result when $\dot{Q}_b+\dot{Q}_c$ is replaced by $U_{tc}(T-T_{ar})$ in Eq. 3.20:

$$U_{tc}(T-T_{ar})+\varrho c\,\frac{dT}{dt}=\dot{Q}_a\ . \tag{3.23 a}$$

Here, U_{tc} (w/m^3°C) is a local tissue cooling coefficient for tissue cooling by all heat transfer mechanisms. It indicates the local energy removal rate (w/m^3) per degree of local temperature rise. Note that if Eq. 3.23 a is divided through by ϱ to be put in terms of SAR (w/kg)

$$\frac{U_{tc}}{\varrho}(T-T_{ar})+c\,\frac{dT}{dt}=\text{SAR} \tag{3.23 b}$$

then the term U_{tc}/ϱ has the units w/kg°C. In the past, several authors have used different nomencla-

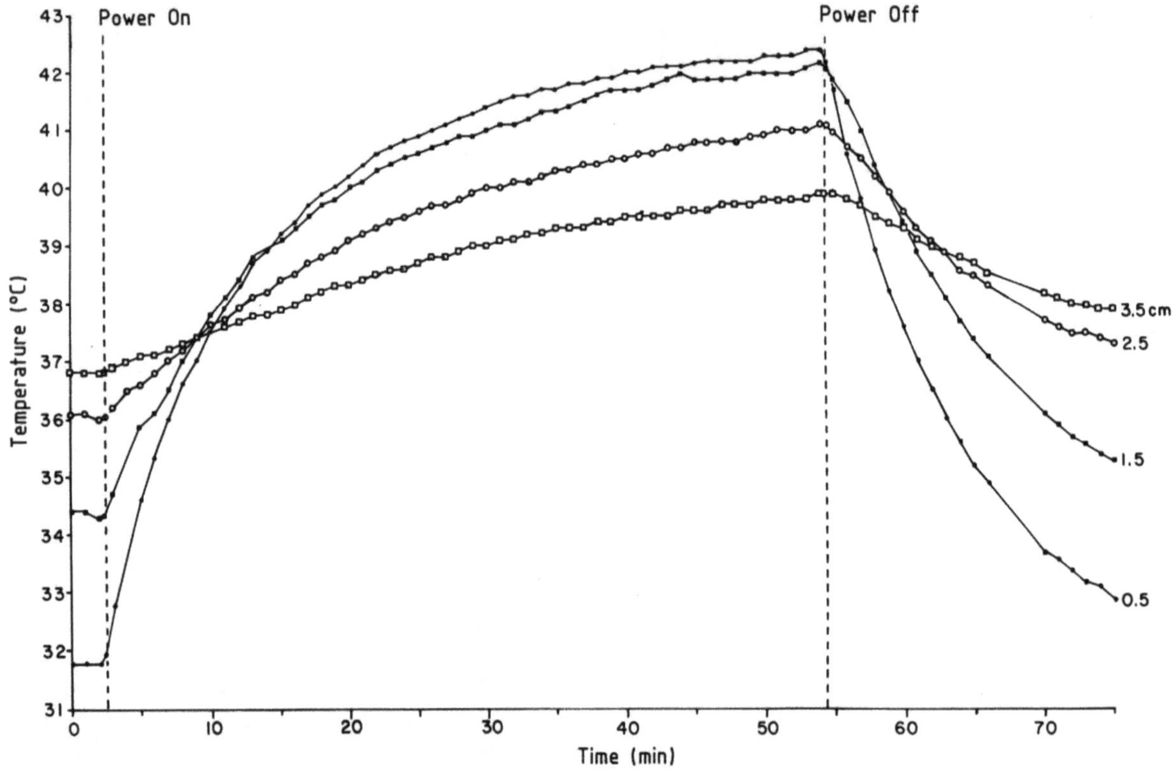

Fig. 3.38. Typical temperature versus time curve for an experiment on a microwave-heated dog thigh with a total absorbed power of 3.1 W and an arterial temperature of 37.4 °C. Temperatures at 1-min intervals are shown for different depths along the applicator axis as listed on the right side. Note the larger initial slopes for the more superficial positions, indicating the larger SAR values at these locations. [115]

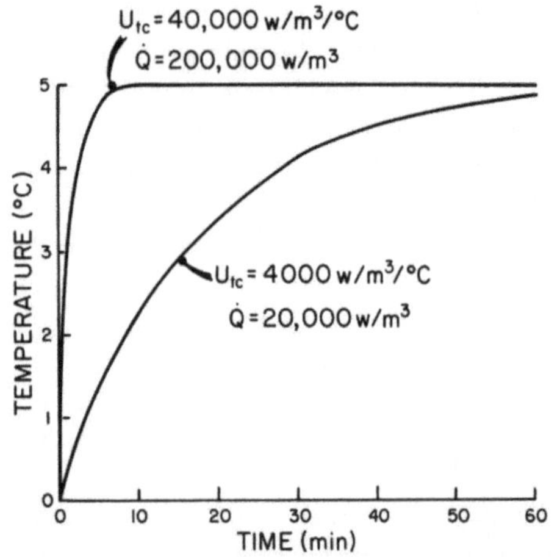

Fig. 3.39. Exponential temperature rise calculated from Eq. 3.24 for two different power levels and blood perfusions

tures for this coefficient, usually including some verbal reference to perfusion (e.g., an effective perfusion, $\dot{W}_e c_b = U_{tc}$, as done by Roemer et al. [115] and PERF = U_{tc}, as done by Lagendijk et al. [72]). It is suggested here that this new nomenclature U_{tc} be adapted to indicate more clearly the nature of this empirical coefficient and specifically to avoid any reference to perfusion. As we will see later, there are some conditions under which U_{tc} can be related to blood perfusion, but these are quite restricted. This overall tissue cooling coefficient is useful for correlative purposes (as is a normal heat transfer coefficient), but its relation to actual tissue perfusion is very tenuous since it is being used to describe both blood flow *and* conduction processes. It should be noted here that values of "perfusion" calculated from thermal washout techniques are actually "effective perfusion" values ($\dot{W}_e$) as defined above [115] or, in the present nomenclature, values of U_{tc}/c_b.

The use of U_{tc} for any quantitative purpose must be very carefully proscribed. For constant T_{ar} and U_{tc} values, and a step increase in $\dot{Q}_a$, the resultant temperature increase is given by

$$T(t) - T_{ar} = \frac{\dot{Q}_a}{U_{tc}} (1 - e^{-t/\tau}) \tag{3.24}$$

where the tissue time constant is given by

$$\tau = \frac{\varrho c}{U_{tc}} . \tag{3.25}$$

Transient temperature profiles for this case are given in Fig. 3.39. Since experimentally obtained curves have the same general shape (e.g., see Figs. 3.37, 3.38), it is tempting to curve fit such data to Eq. 3.24 and obtain experimental τ values and then U_{tc} values from Eq. 3.25. If one does this, one must be careful not to relate U_{tc} (or $\dot{W}_e$ or PERF) to actual perfusions except under circumstances to be described later (since U_{tc} contains both conduction and perfusion effects). The term U_{tc} is really a measure of the ability of the tissue to remove power from some point per degree of local tissue temperature rise; i.e., at steady state from Eq. 3.23a,

$$U_{tc} = \dot{W}_e c_b = \frac{\dot{Q}_a}{T - T_{ar}} \ [\mathrm{w/m^3 \,{}^\circ C}] \tag{3.26}$$

and it thus represents an overall heat transfer coefficient for tissue cooling.

Tissue Cooling

Tissue cooling after power is turned off is also governed by Eq. 3.20 in the general case, but now the source term is zero $[\dot{Q}_a = 0]$. If one again uses the tissue-cooling coefficient approach, the resultant temperature decrease is given by

$$\frac{T(t) - T_{ar}}{T(0) - T_{ar}} = e^{-t/\tau} \tag{3.27}$$

where τ is defined as before, and

$$T(0) - T_{ar} = \frac{\dot{Q}_a(0)}{U_{tc}}. \tag{3.28}$$

Figure 3.40 shows the type of decay one obtains for this equation. Again, the time constant for these decays are given by τ, which is determined by U_{tc}, a quantity dependent on the local conduction process, as well as the local blood perfusion. Thus, measuring the time constant of such a decay does *not* generally give one a measure of the local blood perfusion alone since conduction effects are included – a problem with *all* previous perfusion calculations using thermal washout techniques. The rates of temperature decrease in clinical situations cover a wide range – dependent on both the local blood perfusion and conduction conditions. Figure 3.41 shows such decreases for a clinical patient treatment.

3.2.2.3 Energy Removal – Conduction and Blood Convection

The relative rate of removal of energy by conduction and by blood flow is a topic of importance in understanding and predicting the thermal responses of tumors and one which has motivated several heated discussions in different applications. In attempting to develop an overview of this subject, it is most important to keep in mind the volume of tissue that is being discussed, from the smallest possible volume (a point in space) to volumes as large as a complete tumor.

An Arbitrary Position Inside Heated Tissue

For the smallest scale [a general point inside the heated tissue at some location ($\vec{r}$)], an overall energy balance gives Eq. 3.20. Furthermore, we know that we can describe the conduction effects using Fourier's law. Thus, for uniform thermal conductivity and steady-state (conditions invoked for purposes of simplifying the following discussion)

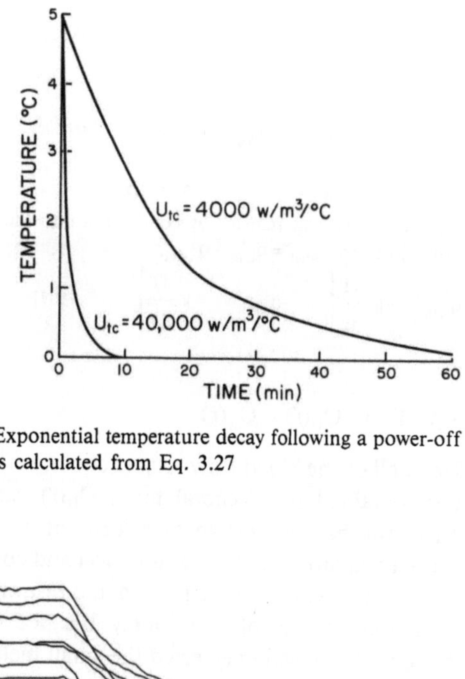

Fig. 3.40. Exponential temperature decay following a power-off transient as calculated from Eq. 3.27

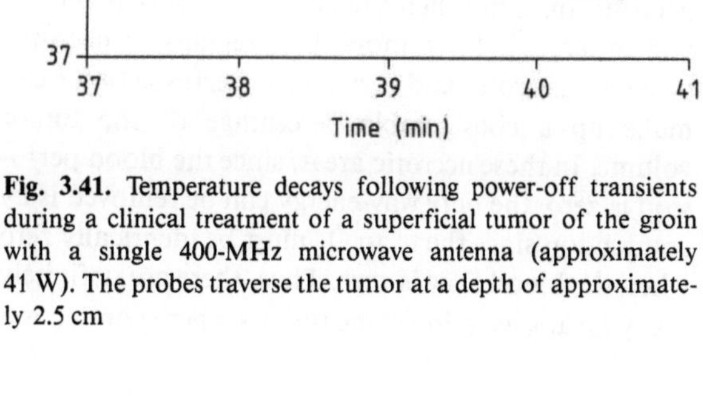

Fig. 3.41. Temperature decays following power-off transients during a clinical treatment of a superficial tumor of the groin with a single 400-MHz microwave antenna (approximately 41 W). The probes traverse the tumor at a depth of approximately 2.5 cm

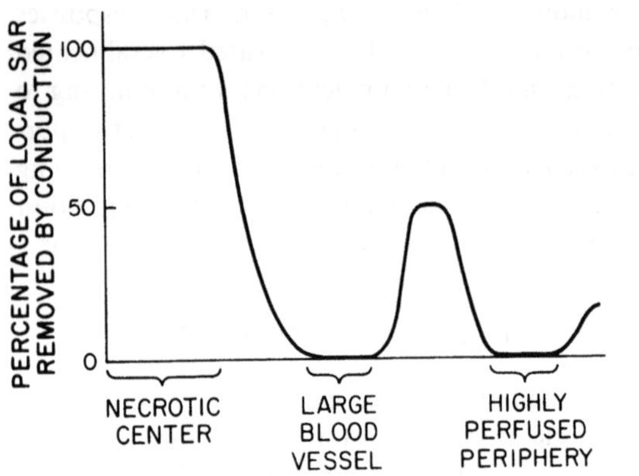

Fig. 3.42. Idealized curve of the percentage of locally deposited energy removed by thermal conduction versus position inside the classical model of a tumor which contains a large blood vessel

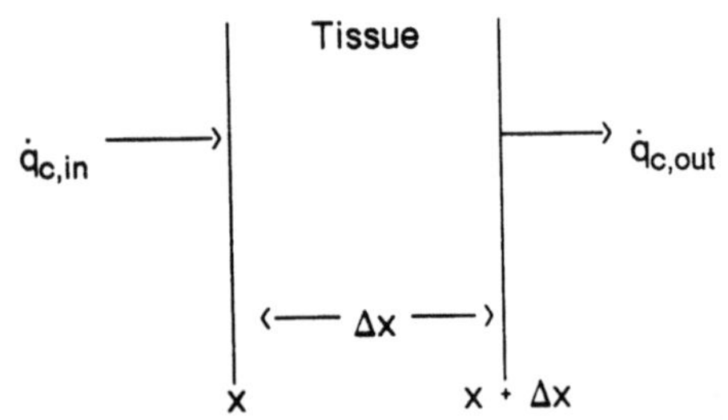

Fig. 3.43. Net heat transfer by conduction into the tissue at a point in space, $\dot{q}_{net} = \dot{q}_{c,in} - \dot{q}_{c,out}$:

$$\dot{q}_{c,in} = -k \left.\frac{dT}{dx}\right|_{x} \; ; \; \dot{q}_{c,out} = -k \left.\frac{dT}{dx}\right|_{x+\Delta x} . \quad [107]$$

$$-\nabla^2 T(\vec{r}) + \dot{Q}_b(\vec{r}) = \dot{Q}_a(\vec{r}) \; . \tag{3.29}$$

Here, all of the blood flow-related cooling effects have been retained in a general term, $\dot{Q}_b(\vec{r})$, so that we have not had to invoke any form of the bioheat transfer equation – our formulation and conclusions are independent of that equation and rest on the fundamental aspects of the energy balance equation. Also, we have again neglected the small metabolic effects. All of the energy input to this point, $\dot{Q}_a$, is either removed by conduction, $-k\nabla^2 T$, or by blood flow effects, $\dot{Q}_b$. There are locations inside of tumors where each one of the cooling terms dominates. For example, it is well known that most tumors have necrotic areas in which the blood perfusion is zero – and in large, bulky tumors these regions of necrotic, or nearly necrotic, and very poorly perfused tissue can make up a considerable percentage of the tumor volume. In these necrotic areas, since the blood perfusion is zero, the *only* way energy can be removed is by conduction since the term $\dot{Q}_b$ must be identically zero when the blood flow is zero. Thus, there are definitely many locations inside some tumors where conduction removes 100% of the locally produced energy. The other end of the spectrum also exists inside of large blood vessels and in areas of high perfusion where blood perfusion provides 100% of the cooling and $\nabla^2 T$ is identically zero. In between these extremes, any distribution of these two variables is possible – and is not known a priori. Figure 3.42 illustrates this range of possibilities for a tumor which follows the classical model of having a necrotic core plus a highly perfused periphery. In this case, we have also shown a large blood vessel being present. To know what this distribution is requires knowledge of two of the variables in Eq. 3.29, for example, the conduction and the power deposition distributions, $-k\nabla^2 T$ and $\dot{Q}_a(\vec{r})$, so that the energy balance equation can be solved for the blood perfusion term, $\dot{Q}_b$. (It is for these reasons that the application of the "thermal washout" measurement of blood perfusion rests on such shaky grounds – no correction is made for the conduction effects, i.e., the term $-k\nabla^2 T$ is simply discarded.) Indeed, to make matters even more interesting than illustrated in Fig. 3.42, it should be noted that both conduction and blood perfusion can carry energy into a given location and act as a source of energy and not a sink, thus giving percentages of removal of less than 0% – i.e., negative numbers. For example, for blood flow, one can imagine a large blood vessel carrying high-temperature blood from a region of high temperature to a region of lower temperature and thus providing additional energy at that location. Likewise, the net flow of energy by conduction can be into a location if $\nabla^2 T \lessgtr 0$. This is possible when one considers in detail the conduction process, which is described by Fourier's law, which says that the rate of conduction of energy per unit area, $\dot{q}_x$ (w/m²), in a specified direction, e.g., x, is given by the product of the thermal conductivity of the tissue, k, and the rate of change of temperature in that direction,

$$\dot{q}_x = -k \frac{dT}{dx} \tag{3.30}$$

so that high thermal conductivities and rapidly changing temperatures give high rates of energy transfer by conduction. The *net* rate of energy transfer by conduction into a point is, however, given by the difference between the conduction into the tissue and the conduction out of the tissue. For the one-dimensional case, this is given by (see Fig. 3.43)

$$\dot{q}_{c,in} - \dot{q}_{c,out} = \left[-k \left.\frac{dT}{dx}\right|_{x} \right] - \left[-k \frac{dT}{dx} \right]_{x+\Delta x} \tag{3.31}$$

where the heat transfer out of the tissue can be approximated by a Taylor series expansion (a linear extrapolation),

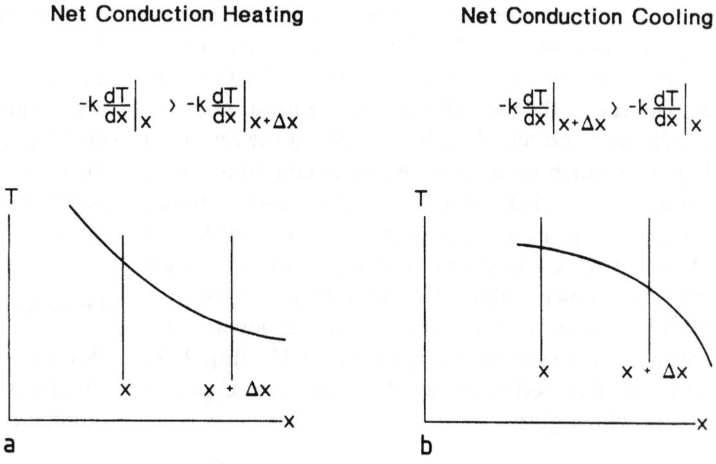

Fig. 3.44a, b. Net rate of energy transfer into the tissue by conduction is governed by the second derivative of the temperature versus position curve: **a** d^2T/dx^2-positive, net conduction is into the tissue; **b** d^2T/dx^2-negative, net conduction is out of the tissue. [107]

$$\left[k\frac{dT}{dx}\right]_{x+\Delta x} = \left[k\frac{dT}{dx}\right]_x + \frac{d}{dx}\left[k\frac{dT}{dx}\right]\Delta x + \dots, \tag{3.32}$$

so that for a constant k,

$$\dot{q}_c = \dot{q}_{c,in} - \dot{q}_{c,out} = \frac{d}{dx}\left[k\frac{dT}{dx}\right]\Delta x + \dots$$

$$= k\frac{d^2T}{dx^2}\Delta x + \dots, \tag{3.33}$$

and so for Δx small, we obtain an equation valid at a point

$$\dot{Q}_{c,in} - \dot{Q}_{c,out} = k\frac{d^2T}{dx^2}. \tag{3.34}$$

Thus, the *net* rate of energy transfer *into* the tissue by conduction is given by the second derivative of the temperature curve. The first spatial derivative, Eq. 3.30, gives the rate of energy transfer across a plane; the second derivative, Eq. 3.34, gives the *net* difference between the transfer into the tissue across a plane from one direction and the transfer out of the tissue in the same direction at an adjacent plane. For three dimensions, we have

$$\dot{Q}_c = \dot{Q}_{c,in} - \dot{Q}_{c,out} = k\frac{d^2T}{dx^2} + k\frac{d^2T}{dy^2} + k\frac{d^2T}{dz^2} \tag{3.35}$$

or, in shorthand notation using the Laplacian operator,

$$\dot{Q}_c = \dot{Q}_{c,in} - \dot{Q}_{c,out} = k\nabla^2 T. \tag{3.36}$$

For the rate of conduction into the tissue greater than the rate of conduction out of the tissue, the net conduction into the tissue is positive (Fig. 3.44a) and thermal energy is added to the tissue; when the opposite is true, the net conduction *into* the tissue is negative and thermal energy is removed from the tissue (Fig. 3.44b).

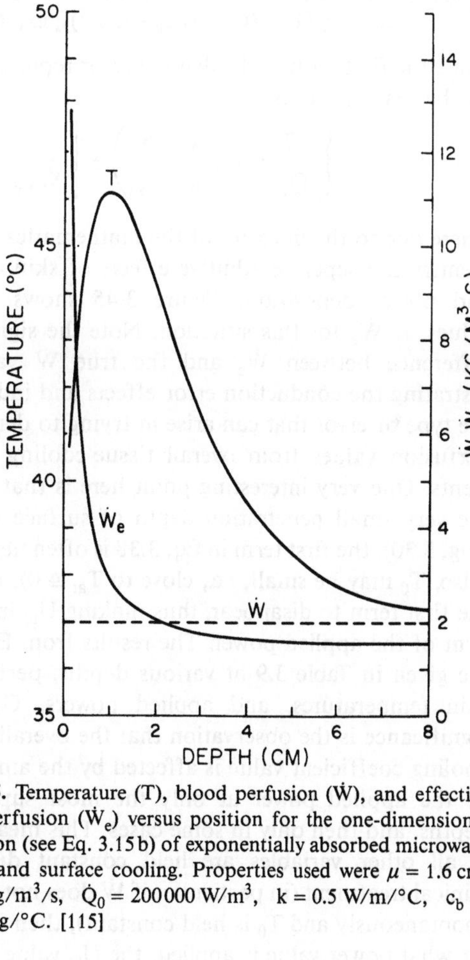

Fig. 3.45. Temperature (T), blood perfusion ($\dot{W}$), and effective blood perfusion ($\dot{W}_e$) versus position for the one-dimensional simulation (see Eq. 3.15b) of exponentially absorbed microwave heating and surface cooling. Properties used were $\mu = 1.6$ cm, $\dot{W} = 2$ kg/m^3/s, $\dot{Q}_0 = 200000$ W/m^3, k = 0.5 W/m/°C, c_b = 4186 J/kg/°C. [115]

To illustrate this point and to show further the pitfalls of using the effective perfusion concept to try to calculate perfusion, consider the skin-cooling case previously described (Eq. 3.15a), with an exponentially absorbed microwave source applied to a homogeneous medium which is cooled on its surface to a temperature T_0 (measured above the arterial temperature, $T_{ar} \triangleq 0$). For this case (Eq. 3.15b), the resultant temperature distribution is shown in Fig. 3.45. One can also calculate the individual energy removal rates for conduction and blood perfusion, giving the results in Fig. 3.46 which show a case where conduction can be adding rather than removing energy from a point, thus giving the negative percentages. These results can also be used to calculate effective perfusion rates using the known values for $T(\vec{r})$ (Eq. 3.15b) and $\dot{Q}(r) = \dot{Q}(0) \exp(-x/\mu)$ (the known exponential absorption of power) in the equation for U_{tc} (Eq. 3.26) with effective perfusion calculated as $\dot{W}_e = U_{tc}/c_b$ as before which gives

$$\dot{W}_e(x) = \frac{U_{tc}}{c_b} = \frac{Q_0 \exp(-x/\mu)}{c_b [T_0 - (Q_0/(\dot{W} c_b - k/\mu^2))] \exp(-x/x_{pn}) + c_b [(Q_0/(\dot{W} c_b - k\mu^2))] \exp(-x/\mu)} \tag{3.37}$$

where the first term in the denominator represents the effect of skin cooling on the temperature. This equation can be rearranged as

$$\dot{W}_e(x) = \frac{U_{tc}}{c_b} = \left\{ \frac{c_b T_0}{Q_0} \exp\left(\frac{x}{\mu} - \frac{x}{x_{pn}}\right) + \left[\frac{c_b}{\dot{W} c_b - k/\mu^2}\right] \left[1 - \exp\left(\frac{x}{\mu} - \frac{x}{x_{pn}}\right)\right] \right\}^{-1} \tag{3.38}$$

where due to the linearity of the mathematics we can identify the separate additive effects of skin cooling and power deposition. Figure 3.45 shows typical values of $\dot{W}_e$ for this situation. Note the significant difference between $\dot{W}_e$ and the true $\dot{W}$ value illustrating the conduction error effects and indicating the type of error that can arise in trying to determine perfusion values from overall tissue-cooling coefficients. One very interesting point here is that due to the very small penetration depth of surface cooling (Fig. 3.30), the first term in Eq. 3.38 is often negligible (also, T_0 may be small, i.e., close to $T_{ar} \triangleq 0$), causing the first term to disappear, thus making U_{tc} independent of the applied power. The results from Eq. 3.38 are given in Table 3.9 at various depths, perfusions, skin temperatures, and applied powers. Of most significance is the observation that the overall tissue-cooling coefficient value is affected by the amplitude of the applied power at only the most superficial depths, and then only in some cases. This means that if all other variables are held constant during a clinical treatment (in particular, if $\dot{W}$ does not change spontaneously and T_0 is held constant), then no matter what power value is applied, the U_{tc} value will remain unchanged. Conversely, if sequential values of U_{tc} do change during a treatment, then those changes must be caused by changes in blood perfusion ($\dot{W}$) regardless of the magnitude of the applied power.

In summary of this section, the major conclusions remain that at any given point in the heated volume the energy removal process can be dominated by either conduction or blood flow (and both of these processes can either add or remove energy from a point) and that one does not generally know the relative magnitudes of these two effects. Historically, this makes the results of thermal washout techniques difficult to evaluate in terms of physiological blood perfusion changes for anything other than qualitative purposes.

Finite Volumes

When one considers finite volumes, one can also have situations which are either conduction or perfusion dominated. For example, for very small heated thermistor probes introduced into the tissue, it is clear that, for many low perfusion cases characteristic of hyperthermia treatments, the removal of energy from the probe is dominated by conduction processes [65]. For even larger volumes such as complete tumors, the relative amount of energy removed will depend on the volume chosen for analysis and the tumor characteristics (Fig. 3.47). For a fixed volume, the total rate of energy removal by conduction is given by the surface integral over the surface area of the volume analyzed

$$\dot{Q}_c = - \oint_{A_{tumor}} k \nabla T \cdot d\vec{A} \tag{3.39}$$

while the rate of energy removal by blood convection is given by a summation of the differences in convected energy between the outflowing venous and incoming arterial supplies, which can be written as

$$\dot{Q}_b = \sum_{vein_j} \dot{M}_j c_b T_{v_j} - \sum_{artery_i} \dot{M}_i c_b T_{ar_i} \,. \tag{3.40}$$

For the example shown in Fig. 3.47, if the volume A is analyzed, all of the energy is removed from the volume by conduction since the blood perfusion is zero everywhere inside the volume, while for volume B, a slight distance away into a highly perfused media where the temperature gradient ∇T is close to zero (so Eq. 3.39 is almost zero), the energy removal is almost all from blood flow. As one makes the volume of analysis larger, one gets farther away from the tumor and into more highly perfused tissue where the temperature profiles are flat and blood perfusion effects

Table 3.9. Tissue-cooling coefficient (U_{tc}) values calculated from Eq. 3.38 for several skin temperatures (T_0), applied powers ($\dot{Q}_0$), and blood perfusions ($\dot{W}$)

W (kg/m³/s)	Q_0 (W/m³)	Tissue-cooling coefficient values (W/m³-°C) Depth (m) 0.01	0.03	0.05
$T_0 = 0\,°C (= T_{ar})$				
0.5	All values	−5880	−2060	−1260
1.0	All values	6590	2940	2310
5.0	All values	23560	18820	18650
$T_0 = -5\,°C$				
0.5	50000	−3820	−1720	−1180
	100000	−4620	−1850	−1220
	200000	−5210	−1970	−1260
	500000	−5590	−2020	−1260
1.0	50000	11970	3280	2390
	100000	8480	3110	2350
	200000	7430	3020	2310
	500000	6890	2980	2310
5.0	50000	44270	19110	18690
	100000	30740	18980	18690
	200000	26710	18900	18690
	500000	24740	18860	18690
$T_0 = +5\,°C$				
0.5	50000	−12770	−2480	−1430
	100000	−8060	−2230	−1340
	200000	−6800	−2140	−1300
	500000	−6220	−2060	−1300
1.0	50000	4540	2690	2230
	100000	5380	2810	2270
	200000	5920	2860	2270
	500000	6300	2940	2310
5.0	50000	16040	18520	18650
	100000	19110	18690	18650
	200000	21130	18770	18690
	500000	22510	18820	18690

dominate. One can, of course, extend the volume farther until one reaches the skin, when conduction inside the nonperfused epithelium dominates again. Clearly, one must be careful to define clearly the region in space one is analyzing.

In general, it is the presence of perfusion in both the tumor and the normal tissue which requires adding significant power to heat a tumor properly, since heating a tissue volume with zero perfusion everywhere would require little power. The ideal analysis of Ocheltree and Frizzell [88] offers an interesting model to study this phenomenon. For practical systems, the amount of power needed to be applied to a given tumor to reach a certain temperature,

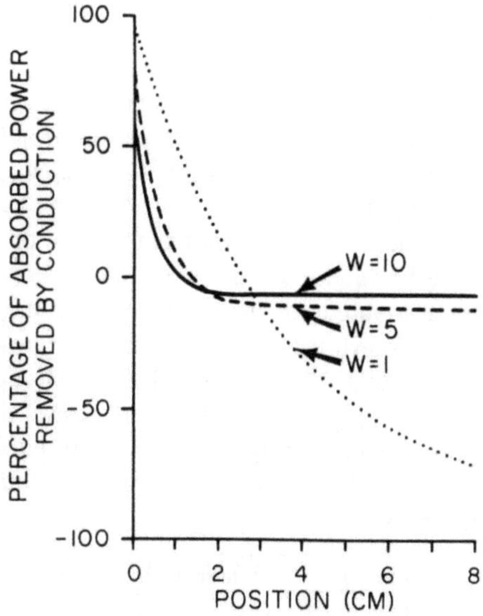

Fig. 3.46. Percentage of energy removed by conduction versus depth into superficial, uniformly perfused tissue heated exponentially and with skin cooling. The normal tissue blood perfusions that were simulated are shown [115]

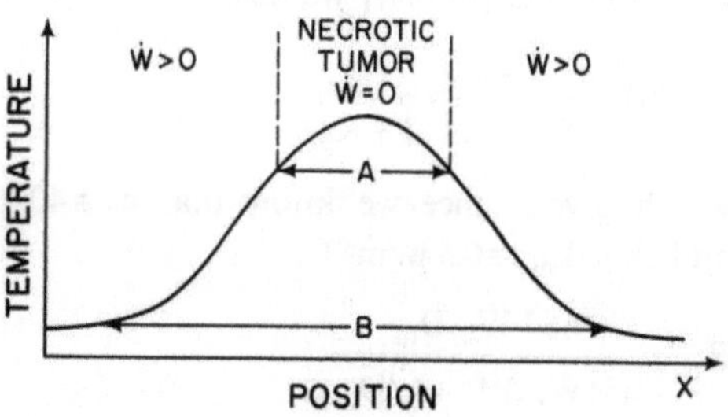

Fig. 3.47. Idealized tumor with necrotic core

or a certain temperature distribution, will be a function of the power distribution pattern of the device being utilized – which can be quite inefficient and deposit considerable power into the normal tissue. In this sense, the analysis fo Ocheltree and Frizzell presents a best-case analysis since their power deposition model is completely conformable and only deposits power where it is needed. For their analysis of a spherical tumor, they determine that the power deposited at the tumor edge, i.e., that power required to overcome conduction effects, is given by

$$P_c = T_{tr}\,[(\dot{W}_{no}c_b k_{no})^{1/2} + k_{no}/r_0]\,4\pi r_0^2 \quad (3.41)$$

while, since the tumor has a flat temperature profile, the power removed by blood flow is just

$$P_b = \int_{V_{tumor}} \dot{W}_{tu}(\vec{r})\,c_b T_{tr}\,dv \quad (3.42)$$

which, for a uniformly perfused case (an overestimation since the necrotic parts of a tumor will not require power), is then

$$P_b = \tfrac{4}{3}\pi r_0^3 \dot{W}_{tu} c_b T_{tr} \ . \tag{3.43}$$

If one wants to, one can consider $\dot{W}_{tu}$ to be an appropriately weighted average blood flow in the tumor. That is, if the total flow to the tumor is $\dot{M}_{tu}$ and the total volume is V_{tumor}, then $\dot{W} = \dot{M}_{tu}/V_{tumor}$. It is interesting here to obtain Eq. 3.43 using an alternative approach which does not require use of the bioheat transfer equation. That is, all blood flow effects can be accounted for by heating all incoming blood to T_{tr}, as previously discussed. The total power required to do this is just $\dot{M}_{tu} c_b T_{tr}$, which again equals $V_{tumor} \dot{W}_{tu} c_b T_{tr}$. For this ideal case, the ratio of power required by blood flow to that required to overcome conduction to the surrounding media is then given as

$$R_p = \frac{P_b}{P_c} = \left(\frac{\dot{W}_{tu} c_b r_0/3}{(\dot{W}_{no} c_b k_{no})^{1/2} + k_{no}/r_0} \right) \tag{3.44}$$

a quantity that can go from zero to values much greater than one. To calculate the percentage of total power that is required to overcome tumor blood perfusion effects $[P_b(\%)]$ we have

$$P_b(\%) = \frac{P_b}{P_c + P_b} = \frac{R_p}{1 + R_p} \tag{3.45}$$

which gives, since we know that $c_b \cong 4000$ J/kg°C and that $k_{no} \cong 0.5$ w/m°C,

$$R_p = \frac{667\, \dot{W}_{tu} D_{tu}}{45 (\dot{W}_{no})^{1/2} + 1/D_{tu}} \ , \tag{3.46}$$

$$P_b(\%) = \frac{667\, \dot{W}_{tu} D_{tu}^2}{1 + 45 (\dot{W}_{no} D_{tu}^2)^{1/2} + 667\, \dot{W}_{tu} D_{tu}^2} \ . \tag{3.47}$$

Figure 3.48 shows the variation of this quantity with the three important variables $\dot{W}_{tu}$, $\dot{W}_{no}$, and D_{tu}. The strong influence of $\dot{W}_{tu}$ on these results is obvious

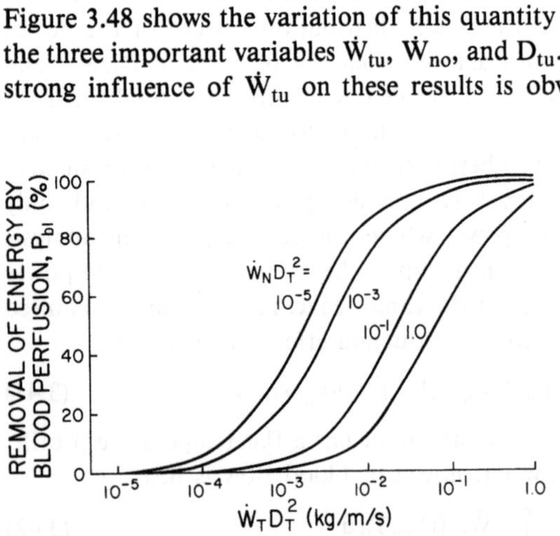

Fig. 3.48. The percentage of the total applied power (needed to heat an ideal spherical tumor to T_{tr}) that is needed to overcome blood perfusion effects (see Eq. 3.47). D_T is the tumor diameter, $\dot{W}_T$ is the tumor perfusion, and $\dot{W}_N$ is the normal tissue perfusion

and in line with clinical observations that small tumor blood perfusion changes seem to require large power changes. For a typical treatment to 42 °C for a 5-cm-diameter tumor with normal and tumor blood perfusions of 1.0 w/m^3-s, we obtain conduction and convection powers of 2.5 w and 1.2 w, respectively, showing the significant role of conduction. These powers, quite low for a typical treatment, also indicate the lack of conformability of typical clinical devices in heating tumors – most of the power goes into the normal tissue where it is removed by normal tissue blood flow or into heating the tumor and its blood supply above the therapeutic temperature when high intratumoral temperatures are reached [109].

3.3 Thermal Dosimetry

For hyperthermia dosimetry, the applications of the above principles can be divided under four main headings [110], which can be thought of as progressing in time through a patient treatment: comparative, prospective, concurrent, and retrospective thermal dosimetry. The goal of comparative thermal dosimetry is to compare the abilities of different heating modalities and configurations to heat properly general classes of patients and tumors. Such comparisons can be done using standardized patient models which contain only the most significant anatomical and physiological features of a range of "typical" patients and the major characteristics of the power deposition patterns. Conversely, in prospective thermal dosimetry (individual patient treatment planning) detailed information is needed regarding the particular patient's anatomy and expected blood perfusion responses so that detailed power deposition patterns can be calculated and used to determine a complete temperature distribution for that patient. The goal of such simulations is to optimize the proposed thermal treatment by maximizing the therapeutic effects of the tumor temperature distribution while minimizing normal tissue damage and patient stress. Concurrent thermal dosimetry (feedback control during a treatment) will involve calculating temperature fields during a treatment and adjusting power deposition parameters (and other variable quantities) to optimize the actual treatments. In present applications, measured temperatures at discrete locations are controlled, while the goal of future treatments is to evaluate and control the complete temperature field. Retrospective thermal dosimetry (post-treatment evaluation of a completed therapy) has as its goal the determination of the complete temperature field (and thermal dose) that was attained during the treatment, based on knowledge of temperatures at the measurement locations. Such data are needed for meaningful clinical evaluations of the equipment's performance and of the heating protocol utilized during the treatment, as well as for determining the efficacy of the hyperthermia treatment.

Because of the relatively advanced stage of radiation therapy and the relatively accurate treatment planning procedures available for that modality, the only area above where strong analogies can be drawn is in the patient treatment-planning process. That is, the equipment selection process (comparative thermal dosimetry), on-line feedback control (concurrent thermal dosimetry), and the retrospective reconstruction of the actual treatment conditions (retrospective thermal dosimetry) are problems which have been essentially solved or eliminated in radiation therapy.

All four areas will be discussed in depth successively, primarily in terms of the need for, and status of, mathematical simulations of treatments. Such simulations are a necessity in this area, just as they are in radiation therapy. The use of complex phantoms (static and dynamic) and animal experiments will also be discussed, but their role, while important and supplemental to simulations, will be limited due to the limitations inherent to these techniques. That is, while phantoms have great value in

1. giving clinical personnel some practical experience in using new equipment,
2. obtaining SAR patterns for relatively simple anatomical geometries, and
3. testing and evaluating feedback control systems

they are much more difficult to work with when one wants to investigate clinically realistic situations, especially when performing parametric studies – something done much better which simulations. Animal experiments have advantages and disadvantages that are similar to those of phantoms and are, at least for purposes of thermal dosimetry, most useful for providing information to improve our simulation capabilities. For these reasons, the following discussion will concentrate on simulation studies as the primary tool to be used in thermal dosimetry.

3.3.1 Comparative Thermal Dosimetry

3.3.1.1 Introduction

The purpose of comparative thermal dosimetry is to determine which power deposition modalities (or configurations for a given modality) are most appropriate for heating certain classes of tumors. This is a general question, which is not restricted to the analysis of which modality or configuration to use for a particular patient. Instead, a broader question is asked, which is concerned with how different heating modalities and configurations compare in their abilities to properly heat general classes of tumors, in various anatomical locations, and for general classes of patients. The overall approach is to determine the power deposition patterns of the various heating systems with respect to the region of interest and then use this information in a numerical formulation of the bioheat transfer equation to calculate the resulting temperature distributions. Since we are interested in general situations, typical standardized values of tissue properties can be used, as can idealized anatomical models of several "average" patients.

The goal of these calculations is to perform an intercomparison of different heating devices and/or of different geometrical configurations for a given device. In such comparisons it is important to have a common basis for evaluating the different devices and configurations and that one be able to evaluate a wide range of clinical conditions. Computer models are ideal for such applications. Once a good program is written, it can be used to rapidly simulate a wide variety of tumors, patients, and heating configurations. Then, the set of clinical conditions simulated for one heating modality/configuration can be repeated *exactly* for all other modalities/configurations that are to be investigated. That is, the comparison has a solid, unchanging, common set of conditions for all evaluations – once the patient/tumor characteristics are set, the *only* things that change are the heating modality characteristics (type, frequency, geometric power deposition, and/or applied power amplitude). This is a very substantial and distinct advantage over the use of clinical trials in which conditions change dramatically from patient to patient and from treatment to treatment for a given patient. Patient trials are also very expensive and time consuming, data acquisition is extremely limited, and obtaining data in a repeatable, reliable manner is a very difficult task. Of course, one may find things in clinical trials that one did not anticipate in the model. Therefore, the interaction of simulations with clinical and experimental situations must be encouraged so that "sufficiently real" patient/tumor models can be developed such that no significant thermal phenomena are left out of the model. Thus, when evaluating simulation results, one must always ask, "is the treatment model 'sufficiently real'?" – a condition which is dependent on the goals one wants to reach. In some cases, relatively simple models will be adequate and adding further detail to the model would only be adding extraneous information and creating additional work. A second way to look at this problem is to realize that, while the simulation model may exclude some detail, that detail is left out for all heating modalities to be studied and if its inclusion does not affect the *relative ranking* of the different modalities/configurations, its inclusion is unwarranted. That is, we are performing a *comparative* study on a scale which may not correspond exactly to reality but which is sufficiently close so that the *relative* performance of the heating system studied can be properly *rank ordered* and that the ranking will be the same as one would find in the clinic. One would like to obtain "absolute accuracy," of course, but "sufficiently real" is adequate in many cases. Thus in the present case, sufficiently real is relative to the ability to be able to properly rank order a set of potential patient/tumor and heating modality/configuration conditions. The rank ordering will then be used to compare the thermal aspects of the devices. Other factors such as expense, clinical considerations, etc., are, of course, also needed in any final decision regarding the choice of which device is best. Therefore, the relative thermal ranking is only one aspect of a larger decision matrix. Nonetheless, the model must be real enough so that the results are approximately what one finds in the clinic. At present, computer simulations of treatments are relatively crude, but, when complemented by experimental results from well-instrumented and carefully performed clinical trials, they have great potential for future use in comparative thermal dosimetry. For comparative thermal dosimetry, we can characterize the two complementary approaches as follows (see also Fig. 3.49):

Computer Simulations. Faster than a speeding bullet when simulating a large number of potential clinical situations and heating modalities in large parametric studies; a basis stronger than a locomotive since the simulations have exactly the same patient/tumor characteristics for all comparative evaluations and one has complete knowledge of all model variables, both independent and dependent; yet not able to leap tall buildings because of limitations on the amount of physiological knowledge that can be put into the model – particularly, knowledge of the blood perfusion responses of tumors.

Clinical Trials. Slower than a sloth's tail in obtaining data since clinical treatments are, by nature, expensive, time consuming, and spaced at long intervals to avoid thermotolerance, and it is difficult to obtain large numbers of nearly identical patients in a trial; a basis less solid than jello pudding since all patients are different, their tumors are different, one knows little if anything about the physiological responses of the patients, and both the applied power and the resultant temperature field are only measured at a few points in the field, leaving large gaps in our knowledge of what we have done to heat the patient, how the patient has responded physiologically to cool her- or himself, and what the resultant temperature

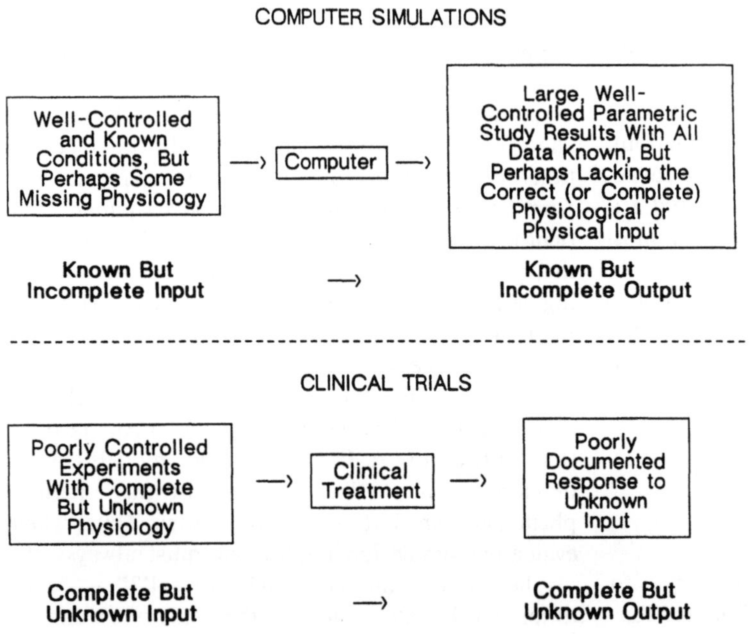

Fig. 3.49. Comparison of strengths and deficiencies of clinical trials and computer simulations when used for comparative thermal dosimetry. Extensive computer simulations complemented by small numbers of clinical trials are preferable to the converse approach

fields are; yet, since it is a real physiological system, it can leap real buildings and none of the patients'/tumors' anatomical or physiological inputs or responses are missing as they might be in simulations.

The results of the computer trials are unambiguous, but their validity can be questioned because of potential missing or incorrect inputs. The results of clinical trials are very ambiguous, and solid conclusions are difficult to reach (or at least can be strongly argued against and are subject to wide interpretation) since there are so many unknowns. Clearly, *for purposes of comparative thermal evaluation* of hyperthermia systems, the deficiencies of and problems with computer simulations are much easier to solve than those of clinical trials, and the simulation approach is to be favored. Yet, very obviously, real clinical trials with devices are needed to perform clinical evaluations of all aspects (not just thermal) of the systems' performances, to evaluate the performances for real situations, and to gather the relevant data for use in simulations. If such trials are performed for purposes of comparative thermal dosimetry, then they should definitely be performed on a limited basis and in conjunction with a comprehensive simulation comparison. This will help avoid the problems present in clinical studies, problems which have arisen in very expensive and time-consuming studies being performed – whose main thermal responses could have been predicted a priori by decent computer simulations (i.e., simulations which have been validated by comparison with experimental, clinical results).

To perform such comparisons (either with simulations or with clinical trials), one needs a common basis for comparison, preferably a single quantitative measure (whose scale can perhaps be divided into ranges or categories). Two such scales have been proposed and utilized, with both approaches being interpretable from a single graph, that of the volume of tumor that is heated to above some minimum acceptable temperature (i.e., some therapeutic level) versus the amplitude of the power applied to the tissue (Fig. 3.50; Table 3.10). For very low applied powers, the tumor temperatures are below therapeutic levels and the volume of tumor reaching the minimum acceptable tumor temperature (T_{tr}) is zero. As power increases, the percentage of tumor reaching T_{tr} becomes finite and, eventually, perhaps 100%. The power is increased continuously until some stopping point is reached. There are three possible reasons for stopping (Table 3.10): the maximum allowable tumor temperature (T_{tu}^{max}) has been reached, the maximum allowable normal tissue temperature (T_i^{max}) has been reached in some normal tissue (i), or the maximum power obtainable from the heating device (Q^{max}) has been reached. Figure 3.50 illustrates the two approaches used; one which measures the percentage of tumor volume above the desired treatment temperature when the stopping point (s_1) is reached, and the second which measures the range of powers that can be applied to give a 100% tumor volume at the treatment

Table 3.10. Stopping conditions for the comparative thermal dosimetry analysis of Fig. 3.50

1. A maximum allowable intratumoral temperature (T_{tu}^{max}) has been reached. This condition is used to simulate conditions present in real clinical treatments. That is, possible overheating of the tumor and possible overheating of surrounding normal tissues are avoided in real treatments (where not all temperatures are measured) by limiting the maximum measured intratumoral temperature
2. A maximum allowable normal tissue temperature (T_i^{max}) has been reached. This temperature can be different in different tissues (i). This condition simulates patient pain and discomfort and possible normal tissue damage
3. A maximum allowable power output for any given device/configuration (Q^{max}) has been reached. This simulates actual hardware restrictions

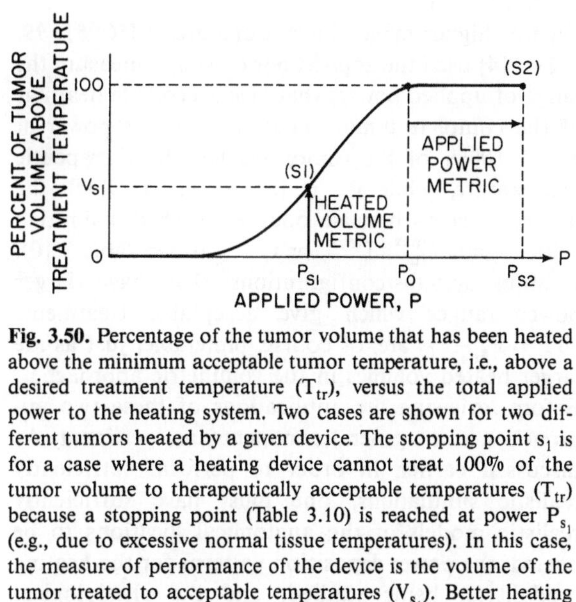

Fig. 3.50. Percentage of the tumor volume that has been heated above the minimum acceptable tumor temperature, i.e., above a desired treatment temperature (T_{tr}), versus the total applied power to the heating system. Two cases are shown for two different tumors heated by a given device. The stopping point s_1 is for a case where a heating device cannot treat 100% of the tumor volume to therapeutically acceptable temperatures (T_{tr}) because a stopping point (Table 3.10) is reached at power P_{s_1} (e.g., due to excessive normal tissue temperatures). In this case, the measure of performance of the device is the volume of the tumor treated to acceptable temperatures (V_{s_1}). Better heating systems will have larger V_{s_1} values. The stopping point s_2 is for a second tumor for which the heating device can heat the complete tumor to therapeutic temperatures (T_{tr}) at a power P_0. For this tumor, the power can be increased further until a stopping point (s_2) is reached. The measure of performance in this case is the range of powers ($P_{s_2} - P_0$) that gives acceptable temperature distributions (100% of tumor volume at or above the desired treatment temperature). Devices that have large acceptable power ranges will have a higher probability of being clinically successful

temperature before the stopping point (s_2) is reached. These approaches are complementary since one works in the range of applied powers that is below that required to obtain a heating volume of 100%, and the other above that power. That is, one approach is useful for situations where the heating systems cannot properly (completely) treat the tumor (point s_1) and the other approach is useful where they can (point s_2). These two complementary approaches give simple, systematic, quantitative, and clinically relevant measures of performance that provide ways of comparing system performances which are superior to the alternative of only reporting temperature or SAR distributions.

The first method has been used by the Dartmouth research group [80, 98–100], who used the volume axis as their measure of performance. The power output is increased until a stopping point (s_1) is reached, and then the volume of tumor heated to acceptable temperatures is measured [that volume at the stopping point (V_{s_1})]. If that volume is less than 50%, the treatment is labeled poor; for volumes between 50% and 75%; fair; between 75% and 100%, good; and for a volume of 100%, excellent. Devices or configurations able to heat more than 100% of the volume cannot be characterized further since they have no metric beyond that point.

For this higher range, the Arizona group [50, 51, 79, 112–114] used the applied power axis to measure the range of applied powers that give acceptable heatings of the complete tumor. That is, P_0 is the power at which 100% of the tumor reaches the therapeutic temperature, while P_{s_2} is the power at which the treatment stops because one has reached a limiting value (again T_{tu}^{max}, T_i^{max}, or Q^{max}, as per Table 3.10). Heating systems/configurations that have larger power ranges which give acceptable treatments ($\Delta P = P_{s_2} - P_0$) are, of course, preferable; just as are larger heated volumes in the volumetric approach.

Before reviewing the applications of these two approaches, some general comments, are pertinent. As discussed earlier, in order to perform sufficiently realistic simulations, one must have sufficiently realistic models of the anatomical locations to be heated, the power deposition patterns for the heating modality(s) being studied, and the physiological responses of the patients, and be able to predict accurately the resultant temperature fields during heating. Currently, we can obtain reasonable anatomies from the sophisticated imaging modalities presently available, although an accurate definition of tumor boundaries remains an unsolved problem for many cases. Second, as seen in Chap. 2, rapid progress has been made in the development of more and more realistic power deposition simulation programs, and that can be expected to continue. Third, there are two areas in which significant effort must be made in the development of an improved bioheat transfer equation: including the effects of blood flow in large vessels; and characterizing the physiological responses of the body to thermal stress, particularly the blood flow responses. While the limitations of the bioheat transfer equation have been discussed earlier (Chap. 1) and will thus not be discussed here (except briefly on p. 186), it is also of interest to note that the rank ordering of systems in these comparative analyses may not be affected by some of these limitations, since they are common to all systems evaluated and may drop out of consideration. This leaves the major problem of simulating the patient's blood perfusion patterns and magnitudes – the bête noire of hyperthermia simulations since these quantities are generally unknown. Fortunately, at least for *comparative* thermal dosimetry, one does not need to know the blood perfusion distribution for a given patient but, instead, just for a typical patient or a set of typical patients. Also, since parametric studies can be performed, a whole range of perfusions can be studied. If one device or configuration is superior for all reasonable perfusions, then the choice of modality is clear, at least for comparative purposes.

While this approach allows one to rank order the heating configurations studied, it is also desirable to be able to relate the results to absolute clinical values as closely as possible. Additionally, it would be useful if one did not have to study a large range of possibilities but, instead, could bracket the possible cases that might occur and simulate the extreme cases. For clinical treatments, these would be the tumor perfusions that were the easiest and hardest to heat (see Fig. 3.51 and [112, 113]). It is useful here, just as before, to have a set of ideals; in this case for the ideal simulation program, as characterized in Table 3.11. The presence or absence of these characteristics can be used to judge the completeness of the models

Table 3.11. Ideal simulation program characteristics for comparative thermal dosimetry

1. Three dimensional
2. Realistic, inhomogeneous tissues
3. Realistic power deposition simulations
4. Best- and worst-case blood perfusion patterns studied for a range of realistic perfusion magnitudes
5. "Improved" bioheat transfer equation used, including:
   a) Large blood vessel effects
   b) Variable arterial blood temperature
   c) Directional effects of blood flow

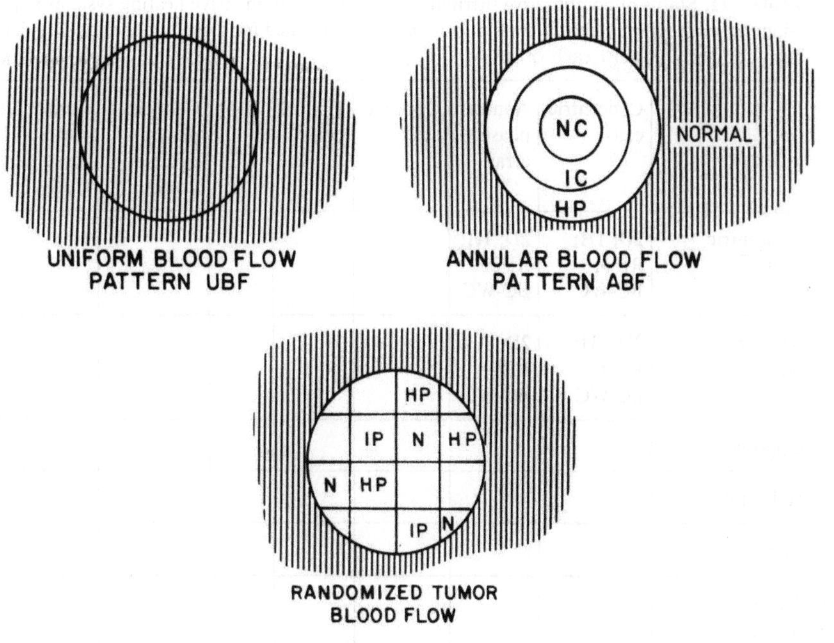

Fig. 3.51. Examples of idealized models of tumor perfusion patterns that are easy (uniform) and hard (annular) to heat properly. Such best- and worst-case situations need to be developed and analyzed for comparative hyperthermia situations. Specifically, these cases need to bracket the actual conditions to be found in tumors. Most real tumors (e.g., a set of randomized tumor blood flows) should have results that fall between the best and worst cases. [110]

reviewed later, although in some cases they are not all necessary as long as the simulations remain "sufficiently accurate" for a given goal. Given these general considerations, we can now review the current state of comparative thermal dosimetry.

3.3.1.2 Current Status of Comparative Evaluations

It is useful here to divide the large number of hyperthermia systems that are presently available into several broad categories that contain the devices designed to heat certain classes of tumors, and to divide these into subclasses where appropriate. Devices in the following categories will be discussed, both in terms of those that have been comparatively analyzed and in terms of intercomparisons that should be performed: regional power deposition systems for the trunk and the extremities, interstitial devices, superficial external applicators, and whole-body hyperthermia systems.

Regional Power Deposition Systems

Trunk

The proper noninvasive heating of deep-seated tumors for the multiple locations where they occur has been the goal in the design and application of many devices because of the frequency of occurrence and importance of these tumors. These include:

1. The Magnetrode concentric coil magnetic induction [136].
2. Application of opposed, Helmholtz pairs of magnetic induction devices [91].
3. The BSD annular phased-array system of multiple, in-phase, concentric microwave antenna [144, 145].
4. The coaxial TEM applicator being developed by Lagendijk [67] and de Leeuw [28].
5. The helical coil device recently developed by Ruggera and Kantor [118].
6. Pairs of opposed capacitor plate electrodes, now available commercially in the Japanese Thermotron system [130].
7. Multiple-electrode capacitor plate electrode systems in a "cross-fire" arrangement proposed by LeVeen et al. [76] and now available commercially in a French three-electrode system [126, 127].
8. Ring electrodes [150].

Also while not truly regional sytems, the following devices have been proposed and/or used for deep-seated tumors of the trunk:

9. The many groups working on multiple-antennae phased-array microwave systems (see Lin [77] for a review of recent developments)
10. Ultrasound systems, either with multiple, stationary transducers (e.g., [37]), or mechanically scanned systems as introduced and used extensively by Lele and his group (e.g., [75]) and also developed and applied at Arizona (e.g., [56]).

Table 3.12. Status of comparative thermal dosimetry for noninvasive heating systems applied to deep-seated tumors of the trunk. Diagonal elements indicate the level of simulations performed for a given modality. Off-diagonal elements show which devices have been compared against each other

	Concentric coils	Annular phased array	Opposed coils	Helical coil	TEM	Capacitive plates: two electrodes	Capacitive plates: three electrodes	Capacitive rings	Phased-array microwaves	Scanned, focused ultrasound
Concentric coils	2D; IH; RPD; BC-WC	2D; IH; RPD; BC-WC								
Annular phased array	2D; IH; RPD; BC-WC	2D; IH; RPD; BC-WC								
Opposed coils										
Helical coil										
TEM										
Capacitive plates; two electrodes										
Capacitive plates; three electrodes										
Capacitive rings										
Phased-array microwaves										
Scanned, focused ultrasound										2D; IH; RPD; BC-WC

1D, 2D, 3D, one, two, or three dimensional; H, IH, homogeneous, inhomogeneous tissue model; SPD, RPD, simplified, realistic power deposition model; IBHTE, improved bioheat transfer equation analysis; BC-WC, best case-worst case blood perfusion models used

Unfortunately, most of the cross comparisons of these devices have not been performed (although they might not be necessary in some cases due to similarities in the power deposition fields), as illustrated in Table 3.12. Here the elements on the diagonal indicate that at least a set of thermal evaluations has been performed for the given device, while off-diagonal elements show which devices have been comparatively evaluated via a thermal analysis, and at what level. Ideally, all elements would be filled with "3D, IH, RPD, IBHTE, BC-WC" to indicate that a fully three-dimensional, inhomogeneous patient model with a realistic power deposition was analyzed with an improved bioheat transfer equation, for a range of blood perfusions from a best-case to a worst-case model. One only needs to take a glance at this table to recognize the newness of the hyperthermia field, and even more so of hyperthermia simulations. The reason for this situation is obvious – due to the recent and rapid development of hyperthermia, the basic tools for performing the simulations have not been developed, particularly three-dimensional power deposition patterns for inhomogeneous tissues, improved bioheat transfer equations, and knowledge of clinical blood perfusion responses. The results are also obvious in the clinical environment – wide-ranging claims for the thermal performances and efficacy of many systems, with no common, valid method of comparing them. That is, since the systems' thermal analyses have been done clinically with all of the in-

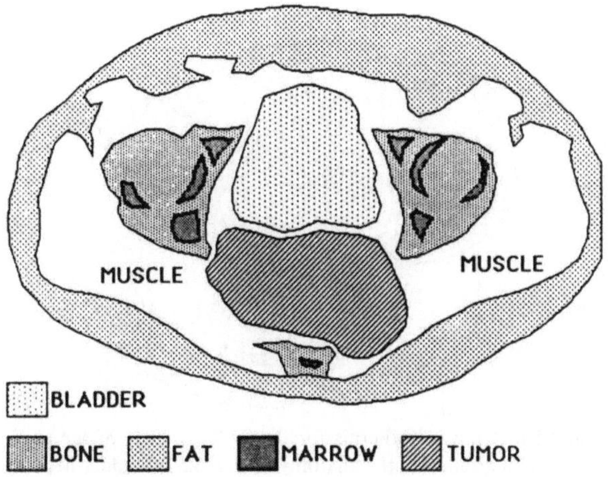

Fig. 3.52. Two-dimensional pelvic model used in comparative thermal dosimetry analysis of concentric coil and annular phased-array systems. [142]

herent unknowns, we are burdened by the unknown-input, unknown-output problem of clinical trials, as illustrated in Fig. 3.49.

Two regional systems have been extensively evaluated, and these are, not unexpectedly, the two devices which have had the most extensive clinical applications – the magnetrode concentric coil device [136] and the BSD annular phased-array system [144, 145]. The initial simulations of these two devices were one-dimensional, analytical [137], and numerical studies [50, 51] which clearly showed the major relative strengths and weaknesses of the two systems. Recently, these one-dimensional analyses have been extended to two-dimensional simulations using much more complex models of patient anatomies for several pelvic, abdominal, and thoracic tumors [100, 142]. A brief review of part of their studies follows to illustrate the types of comparisons that have been and can be performed. One site studied extensively with these models was a two-dimensional, inhomogeneous, tumor-bearing, pelvic cross-section (Fig. 3.52). Realistic finite element-based power deposition patterns were generated for this inhomogeneous tissue for both the concentric coil (CC) and annular phased-array devices (AA). The resultant temperatures were calculated for a wide variety of blood flows, and the tumor volume heated to the desired treatment temperature was determined when the maximum allowable power was reached (point s_1 of Fig. 3.50). The limiting temperatures used were $T_{tu}^{max} < 60\,°C$, $T_{fat}^{max} = T_{mus}^{max} = T_{bone}^{max} = 44\,°C$; $T_{viscera}^{max} = 42\,°C$. Therapeutic tumor temperatures of both 42 °C and 43 °C were evaluated. The HEP (hyperthermia equipment performance) ratings of poor (P), $V_{s_1} < 50\%$; fair (F), $50\% < V_{s_1} < 75\%$; good (G), $75\% < V_{s_1} < 100\%$; and excellent (E), $V_{s_1} = 100\%$ were used. Three possible states of the bladder were evaluated: filled with static urine, flushed with non-ionized water which was not temperature controlled, and flushed with non-ionized water which was kept at 42 °C. The SAR and temperature patterns for the latter case are shown in Figs. 3.53–3.56 (p. 162).

Table 3.13 shows the results for the cases analyzed, including a listing of the conditions which caused the applied power to be limited (point s_1, Fig. 3.50). The basic comparative conclusion from their studies was that the annular array produced better ratings than the concentric coil in almost all cases. Also, the ratings for the annular array were generally low, indicating that it would have trouble properly heating deep-seated tumors. It is interesting to note that this basic conclusion is the same as that drawn from the simpler one-dimensional studies. However, the cur-

Table 3.13. HEP ratings for Fig. 3.52 (pelvic with bladder); flushed bladder held at 42 °C

Perfusion rates (ml/100 g/min)						Ratings				Power level	
FT	MU	BO	MA	BL	TU	CC		AA		CC	AA
						42 °C	43 °C	42 °C	43 °C		
03+	2.7*	0	2	0	0	P	P	G	G	2.2	3.1
*+					5	P	P	P	P	2.2	5.0
*+					15	P	P	P	P	2.2	5.0
5+	15*	2	12	0	0	F	P	G	F	7.8	5.5
+	*				5	P	P	G	F	7.8	16.8
+	*				15	P	P	P	P	7.8	26.2
15+	54	5	45	0	0*	F	F	G	G	21.3	10.4
+	*				5	P	P	G	G	21.3	26.5
+	*				15	P	P	G	F	21.3	46.7

FT, fat; MU, muscle; BO, bone; MA, marrow; BL, bladder; TU, tumor; *, AA-limiting tissue; +, CC-limiting tissue

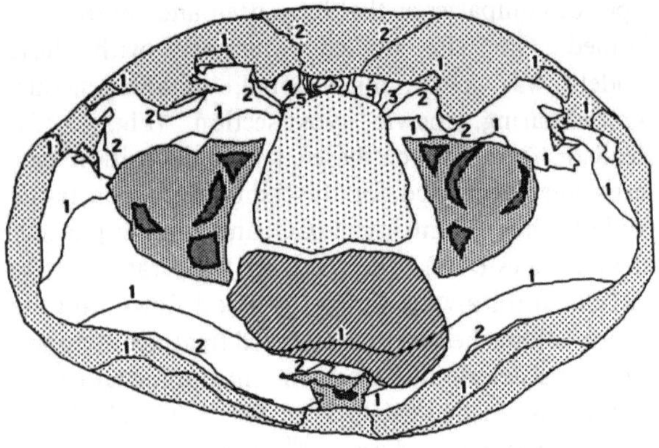

Fig. 3.53. Iso-SAR contours for the concentric coil applied to the anatomy of Fig. 3.52; bladder filled with non-ionized water at 42 °C. [142]

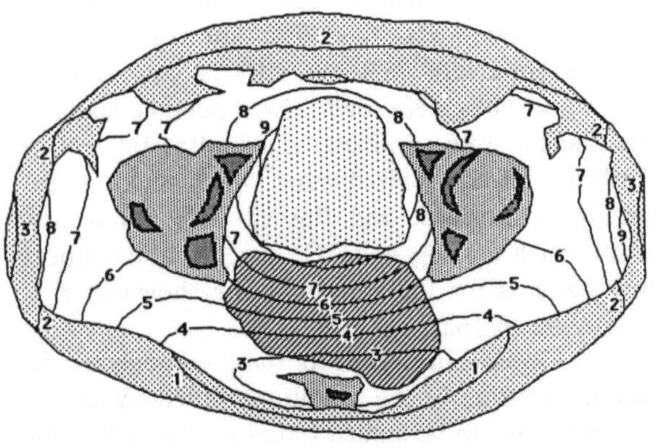

Fig. 3.54. Iso-SAR contours for the annular phased array applied to the anatomy of Fig. 3.52; bladder field with non-ionized water. [142]

rent two-dimensional results shed light on many other aspects of the problem and extend the one-dimensional studies. The results of this comparison, plus a comparison with clinical observations using these two devices, is summarized below. This comparison clearly illustrates that these simulations can be powerful (and fast and efficient) tools for comparative evaluations of devices since they seem to be able to reproduce general clinical trends. (Here these authors refer to an ARD, absorption rate density, where $ARD = \varrho SAR = \dot{Q}_a$).

Clinical Observation. Deep-seated heating with concentric coils has been therapeutically ineffective mainly because of inability to deposit power at depth. As a result, attempts at deep heating have often resulted in higher temperatures in the superficial normal tissue than in the deeper tumor. Annular arrays have produced broader, deeper regional heating than concentric coils, but heating patterns have often been unpredictable.
Theoretical Result. Calculated ARD distributions for a concentric coil (Paulsen et al. [100]) have shown little deep power deposition with large relative energies absorbed in the normal tissue near the body surface, while for an annular array (Paulsen et al. [100]) they have shown broad energy absorption across

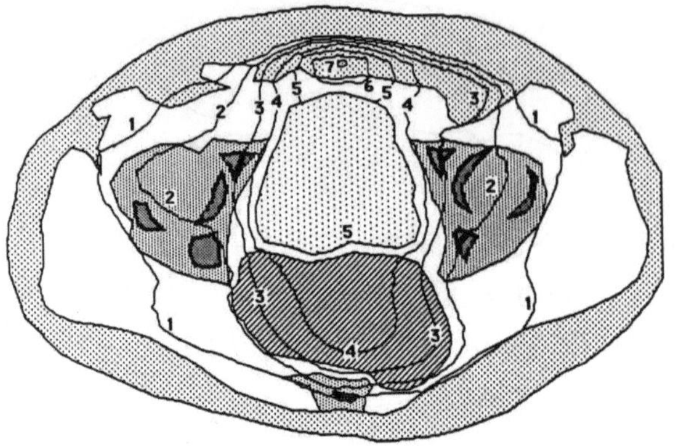

Fig. 3.55. Relative isotherms for the SAR patterns of the concentric coil applied to the anatomy of Fig. 3.52; bladder held at 42 °C. [142]

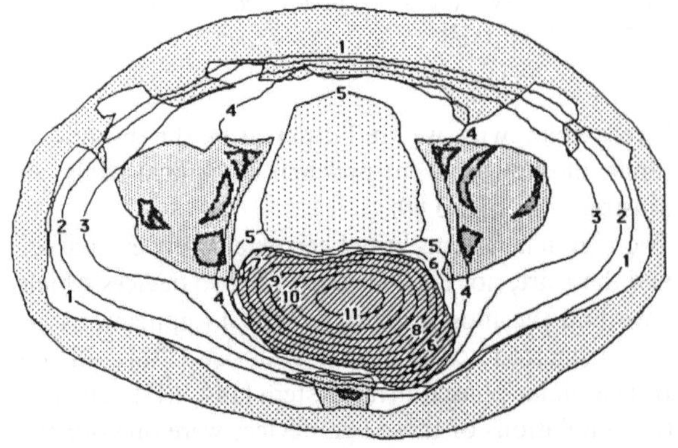

Fig. 3.56. Relative isotherms for the SAR pattern of the annular phased array applied to the anatomy of Fig. 3.52; bladder held at 42 °C. [142]

most body cross-sections, including significant power deposition at depth (e.g., cf. Fig. 3.53 and 3.54).

Clinical Observation. Concentric coils have been ineffective for tumors in the central pelvic region because of inability to deposit energy at depth and the occurrence of severe sacrococcygeal pain in the patient. Annular arrays, on the other hand, have shown the most promise in the pelvic region. Central pelvic temperatures of 41 °C have been readily achieved; however, tumor temperatures of 43 °C have been difficult to obtain and maintain (perhaps due to conservative treatment protocols).
Theoretical Result. The HEP ratings here (see Table 3.12) and in Paulsen et al. [100] have demonstrated that an annular array performs markedly better than a concentric coil in the pelvic region. Furthermore, the annular array has produced its best HEP ratings in this body section, while the performance of the concentric coil has remained relatively ineffective. Out of 66 total cases using the 43 °C threshold, the annular array produced HEP ratings of 32 P, 13 F, and 21 G; whereas, the concentric coil produced ratings of 58 P, 7 F, and 1 G.

Clinical Observation. In the abdomen, annular arrays have appeared only slightly superior to concentric coils; however, both devices have shown major limitations in this body section.
Theoretical Result. In the abdomen, an annular array has produced HEP ratings [100] that are only somewhat better than those of a concentric coil, but neither device's ratings have been

very favorable. In 30 cases using the 43 °C threshold, the annular array received HEP ratings of 18P, 12F, and 0G; whereas the concentric coil received ratings of 25P, 5F, and 0G.

Clinical Observation. Temperature distributions in large pelvic or abdominal tumors have seldom been uniform even though temperature elevation at depth has been achievable with an annular array.
Theoretical Result. The large number of fair and poor HEP ratings has indicated that ther thermal profiles produced by these devices have significant thermal gradients in tumors which often make temperature distributions therapeutically nonuniform [142 pp. 435–437].

Further studies are needed in order to draw firmer conclusions with improved models, but one can see that the models can be used to perform clinically useful comparisons and evaluations. Indeed, there are now three clinical papers which present comparative results for these two devices [42, 90, 122], and the major conclusions of these clinical studies were previously predicted by the simulations.
Two major extensions of these simulations that would be useful would be go to three dimensions, a task which is presently being undertaken (K. Paulsen 1987, personal communication) and possibly to account for preheating of blood in the servicing vessels before it reaches the tumor. Some modeling of three-dimensional effects has been performed for whole-body models of annular array heating systems, primarily to study the effects of "aberrant heating" (e.g., see [47]), i.e., local pain at locations where electric fields are constrained and/or leave the body normal to the tissue. Samulski et al. [120] also discuss the clinical limitations placed on the applied power which can occur because of this phenomenon. If this feature were incorporated in the model, the result would be a potential lowering of the ratings for the annular array system, causing even poorer performance. Similarly, the effects of neglecting three-dimensional heat transfer are that only the plane which is located in the center of the power deposition field is analyzed and the effects of both lowered power deposition away from this plane and heat transfer in the axial direction are neglected. That is, the two ends of a tumor along the axis of the body tend to be colder than the tumor center, and thus a three-dimensional model which included these would need higher powers in order to heat properly a given volume of the tumor. These higher powers would cause higher temperatures at all locations, possibly causing treatment termination at lower heated volumes and thus giving lower HEP ratings for both the annular phased array and concentric coil devices.
These basic three-dimensional effects have been studied by Chen et al. [21] in a simple three-dimensional, inhomogeneous patient model subject to uniform heating. The model used is illustrated in Fig. 3.57, and it has been used to compare three- and two-dimensional simulation predictions. Three-dimen-

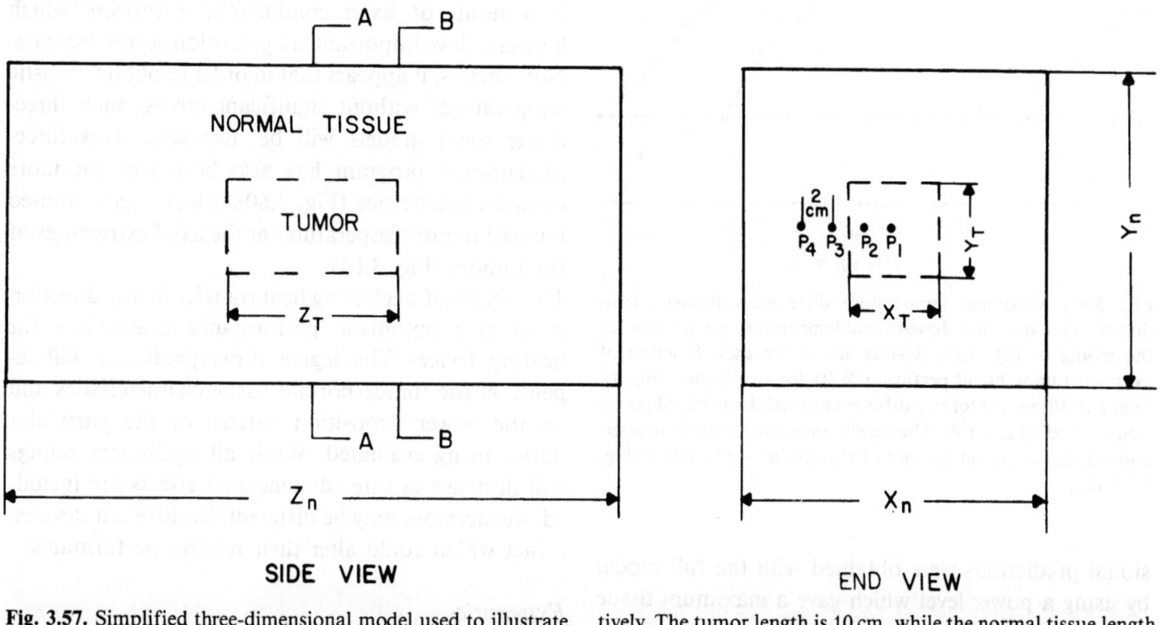

Fig. 3.57. Simplified three-dimensional model used to illustrate the effects of axial conduction. The tumor and normal tissue are uniformly perfused at different values, and all of the tissue is heated uniformly. The tumor and normal tissue are rectangular parallelepipeds with heights and depths of 6 and 20 cm, respectively. The tumor length is 10 cm, while the normal tissue length is 40 cm. All external surfaces of the normal tissue are assumed to be at 37 °C. P1–P4 indicate the locations of the axial temperature profiles shown in Fig. 3.58. [21]

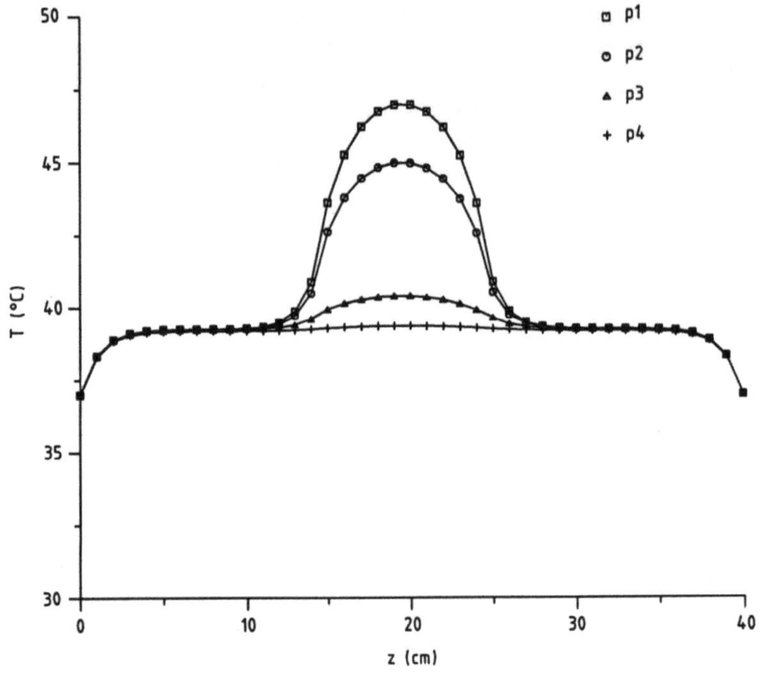

Fig. 3.58. Temperature versus axial position for the necrotic, 10-cm-long tumor of Fig. 3.57 with normal tissue perfusion of 1 kg/m^3/s. The temperature profiles for the central axis through the tumor (P 1) and for parallel lines offset from that axis by 2-cm increments (P 2 → P 4) are shown. [21]

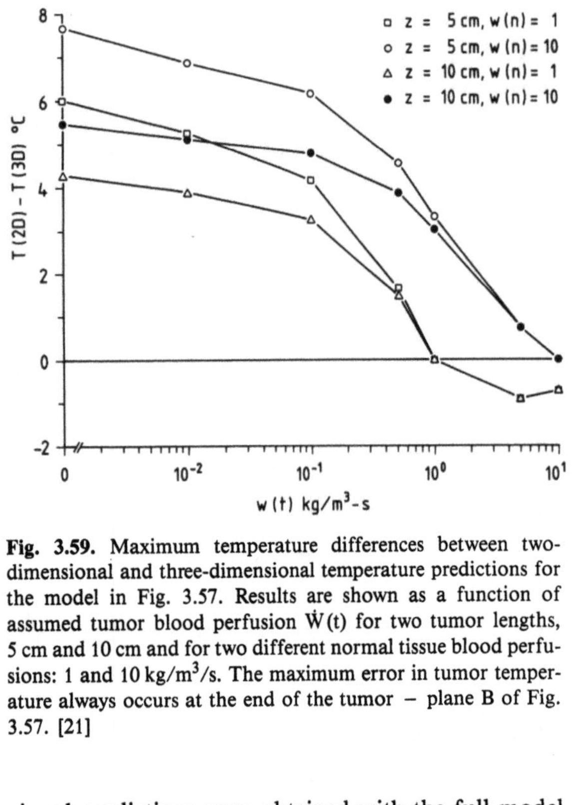

Fig. 3.59. Maximum temperature differences between two-dimensional and three-dimensional temperature predictions for the model in Fig. 3.57. Results are shown as a function of assumed tumor blood perfusion $\dot{W}$(t) for two tumor lengths, 5 cm and 10 cm and for two different normal tissue blood perfusions: 1 and 10 kg/m^3/s. The maximum error in tumor temperature always occurs at the end of the tumor – plane B of Fig. 3.57. [21]

sional predictions were obtained with the full model by using a power level which gave a maximum tissue temperature of 47 °C (i.e., a 10 °C temperature rise above an arterial temperature of 37 °C; see Fig. 3.58). The two-dimensional simulations were done for the central plane (A) of Fig. 3.57, using all of the same properties as in the three-dimensional case, including the applied power level. Figure 3.59 shows the differences between the predictions of the two-dimensional model and the three-dimensional model for the end of the tumor (B, Fig. 3.57). Significant errors can be seen in the two-dimensional results for the end of the tumor, especially for poorly perfused tumors. This is a result of axial conduction, a process which becomes less important as perfusion levels increase. Nonetheless, it appears that in order to obtain realistic temperatures without significant errors, such three-dimensional models will be necessary. This three-dimensional program has also been run for more complex geometries (Fig. 3.60), which again showed lowered tumor temperatures at the axial extremities of the tumors (Fig. 3.61).

The effects of neglecting heat transfer in any direction is to give optimistic performance predictions for heating devices. The degree of overprediction will depend on the tumor/normal tissue characteristics and on the power deposition pattern of the particular device being evaluated. While all equipment ratings will decrease as three-dimensional effects are included, the decrease may be different for different devices, a fact which could alter their relative performance.

Extremities

The variety of systems applicable to regional heating of the extremities include all of the devices mentioned above, and modifications thereof. Again, a few of

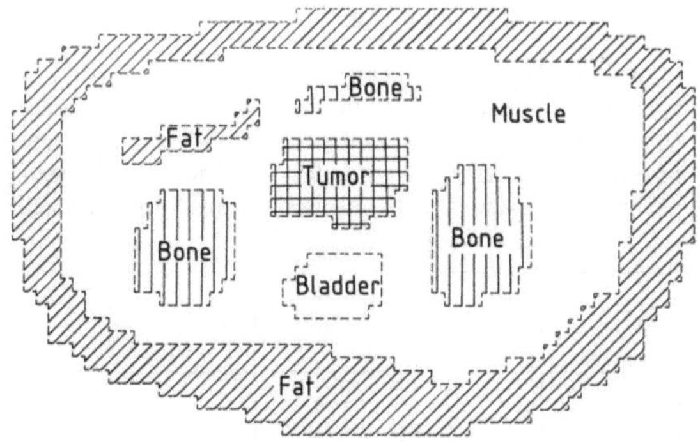

Fig. 3.60. Digitized CT scan of cross section of a pelvic tumor. Eleven such sequential scans were taken at 1-cm intervals along the axis of the body to construct a three-dimensional finite difference model of the patient. The tumor extended for 6 cm along the body axis. [21]

these approaches have been analyzed individually, but no cross comparisons are available.

Local Hyperthermia Systems

It is convenient here to divide heating systems into noninvasive and interstitial techniques.

Noninvasive Approaches

Here, a variety of approaches have been proposed and many used in clinical settings. These systems differ from the above regional/extremity systems only in that smaller volumes of tissue are heated. They include:

1. Single, stationary mirowave antennae with a variety of field shapes which depend on the particular antenna used.
2. Multiple stationary microwave antennae [52].
3. Single or multiple microwave antennae that are mechanically scanned [74].
4. Single, planar ultrasound systems.
5. Multiple stationary planar ultrasound systems [146].
6. Scanned planar [143] and focused [56, 75] ultrasound systems.
7. Two-electrode RF plate systems.
8. Multiple-elecrode external RF systems [76].

Table 3.14 illustrates the status of thermal modeling for these systems. One can see here the paucity of information for these devices, with very little analysis of individual modalities and no cross comparisons. Thus, many different institutions use a variety of different devices and configurations, with an even wider variety of claims for relative performance. Since there is no common basis for comparison of these claims

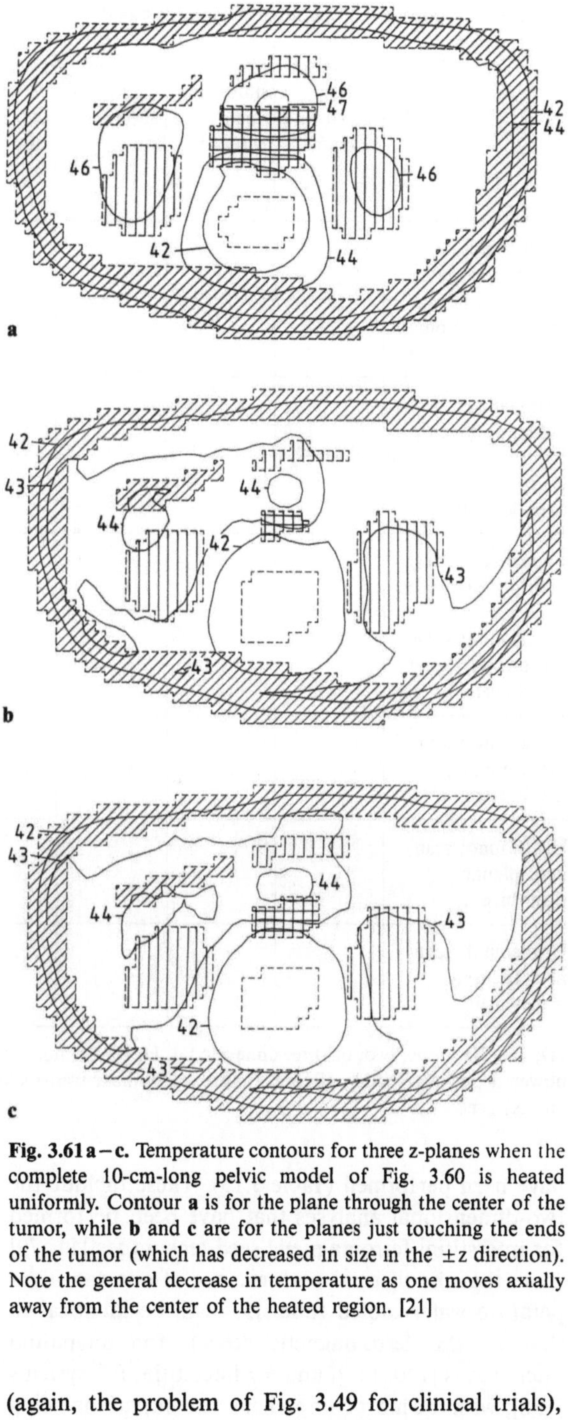

Fig. 3.61 a – c. Temperature contours for three z-planes when the complete 10-cm-long pelvic model of Fig. 3.60 is heated uniformly. Contour **a** is for the plane through the center of the tumor, while **b** and **c** are for the planes just touching the ends of the tumor (which has decreased in size in the ±z direction). Note the general decrease in temperature as one moves axially away from the center of the heated region. [21]

(again, the problem of Fig. 3.49 for clinical trials), one cannot comparatively evaluate them or make very valid judgments of their relative thermal performance.

Interstitial Systems

For interstitial systems, which have an even more highly focused power deposition pattern than the systems described above, several thermal analyses

Table 3.14. Status of comparative thermal dosimetry for noninvasive hyperthermia of superficial, localized tumors

	Single stationary microwave antenna	Multiple stationary microwave antenna	Scanned microwave antenna	Capacitive plates: two electrodes	Capacitive plates: multiple electrodes	Ultrasound: single stationary, planar transducer	Ultrasound: multiple stationary transducers	Ultrasound: scanned, planar transducer	Ultrasound: scanned, focused transducer
Single stationary microwave antenna									
Multiple stationary microwave antenna									
Scanned microwave antenna									
Capacitive plates: two electrodes									
Capacitive plates: multiple electrodes									
Ultrasound: single stationary, planar transducer									
Ultrasound: multiple stationary transducers									
Ultrasound: scanned, planar transducer									
Ultrasound: scanned, focused transducer									3D; IH; RPD; BC-WC

1D, 2D, 3D = one, two, or three dimensional; H, IH, homogeneous, inhomogeneous tissue model; SPD, RPD, simplified, realistic power deposition model; IBHTE, improved bioheat transfer equation analysis; BC-WC, best case-worst case blood perfusion models used

have been performed (Table 3.15). These include the two-dimensional analyses that have been performed for interstitial ferromagnetic seed techniques [11, 79] (note that the thermal performance of constant-temperature water-cooled tubes [53] will be identical to that of the ferromagnetic seeds), for interstitial microwaves [140, 141], and for interstitial RF systems [138], with the most comprehensive comparison being the recent study by Mechling and Strohbehn [80], who comparatively analyzed the behavior of ferromagnetic seeds, interstitital LCF, and interstitial microwave antennae in a two-dimensional study of both homogeneous and inhomogeneous tumors. Figure 3.62 illustrates the geometry of the implants used in part of this latter study, while Table 3.16 illustrates the studies' results for homogeneously perfused tissues, again in terms of HEP ratings, with a therapeutic temperature of 43 °C, a maximum allowable tumor temperature of 60 °C, and a maximum allowable normal tissue temperature of 44 °C. Here, one can see that all three systems perform well at low blood perfusion rates, with all performances decreasing as blood perfusion increases and with the microwave system keeping its high ratings for more cases of increased perfusion. To obtain the same rating for all systems at a given high blood perfusion would require a higher density of implants for ferromagnetic and RF systems. Thus, in this case, it is quite critical to know the tumor blood perfusion characteristics if one is to refine these ratings and determine which of these modalities are acceptable (although the required implant density may be determined by clinical considerations). For these interstitial systems, the three-dimensional characteristics will be

Table 3.15. Status of comparative thermal dosimetry for interstitial devices

	Constant temperature sources (ferro-magnetic seeds; heated tubes): single temperature for all sources	Interstitial RF systems: single fre-quency, constant power for all elec-trodes	Interstitial microwaves: single fre-quency and phase, con-stant power for all elec-trodes	Constant temperature sources: variable temperature sources at different locations	Interstitial RF systems: independent control of electrode power and frequency	Interstitial microwa-ves: phase and am-plitude controlled
Constant temperature sources (ferromagnetic seeds; heated tubes): single temperature for all sources	2D; IH; RPD; BC-WC	2D; IH; RPD	2D; IH; RPD			
Interstitial RF systems: single frequency, con-stant power for all electrodes	2D; IH; RPD	2D; IH; RPD	2D; IH; RPD			
Interstitial microwaves: single fre-quency and phase, constant power for all electrodes	2D; IH; RPD	2D; IH; RPD	2D; IH; RPD			
Constant temperature sources: variable tem-perature sources at different locations						
Interstitial RF systems: independent control of electrode power and frequency						
Interstitial microwaves: phase and amplitude controlled						

1D, 2D, 3D, one, two, or three dimensional; H, IH, homogeneous, inhomogeneous tissue model; SPD, RPD, simplified, realistic power deposition model; IBHTE, improved bioheat transfer equation analysis; BC-WC, best case-worst case blood perfusion models used

very important since the power deposition control along the implant axis may be quite difficult for both RF and microwave systems, whereas the constant temperature sources will have good temperature control along their axis, thus possibly improving their relative ratings in any three-dimensional comparison. Thus, a three-dimensional analysis is needed to complete this comparative analysis, especially for irregularly shaped tumors where variable-length implants will be needed. Such an analysis also needs to include the effect of large blood vessels, something not considered in any previous analyses of interstitial techniques. Additionally, there are several nonthermal factors to be considered, as discussed by Strohbehn and Mechling [139].

Whole-Body Hyperthermia

For systems attempting to produce whole-body hyperthermia, there are two major heat transfer considerations. The first concerns the temperature distribution inside the body. That is, while the goal of these treatments is to produce a uniform temperature inside the body at the highest possible value without causing normal tissue damage (usually 41.8 °C), nonetheless, there are generally small temperature differences from organ to organ (Fig. 3.29 and 3.63). While these differences are small, they can be quite important due to their proximity to critical tissue temperatures. In order to calculate these differences for the whole body, one needs a whole-body model which can determine the temperature distributions inside various significant organs. This requires use of a whole-body temperature regulatory model similar to those previously developed for various thermoregulatory and environmental studies, such as the models of Stolwijk and Hardy [135], Wissler [157], and Gordon et al. [43]; e.g., see Figs. 3.64 and 3.65. Charny et al. [16] have recently used an extension of these models to calculate temperature distribution during regional hyperthermia with the APAS system. Figure 3.66 illustrates some of their temperature distribution and blood perfusion results from a simulated treatment. In addition to calculating internal temperatures, such models can also be used to perform comparative analyses of different whole-body heating modalities, particularly to solve for rates of increase in temperature, a potentially important consideration in these devices both to reduce overall treatment time and possibly avoid the development of thermotolerance during the initial heating period – a speculative problem at present [48]. These rates are dependent on the heating modality, just as are the internal temperature distributions.

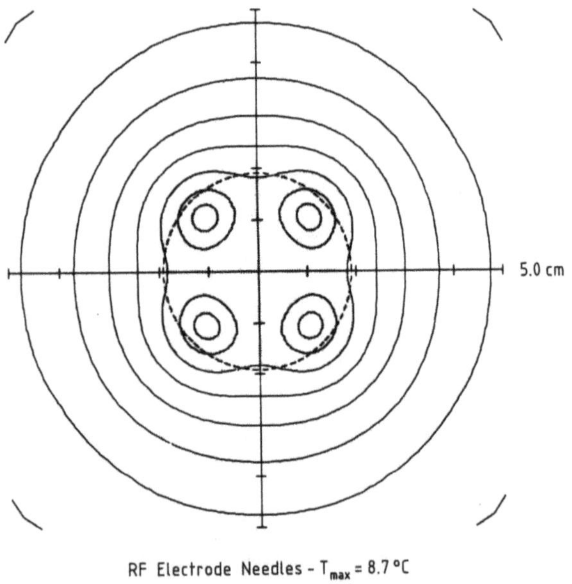

Fig. 3.62. Temperature distribution for rf needles implanted in a 2×2-cm-square array inside a uniformly perfused tissue with a blood perfusion rate of 2.5 ml/100 g/min. Isotherms at 1 °C intervals are shown, starting with the 8 °C rise around each electrode. [139]

There are four basic methods that have been used for inducing whole-body temperatures (see van der Zee et al. [149] for a recent review):

1. Fever induced by using toxins to increase metabolic activity and elevated temperatures.
2. Transcutaneous methods which use convective and radiative heat transfer from a controlled exterior environment to the skin to transfer energy into the body (these include water baths, water suits and blankets, hot air chambers, molten wax baths, and radiant heating devices).
3. Extracorporeal blood heating in which blood is removed from the body via a femoral arterial-venous shunt, passed through a heat exchanger to

Table 3.16. HEP ratings for three interstitial hyperthermia systems. [139]

Blood flow (ml/100 g/min)	Seed Spacing (cm)			RF Spacing (cm)			Antenna Spacing (cm)		
	1	2	3	1	2	3	1	2	3
a) *Device diameter – 1 mm*									
0.0	E	E	E	E	E	E	E	E	E
2.5	E	G_N	G_N	E	E	F_N	E	E	G_N
5.0	E	G_N	P_N	E	G_N	P_N	E	E	G_N
10.0	E	G_T	P_T	E	F_N	P_N	E	E	G_N
20.0	G_T	P_T	P_T	E	P_N	P_N	E	E	F_N
50.0	F_T	P_T	P_T	G_N	P_N	P_N	E	G_T	P_N
100.0	P_T	P_T	P_T	G_N	P_T	P_T	E	G_T	P_N
b) *Device diameter – 2 mm*									
0.0	E	E	E	E	E	E	E	E	E
2.5	E	G_N	G_N	E	E	F_N	E	E	G_N
5.0	E	G_N	P_N	E	G_N	P_N	E	E	G_N
10.0	E	G_N	P_N	E	F_N	P_N	E	E	G_N
20.0	E	F_T	P_T	E	P_N	P_N	E	E	F_N
50.0	F_T	P_T	P_T	G_N	P_N	P_N	E	G_T	P_N
100.0	P_T	P_T	P_T	G_N	P_N	P_N	E	G_T	P_N

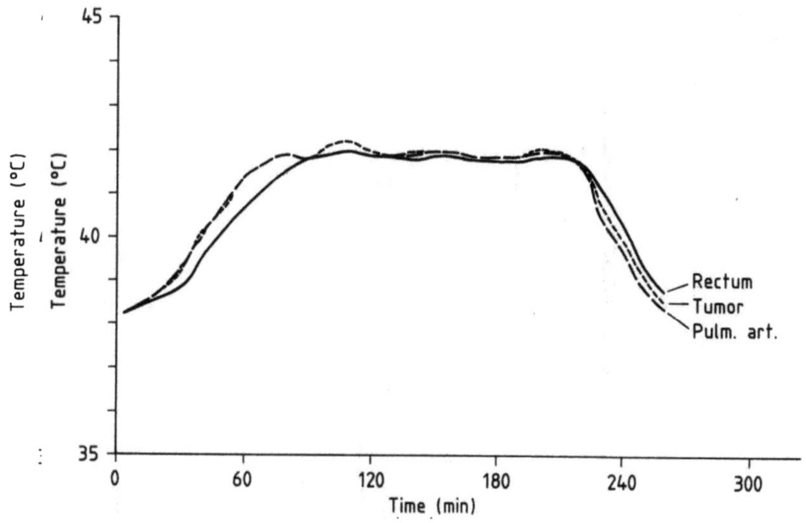

Fig. 3.63. Example of a time-temperature plot for human whole-body hyperthermia. Note that the rectum temperature lags behind the other temperatures. [149]

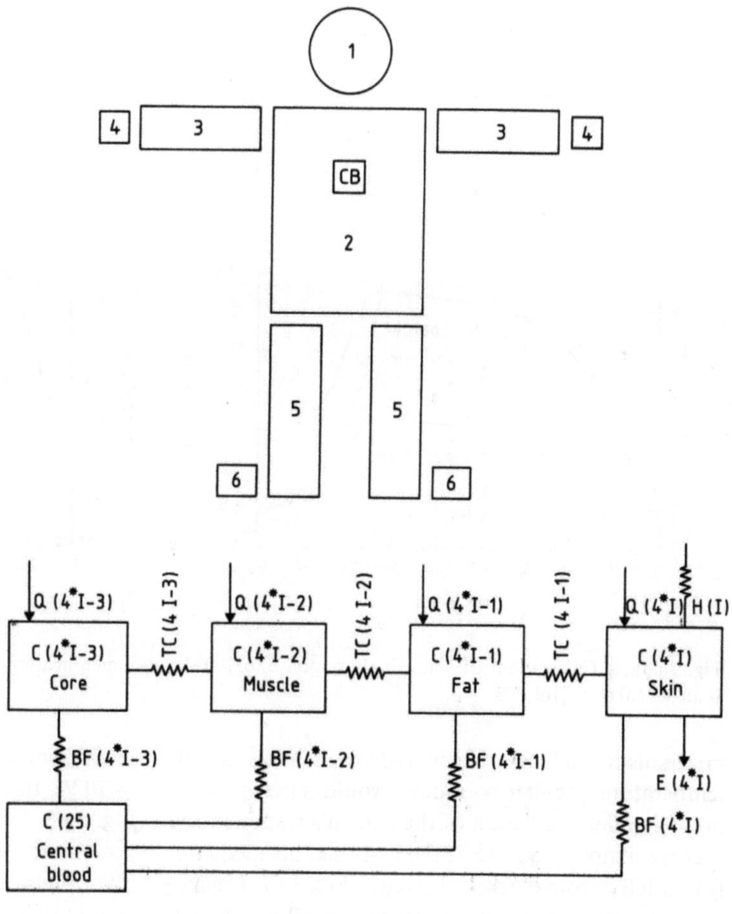

Fig. 3.64. The six segments of the controlled system for a whole-body thermal model and the arrangement of thermal nodes within one segment. [134]

increase its temperature, and returned to the body via the venous shunt.

4. The use of the previously described regional heating devices to deposit large amounts of power into the body and thus rapidly increase temperatures.

To compare the relative heating rates possible with these methods, a very simple lumped capacitive analysis can be used, as illustrated in Fig. 3.67. For the febrile method, the person will be insulated against energy losses, and the increase in metabolism due to increased temperature will be the basic

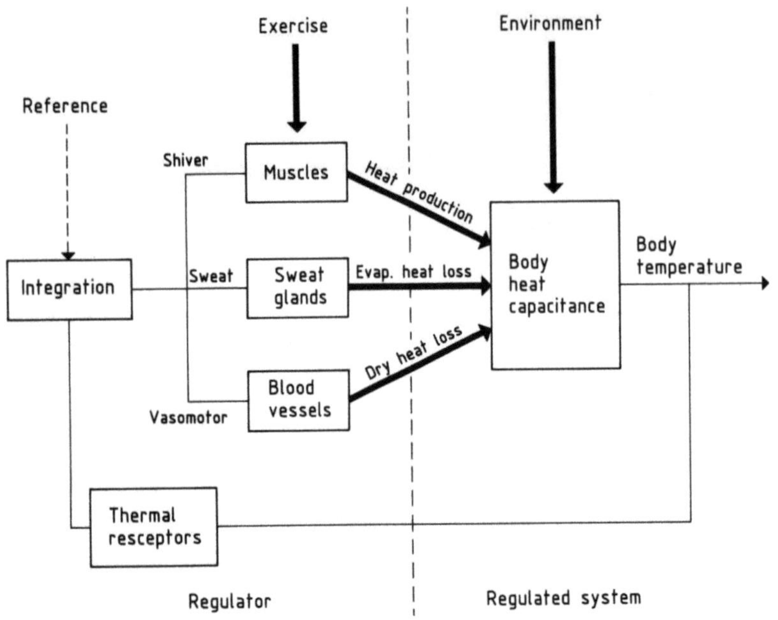

Fig. 3.65. Simplified block diagram of the human thermoregulatory control system used in Fig. 3.64. [134]

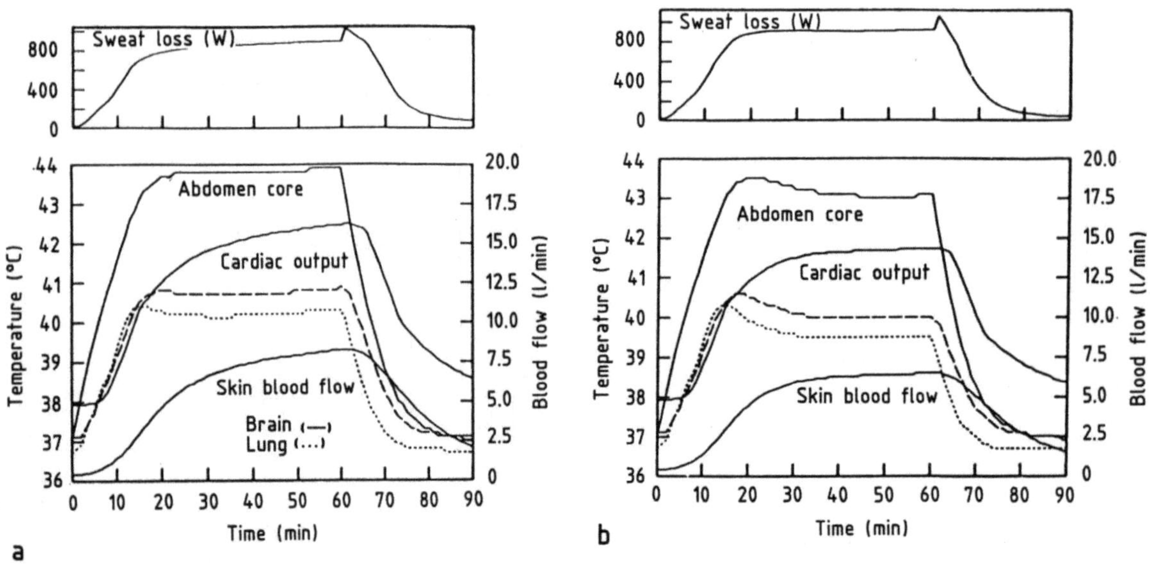

Fig. 3.66a, b. Calculations of whole-body response to 1000-W abdomen heating with no spray cooling: **a** air velocity at 0.6 m/s; **b** air at 1.0 m/s. [16]

mechanism producing the hyperthermia. While a full-temperature regulatory model would give a much more detailed prediction of the person's response, the average temperature rise of the body can be adequately predicted from the model given in Fig. 3.67. Neglecting all energy losses, the equation describing the average body temperature contains just two terms, energy storage and metabolism:

$$Mc\,\frac{dT_{ave}}{dt} = \dot{Q}_m(T_{ave}) = \dot{Q}_m(T_{ba}) \times 1.07^{(T_{ave}-T_{ba})/0.5} \,. \tag{3.48}$$

For an average person of mass $M = 70$ kg and a resting metabolism at 37 °C of $\dot{Q}_m(T_{ba} = 37\,°C) = 70$ W, the rate of temperature increase is given in Fig. 3.68. For the regional heating devices, additional power can be added to the body, thus increasing the rate of temperature rise. For this case, the whole-body energy balance becomes

$$Mc\,\frac{dT_{ave}}{dt} = \dot{Q}_m(T_{ave}) + \dot{Q}_a \,. \tag{3.49}$$

If 1000 W of power is applied continuously (a number which is within the capabilities of these devices and is used in clinical practice for regional power deposition), then the results in Fig. 3.68 are obtained, indicating the greatly increased rate of temperature increase obtainable with this approach. Again, one would turn the power off at 42 °C and use some cooling method to balance the increased metabolism with some increased heat transfer from the body – a consideration not to be discussed at this point. However, the price one must pay for this increase in speed is the highly nonuniform internal temperature distribution inside the body, with significantly elevated temperatures in the region where power is deposited. This not only presents several significant clinical considerations, but will also limit the amount of power one can place in the body to avoid excessive temperatures in the heated region, particularly as one approaches the final treatment temperature. Such thermal details can, hopefully, be obtained using the whole-body and regional three-dimensional models previously mentioned.

The extracorporeal technique would also obey Eq. 3.49 and have an average temperature response similar to the regional heating devices, with $\dot{Q}_a$ being the power applied to the blood. In this case, the powers that can be deposited are smaller and are limited by the increase in temperature of the blood as it passes through the heat exchanger

$$\dot{M}_b c_b \Delta T_b = \dot{Q}_a \ . \qquad (3.50)$$

For an allowable 5 °C rise of the blood in the heat exchanger and up to 2 L/min blood flow diverted, this gives $\dot{Q}_a \cong 600$ W, showing the lower powers used by this method compared with the regional devices and thus the subsequent relatively longer heating times required. Heating times to reach 41.5 °–42 °C have been reported to be between 30 and 90 min, consistent with the results of Fig. 3.68 [97].

Finally, for the transcutaneous systems, the energy balance equation becomes

$$M c \frac{dT_{ave}}{dt} = \dot{Q}_m(T_{ave}) + (UA)_{sk}(T_{env} - T_{ave}) \ , \qquad (3.51\,a)$$

where the average heat transfer coefficient from the environment to the skin area (A_{sk}) is given by U_{sk}, a factor which depends on the particular device being used. If one models the radiant heating device with an exposed skin surface area of 1.2 m^2 and utilizes standard convective and radiative heat transfer coefficients of $h_{conv} = 4.0$ w/m^2°C and $h_r = 5.9$ w/m^2°C, then one obtains

$$M c \frac{dT_{ave}}{dt} = \dot{Q}_m(T_{ave}) + (hA)_r(T_r - T_{ave}) + (hA)_{conv}(T_{air} - T_{ave}) \ . \qquad (3.51\,b)$$

For typical conditions of this device ($T_r = 65$ °C, $T_{air} = 55$ °C [54]), the resulting variation of the average temperature of the patient with time is given in Fig. 3.68. One can see a significant increase in heating rate compared with the fever approach, but this method is still much slower than the use of regional power deposition methods. This time difference could be significant from the patient management view and/or the development of thermotolerance, as previously discussed. In any case, the modeling approach can clearly be applied here to evaluate comparatively the relative heating rate capabilities of these different devices using a standard, common model. The larger, whole-body temperature regulatory models can be used to refine and extend these results, as has been initiated by Charny et al. [16].

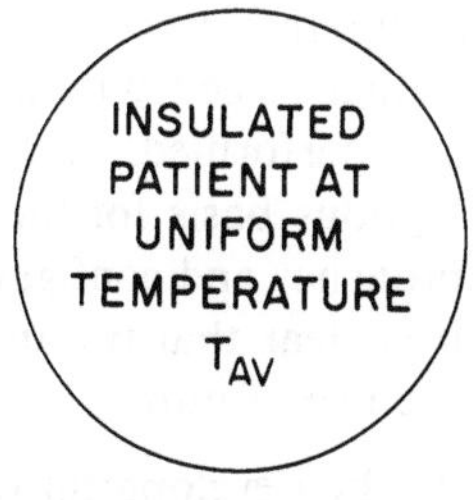

Fig. 3.67. Simple thermal model of insulated patient at some average temperature (T_{ave}) undergoing whole-body hyperthermia

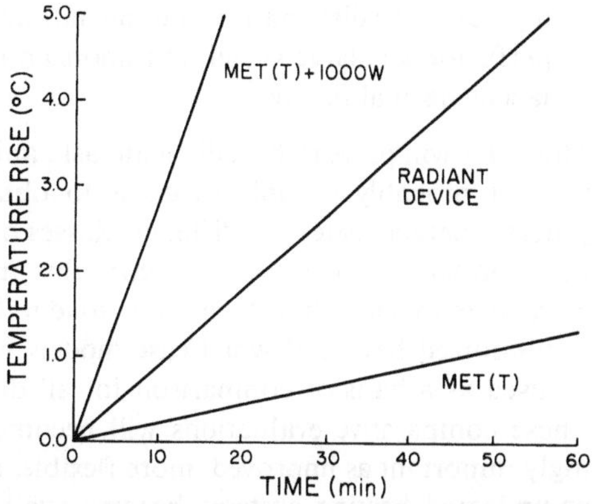

Fig. 3.68. Temperature versus time curves for relative heating rates otained by metabolism alone, i.e., the febrile method labeled MET (Eq. 3.48); by that metabolic response plus regional heating of 1 kW (Eq. 3.49); and by the radiant heating device Eq. 3.51 b) all for the idealized patient of Fig. 3.67

3.3.1.3 Conclusions

It is clear that while a great variety of technical problems need to be solved in this area, the comparative thermal analyses of different systems can still make a very valid contribution to hyperthermia in a manner which has several characteristics superior to what can be obtained from clinical trials. These two modes of comparative evaluations are very complementary, and both are needed for a thorough evaluation. Once they are performed, such analyses can add an unambiguous basis for thermally comparing different approaches and configurations. For valid model results, it is clear that two important steps must be taken in the near future

1. the development of three-dimensional models for inhomogeneous tissues for both power deposition and temperature distribution calculations and
2. the acquisition of significantly more information regarding the distribution and magnitude of blood perfusion and large vessels in tumors and their adjacent normal tissues.

The latter will prove to be a difficult task, and the best we will probably be able to do is to obtain some general characteristics for different classes of tumors. For comparative thermal dosimetry, this may, however, give us enough information to develop some standardized best- and worst-case models which can be used as a basis of comparison for all devices.

These comparative evaluations will become increasingly important as improved, more flexible, and more complicated heating systems become available. The use of these systems will involve making more decisions regarding the number, placement, relative orientations, and types of applicators to be used – decisions which will be too difficult to make without the assistance of computerized, comparative thermal dosimetry calculations. These calculations will need to include a method of comparatively evaluating different possible power deposition patterns for a given device, as was done for the analysis of Fig. 3.50.

3.3.2 Prospective Thermal Dosimetry

3.3.2.1 Introduction

Once a comparative evaluation is completed and a heating modality has been chosen for a particular patient, individual treatment planning becomes important. The basic concepts remain the same as in the previous category, except that the specific characteristics of the particular individual patient are now needed, rather than those for a generalized, typical patient. Parametric analysis can be used for tailoring the treatment to that patient rather than for comparing the general features of various modalities.

Several separate tasks are important. The first is to locate the tumor and the general anatomical features of the surrounding normal tissues through use of CT scans or other imaging techniques. Typical thermophysical property values from the literature can be assigned to the normal tissues. Properties of tumor tissues can be estimated based upon information that might be available on its constituents, such as the concentration of water or lipids. The power deposition pattern then must be determined for the region to be treated using the methods previously discussed (Chap. 2). In treatment planning, the actual blood flow in the normal tissues, as well as in the tumor, that *will be present* during the hyperthermia treatment must be known. Finally, the above information must be used in a temperature-solving routine that is flexible and can be easily used to assist clinical personnel in making the pretreatment decisions. The largest unknown in all of the above is the blood flow to be present during the treatment. Even though this information is generally unavailable, it still might be possible to use techniques such as the bracketing case tumor model concept (Fig. 3.51) of simulating easy- and hard-to-heat tumor and tissue situations to establish if the power deposition technique in question has a reasonable chance of producing an acceptable treatment of the tumor.

It is significant to note here that the concept of planning implicitly involves both having choices and having the techniques and tools available to assist in making these choices – two luxuries that hyperthermia has generally been lacking. That is, most equipment previously utilized has had a fixed, inflexible power deposition field which was always oriented with respect to the patient in a relatively well circumscribed manner – with only a small degree of allowable variation. For example, the patient was placed inside a regional power deposition device, such as the annular array, with the tumor located in the center of the device and, perhaps, the patient was moved around slightly. Similarly, for superficial microwave treatments, the antennae centerline was aligned, approximately, with the tumor center. Once this orientation was performed, power could be turned on and the power amplitude increased until patient tolerance levels, or maximum acceptable tumor temperatures, were reached. Thus, there was not really much planning to be done, and patient treatment planning was essentially superfluous.

Fortunately, newer hyperthermia treatment modalities are becoming increasingly flexible and, of course, complicated. For optimal treatments, implanted multiple-electrode RF, multiple-antennae microwave, and ferromagnetic seeds or constant-temperature water tube systems need to have the numbers, lengths, locations, and relative strengths of the needles calculated ahead of time for irregularly shaped three-dimensional tumors. This is particularly true for treating tumors adjacent to critical internal tissues, such as for brain tumors. Likewise, scanned focused ultrasound systems, phase- and amplitude-controlled multiple-antennae microwave systems, multiple-transducer ultrasound systems, and multiple-electrode RF systems all require similar decisions. If these treatments are to be optimized for the patient's benefit, then they need to be planned, and such planning can only be done using large, computerized treatment simulations.

The analogy with radiation treatments is obvious in terms of the need. As hyperthermia matures as a treatment modality, such patient treatment planning will become routine, just as it is for radiation therapy. However, the analogy is flawed when one considers the complexity of the problem. For radiation treatments, one need only calculate the energy deposition characteristics. For hyperthermia, however, a two-step process is involved. First, the power deposition characteristics must be determined (as in radiation therapy) and then the tissue energy removal characteristics must be determined. The difference between these two separate effects gives the final resultant temperature field. For hyperthermia, not only is the determination of the energy deposition pattern more difficult than for most radiation calculations – because of the presence of numerous important tissue inhomogeneities and the need to consider the wave nature of the applied power – but the second step is also very involved. This step, determining the energy removal rate in the tissue, is difficult because it involves being able to predict, a priori, the physiological response of the organism to the treatment – in particular, one must know what the patient's blood flow *will be* during the treatment, not just its value at the beginning of the treatment (a more tractable task). Finally, as was discussed in Chap. 1, the fundamental basis of the equation commonly used to calculate the final temperatures (the Pennes bioheat transfer equation) has several limitations and it needs to be improved and/or augmented in the future. If hyperthermia is to become a commonly utilized modality and if it is to be used in the best possible manner for the patient, then the above difficult tasks must be performed. The following sections will discuss each of them in turn.

3.3.2.2 Simulation Requirements

Ideal Treatment Planning Program

An ideal system would know the tumor and normal tissue anatomy to within some acceptable accuracy, say ±1 mm, and the thermophysical properties to say within ±1%. Also, the tissue blood perfusion rate would be known to the same accuracy (as a function of temperature during a treatment), as would the location of and blood flow rate in all relevant major vessels. All of this information would be entered into the computer program automatically from a series of closely spaced, high-resolution CT or MRI scans which would automatically identify all tissue boundaries and assign the appropriate properties. All temperature calculations would then be done automatically by an optimization routine which would determine the optimal heating system configuration for the patient using a new form of the bioheat transfer equation which has been proven to predict accurately temperature fields inside living tissues. Of course, real life in the clinic is presently quite different than this, as described in the following.

Current Status of Practical Systems

Tissue Anatomy

The process of simulating a treatment for a given individual requires that one know the anatomy of the tumor and the adjacent normal tissues that will be significantly affected by the hyperthermia treatment and/or that will significantly affect that treatment. In some cases, the ideal can be approached quite closely, with clearly defined organ and tumor boundaries present on sequential ultrasound, CT, or MRI scans – small, infiltrative fibers cannot, of course, be seen. In principle, therefore, for some tumors one can do a reasonably good job of obtaining the three-dimensional boundaries between the tumor and normal tissues – although the correlation of actual tumor morphology and imaging characteristics is not always exact (e.g., see [13]). The identification of such tumor boundaries must still be done visually, since reliable tissue boundary or tissue characterization algorithms are not generally available at present, although this is an active area of research for all diagnostic modalities. On the other hand, some tumor boundaries are difficult to see with any existent modality, and they can only be estimated by palpation, at best. Thus, while current clinical methods of tumor and normal tissue boundary identification range from palpation to sequential CT, MRI, or ultrasound scans, the current highly developed status of the latter methods and their potential for future development means that the tissue boundary recognition problem will essentially be solved. Considerable work remains to be done to automate that process, but this is a requirement for many applications other than hyperthermia and is an area of active research. Thus, this problem will be solved in a relatively rapid manner due to its fundamental importance to a wide variety of medical applications. Already in hyperthermia, several research groups can perform calculations for two-dimensional inhomogeneous tissues, with some programs able to calculate temperature profiles for three-dimensional anatomies reconstructed from sequential CT scans (e.g., Fig. 3.61). The latter program [21] requires the operator to trace the individual tissue organ boundaries on the sequential CT scans. The program then automatically assigns standard tissue thermophysical properties to each organ – values which can be changed interactively by the operator. This type of program is currently being used for the three-dimensional calculation of temperature distributions for ferromagnetic curie-point seeds [20] and for scanned, focused ultrasound [83], both of which are flexible heating modalities that can benefit greatly from treatment simulations.

Power Deposition Characteristics

The power deposition patterns to be present in patients can be determined in four ways: through the use of tissue-equivalent phantoms, computer simulations of patients, animal experiments, and/or using data obtained from the patients themselves. The use of phantoms and computer simulations has been discussed previously (Chap. 2) and will only be discussed briefly here to give an overview of their characteristics. Table 3.17 summarizes the abilities, difficulties, and potentials for these different methods when applied to patient treatment planning. It is clear from a consideration of these factors that while homogeneous phantoms can give one a good understanding of the basic or fundamental SAR distribution for a given device and are useful for gaining experience with the system's performance, they lack both the anatomical property accuracy and the flexibility characteristics needed for investigating many different situations in parametric studies. While they will remain invaluable tools for basic studies of the actual characteristics of a given piece of hardware for use in hands-on tests of those systems and their associated feedback control systems and software, their use for patient treatment planning is closely circumscribed – i.e., they will be useful tools for providing test cases for calibrating the computer simulation programs.

By far the two most promising approaches for use in patient treatment planning are computerized simulations and actual patient tests. These two approaches should, of course, be closely integrated in order to optimize the patient's treatment planning process since experimental data from patients can be used to great advantage in developing and improving the simulation programs. Before discussing these interactions in depth, we should first note that it is common practice for external beam radiation treatments to use a simulator to perform a "simulation" treatment (i.e., to obtain the exact patient and tumor geometry for the treatment machine and patient orientation that will be used clinically) prior to an actual treatment, in order to obtain information directly from the patient which will allow an improved radiation treatment. The same process is desirable with hyperthermia treatments when one has an externally applied heating modality for which planning is necessary (as with radiation, for interstitial techniques this process would be too traumatic for the patient). To perform such a hyperthermia "simulation treatment", one would place the patient in the system to be used and

1. apply the transient, low-level power amplitude to obtain SAR levels at the locations where sensors are located (if possible, these positions should be chosen in an optimal sense so that they can provide the most information) and
2. repeat this process for as many different transducer/applicator characteristics (number, frequency, orientation, etc.) as are needed to obtain

Table 3.17. Rank ordering of techniques for determining patient SAR distributions

Lowest									Highest
Anatomical accuracy	Homogeneous static phantom	→	Animal	→	Inhomogeneous static phantom	→	Computer simulations	→	Patient
Property accuracy	Homogeneous static phantom	→	Inhomogeneous static phantom	→	Animal	→	Computer simulations	→	Patient
Flexibility for investigating different possible system configurations	Patient	→	Animal	→	Homogeneous static phantom	→	Inhomogeneous static phantom	→	computer simulations

the information required to calibrate the patient model.

This computerized patient model would then be used to plan the treatment for that patient.

These "simulation treatments" can also be used to obtain information regarding the patient's reaction to the treatment (primarily pain) and the tissue-cooling coefficient, as discussed later. The uses of such "simulation treatments" are summarized in Table 3.18. For our present purposes, we will primarily discuss their use in obtaining SAR data for patient treatment planning.

The use of transient applications of power is required in order to obtain SAR data from patients, with calculations based on measurements of transient temperature data taken from temperature transducers located in a heated tissue region. Conservation of energy can be applied in such an analysis [115], and the bioheat transfer equation is not needed. If we consider a step change in applied power at time t, from a value of $\dot{Q}_a(t^-)$ at time t^- just before the step change to a value of $\dot{Q}_a(t^+)$ immediately after the step change, an energy balance at the instant before the change in power is given by

$$\dot{Q}_m(t^-)+\dot{Q}_a(t^-)=\dot{Q}_c(t^-)+\dot{Q}_b(t^-)+\varrho c\,\frac{dT(t^-)}{dt} \tag{3.52}$$

and the same equation holds at the instant following the power change, with all terms evaluated at time t^+,

$$\dot{Q}_m(t^+)+\dot{Q}_a(t^+)=\dot{Q}_c(t^+)+\dot{Q}_b(t^+)+\varrho c\,\frac{dT(t^+)}{dt}\,. \tag{3.53}$$

In these equations, $\dot{Q}_c(t)$ is the net conduction of energy out of the region, $\dot{Q}_b(t)$ is the net removal of energy out of the region due to blood perfusion, $\dot{Q}_a(t)$ is the local absorbed power density, $\dot{Q}_m(t)$ is the local metabolic rate, and the remaining term is the energy storage rate. Combining these equations gives

$$\begin{aligned}\dot{Q}_a(t^+)-\varrho c\,\frac{dT(t^+)}{dt}-\left[\dot{Q}_a(t^-)-\varrho c\,\frac{dT(t^-)}{dt}\right]\\ =\dot{Q}_c(t^+)+\dot{Q}_b(t^+)-\dot{Q}_m(t^+)\\ -[\dot{Q}_c(t^-)+\dot{Q}_b(t^-)-\dot{Q}_m(t^-)]\,.\end{aligned} \tag{3.54}$$

It can be assumed that the conduction, convection, and metabolic terms are equal for short times just before and after the power step; that is,

$$\dot{Q}_m(t^+)=\dot{Q}_m(t^-)\,,\quad \dot{Q}_c(t^+)=\dot{Q}_c(t^-)\,,\quad \dot{Q}_b(t^+)=\dot{Q}_b(t^-) \tag{3.55}$$

Table 3.18. Information gained from patient "simulation treatments"

Measured quantity	Use
$SAR(\bar{r}_i)$	Use measured $SAR(\bar{r}_i)$ at several discrete locations as input to a computer simulation of the patient in order to calibrate the model for that patient
Patient reaction	Determine possible locations of patient pain and/or discomfort
Tissue-cooling coefficient	Determine tissue-cooling coefficient at low power levels for use in computer model of patient

which reduces Eq. 3.54 to the general result given below:

$$\dot{Q}_a(t^+)-\varrho c\,\frac{dT(t^+)}{dt}=\dot{Q}_a(t^-)-\varrho c\,\frac{dT(t^-)}{dt}\,. \tag{3.56}$$

The two temperature slopes can be determined experimentally, so if either $\dot{Q}_a(t^+)$ or $\dot{Q}_a(t^-)$ is known, the other value can be determined from Eq. 3.56.

Two special cases of Eq. 3.56 are important. The first is a power-on transient in which the subject is initially in a resting, steady-state condition so that

$$\frac{dT(t^-)}{dt}=0 \tag{3.57}$$

with no power initially applied; that is, $\dot{Q}_a(t^-)=0$. Then, Eq. 3.56 reduces to the familiar expression

$$\dot{Q}_a(t^+)=\varrho c\,\frac{dT(t^+)}{dt} \tag{3.58}$$

which gives the linear variation in temperature for short periods following the application of power. Linearity breaks down, of course, when temperature differences become large enough for thermal conduction and perfusion effects to become significant. [Note also that the special case (Eq. 3.58) can also be derived separately from the general energy balance (Eq. 3.53) if one assumes the applied power and transient terms are much larger than the conduction, blood convection, and metabolic terms.] If the tissue was not in an initial steady state, then Eq. 3.56 would reduce to [again for $\dot{Q}_a(t^-)=0$]

$$\dot{Q}_a(t^+)=\varrho c\,\frac{dT(t^+)}{dt}-\varrho c\,\frac{dT(t^-)}{dt}\,. \tag{3.59}$$

The second common case is a power-off transient for which the tissue is in an initial steady state, so that

$$\frac{dT(t^-)}{dt}=0\,. \tag{3.60}$$

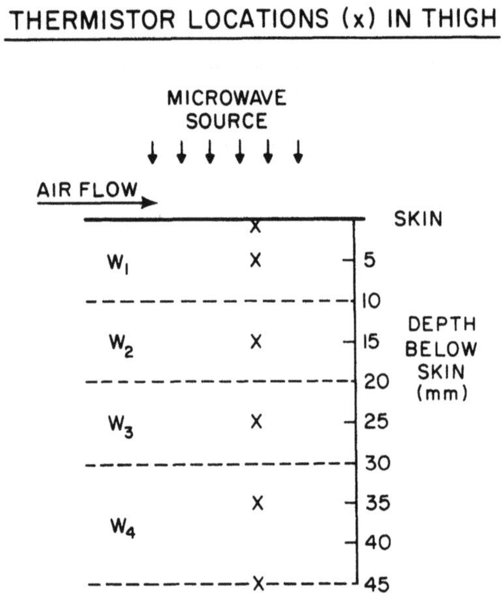

Fig. 3.69. Schematic diagram of experimental arrangement used to measure SAR values at different depths. The thermistors were located along the centerline of the applicator. [115]

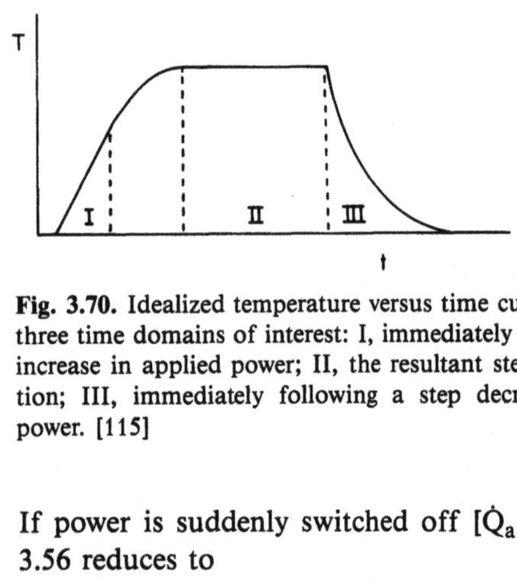

Fig. 3.70. Idealized temperature versus time curve showing the three time domains of interest: I, immediately following a step increase in applied power; II, the resultant steady-state condition; III, immediately following a step decrease in applied power. [115]

If power is suddenly switched off [$\dot{Q}_a(t^+) = 0$], Eq. 3.56 reduces to

$$\dot{Q}_a(t^-) = -\varrho c \frac{dT(t^+)}{dt} \qquad (3.61)$$

which allows the applied power to be calculated from the initial slope of the decaying temperature curve. Again, if the initial state is not quite steady, Eq. 3.56 gives

$$\dot{Q}_a(t^-) = -\varrho c \frac{dT(t^+)}{dt} + \varrho c \frac{dT(t^-)}{dt} . \qquad (3.62)$$

This theory, stating that the local SAR values can be determined from either a power-on step (Eq. 3.59) or a power-off step (Eq. 3.62), has been experimentally evaluated using an external microwave applicator on dog thighs (Fig. 3.69). An idealized transient tempera-

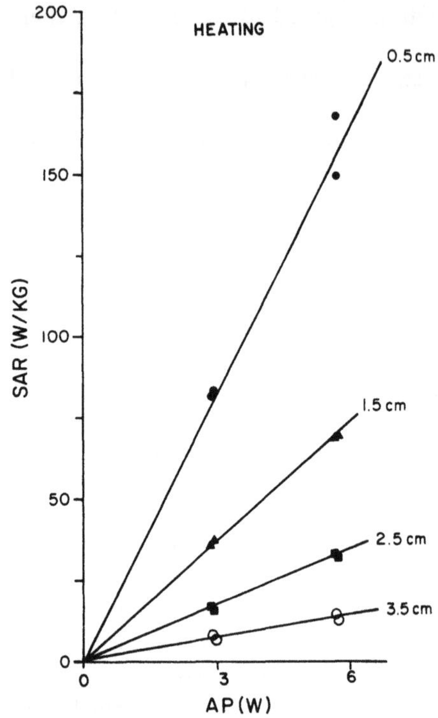

Fig. 3.71. Correlation of local SAR values versus net applied power (AP) for a step increase in power (heating). ○, 3.5 cm; ■, 2.5 cm; ▲, 1.5 cm; ●, 0.5 cm deep from skin surface. [115]

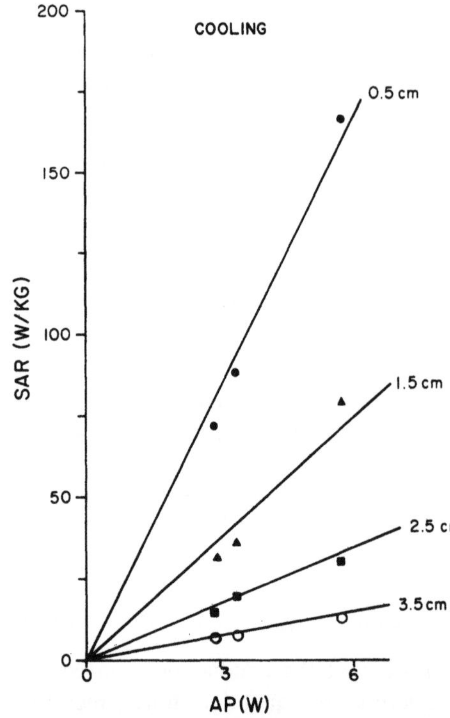

Fig. 3.72. Same experiment as in Fig. 3.71 but for a step decrease in power. The straight-line least squares fits to the heating data from Fig. 3.71 (*solid lines*) are superimposed on the cooling data (*symbols*) for each of the four positions. [115]

ture trace is given in Fig. 3.70 for a step function in power applied to the thighs, kept on until steady state is reached, and then abruptly turned off. Figure 3.38 shows typical experimental results for several depths along the applicator axis. One can calculate the SAR values at each depth from Eqs. 3.59 and 3.62 and plot the results as a function of the amplitude of the total applied power. The results should give a straight line for each temperature sensor, with the slope dependent on the depth of the sensor (which determines the relative magnitude of the SAR for a given total applied power). This occurs, as seen in Fig. 3.71, for the step increase in power (Eq. 3.59) and in Fig. 3.72 for the abrupt power turn-off (Eq. 3.62), with both equations giving the same result, i.e., the same slope of the line for each temperature sensor. These results experimentally verified the previously developed theory.

The slope of each line in Figs. 3.71 and 3.72 reflects the amount of SAR present at a given location per unit of total applied power. Griffiths et al. [44] have used this slope (q) as a normalized SAR value, where since the curves are linear and go through the origin

$$q(\vec{r}) = \frac{SAR(\vec{r})}{AP(W)} \,. \tag{3.63a}$$

Note that the slope of the curve (q) can also be obtained directly from a power change Δ AP during a treatment

$$q(\vec{r}) = \frac{\Delta SAR(\vec{r})}{\Delta AP(W)} \tag{3.63b}$$

where Δ SAR can be obtained directly from Eq. 3.56 as

$$\Delta SAR = \frac{\Delta \dot{Q}_a}{\varrho} = c \left[\frac{dT(t^+)}{dt} - \frac{dT(t^-)}{dt} \right] \tag{3.63c}$$

and Δ AP can be measured independently. This variable allowed them to comparatively evaluate the performance of different configurations of a capacitive heating system at two different sites. Their results are shown in Fig. 3.73 for several different step changes in power on a given patient. All power changes should

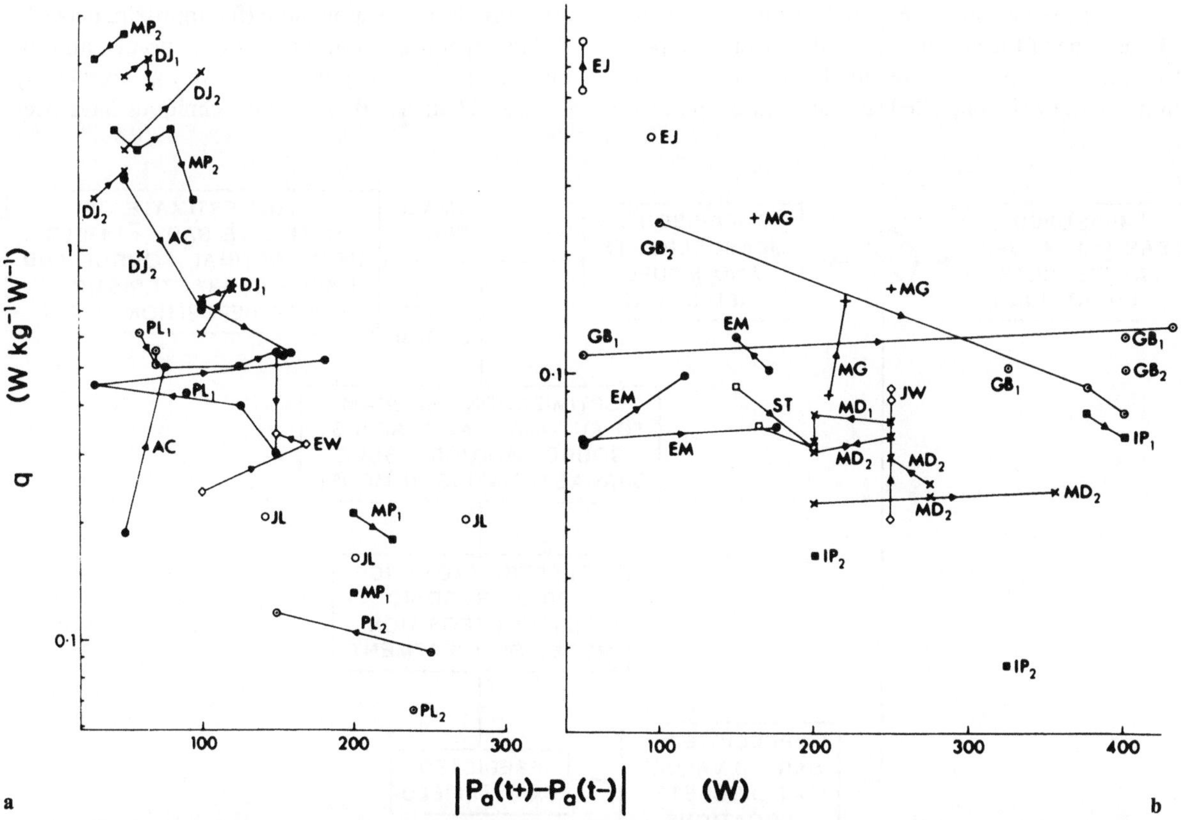

Fig. 3.73a, b. SAR values per watt of applied power (W/kg-W) versus the change in applied power $[P_a(t^+) - P_a(t^-)]$ for patients being heated by capacitive heating of **(a)** superficial tumors and **(b)** axillary tumors [44]. Patient initials are shown once for each treatment. *Suffixes 1* and *2* represent different applicator configurations for the same site, except for patient MP, where *1* and *2* represent separate sites. The superficial and axillary tumors had "representative SAR" values of 89 and 30 W/kg, respectively. Note the scale change between **a** and **b**

give the same value of q for a fixed position of a temperature sensor and a fixed applicator configuration; i.e., the slope of each curve in Fig. 3.71 and 3.72 does not change with applied power. Thus, in Fig. 3.73, any variation from a horizontal line shows that the experimental conditions have changed. One can also use this approach comparatively to evaluate different heating modalities (and, of course, configurations) for a fixed thermocouple position, since the higher the q value for a given device, the better its relative penetrating ability. That is, two devices may both be able to obtain a given SAR value at a fixed depth, but if one device requires a total power of 1000 W to do this and the other requires only 100 W (i.e., its q value is ten times higher), them the second device is clearly more promising since it will probably not result in as many patient complications. This is a very useful tool for comparative thermal dosimetric analysis of different devices, and its use is encouraged for more applications. The use of the q concept, i.e., SAR per unit of total applied power, normalizes the total applied power and allows different devices to be compared on a common basis.

Clear step changes in power and the proper evaluation of the slope of the increasing and decreasing temperature curves are, of course, required to do these calculations. In the well-controlled environment of the above animal experiments (Fig. 3.69), the step increase temperatures were generally fit to a straight line using data from a 40-s period and a linear least squares fit. (The 40-s time period was a good compromise between two little data and too long a time period – which would have introduced cooling artifacts.) The first data point after the step increase in power was neglected to eliminate artifacts. This was possible since it is the slope of the line that is important. A straight-line fit was similarly made to the slowly changing temperatures just prior (30 s) to the power increase in order to calculate the temperature slope at time t^- in Eq. 3.59. For the power-off calculations, the slowly changing slopes (at t^-) could generally be fit to a straight line, but the temperatures following the power-off dropped rapidly and had considerable curvature after a short period. This curvature is to be expected since the heat transfer conditions are changing rapidly and there was generally a much higher blood flow level at the end of these experiments than at the start. This, of course, is not a problem since it is the *initial slope* immediately after the power-off that is important. To adjust for this curvature, the data were fit to an exponential (for approximately 40 s of data, again ignoring the first data point), and the initial slope of the exponential curve was used in Eq. 3.62 for dT/dt ($t = 0^+$). These techniques have been

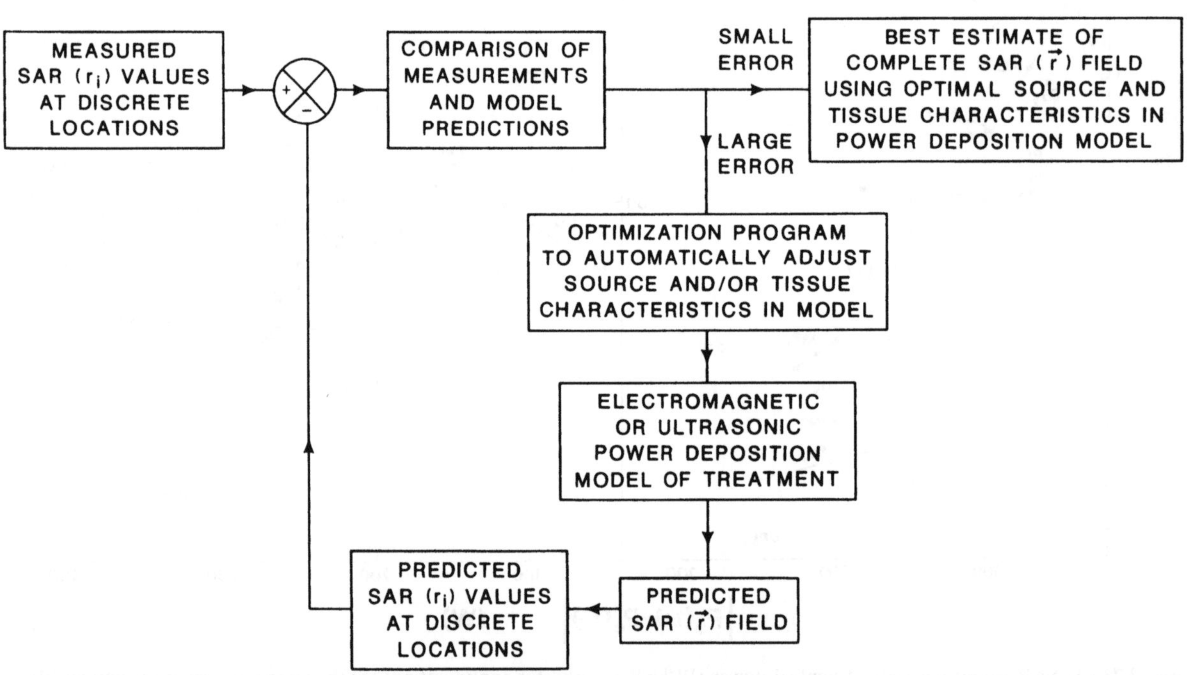

Fig. 3.74. Block diagram showing the proposed complementary use of SAR($\vec{r}_i$) data at discrete locations from actual and/or "simulation treatments" on patients, and computer simulations to predict complete SAR($\vec{r}$) patterns for use in patient treatment planning. The unknown parameters of the patient and/or the source models are automatically adjusted to force the model to agree with the measured data

modified by Cetas et al. [15] for an evaluation of clinical data.

Now, returning to the use of these clinical patient data for treatment planning, one can take the measured SAR (and q) data for different locations and configurations and use them iteratively to improve one's patient models, as outlined in Fig. 3.74. The goal of this process is to use the known individual patient anatomy plus the known distributions of SAR at a few points, SAR($\vec{r}_j$), to calibrate the general patient and source models to the individual patient treatment configuration. The parameters to be adjusted in the general patient model will depend on the power deposition modality used, but could involve the reflection coefficients at boundaries, assumed boundary conditions, the source strength and geometry, and/or the distribution of physical properties. To make this process most useful, the locations where SAR is to be measured will need to be chosen carefully in an optimal sense so that the most useful information is obtained for calibrating the model. Figure 3.18 shows the results of using such model adjustments to force the model predictions to agree with the experimental results from a phantom.

Blood Perfusion Measurements

The predictive abilities of any patient treatment simulations will depend strongly on how well the blood perfusion is known for the patient. Again, two levels of prediction are relevant. First, one could attempt to answer questions in an absolute sense (for example: What will be the *exact* temperatures in the patient for this proposed treatment configuration?), or, in a slightly less demanding (but still absolute) sense, one might ask. What are the probabilities of this device/configuration properly heating this patient's tumor? Second, one might only propose to answer a relative question regarding the rank ordering of different heating system configurations to find the best configuration among a range of possibilities. Table 3.19 summarizes these three options plus the associated requirements that they pose on the need for obtaining blood perfusion measurements. Also listed are the uses to which the model results might be put. Thus, there is a range of possible levels of knowledge of blood perfusion which have clinical relevance. It is most important to note that it is the blood perfusion and flow *during* the hyperthermia treatment that is important – not just the flow *before* the treatment. This is extremely important since pretreatment measurements, which are much easier to obtain, could be used *if the blood perfusion did not change during the treatment.* Unfortunately, this does not always seem to be the case, as the existing (sparse) reviews of blood flow during hyperthermia seem to show.

There are several recent, comprehensive reviews of the extensive experimental research that has been done on the effect of hyperthermia on normal and tumor tissue blood perfusion, with Emami and Song [35], Gerweck [40], Jain and Ward-Hartley [57], Reinhold and van den Berg-Blok [105], Song [129], and Reinhold and Endrich [104] providing the latest summaries of the state of our knowledge concerning perfusion changes. These data come almost exclusively from experimental animal studies. Clinically, little is

Table 3.19. Blood flow knowledge requirements for various levels of patient treatment planning

Modeling level	Required blood flow knowledge	Prediction uses
Absolute (exact):		
Accurately predict actual temperatures for potential treatment configuration	Accurate absolute knowledge of actual blood flow distribution and magnitudes	Decide on whether or not treatment will be successful and if (and how) it should be performed
Absolute (limits):		
Accurately predict temperatures for best- and worst-case patient blood perfusion cases – i.e., for the easiest and hardest to heat perfusion patterns and magnitudes	Knowledge of range of blood perfusion patterns and magnitudes to be expected for this patient	Rank order the possible heating configurations by determining their ability to treat properly the easiest and hardest to heat cases. Eliminate configurations that will not heat the easiest case and retain those that can properly heat the hardest to heat case
Relative:		
Predict the temperature distribution for a given set of reasonable blood flow conditions that can be expected to occur for this patient	Reasonable distributions and magnitudes	Rank order the possible heating configurations and use the "best" method for the actual treatment to see what happens

known concerning tumor perfusion changes during human patient hyperthermia treatments, and our quantitative (and, indeed, qualitative) knowledge of normal tissue perfusion changes under high-temperature thermal stresses during treatments also remains meager (see p. 139). Thus, considerable work must be done in this area. In addition to gathering data on an individual patient before a treatment, we must also be able to predict a priori what that particular patient's blood flow response will be if absolute predictions are to be made.

The ability to predict tumor and normal tissue perfusion responses is clearly not available at present and will require extensive experimental work if it is ever to be achieved. In the best situations, one might only see that a given patient has a high probability of having a certain response and thus be able to do a best case/worst case type of analysis based on the expected patient response. In any case, a large data base will need to be developed initially. This will need to be based on tumor perfusion responses during hyperthermia, so it is reasonable here to review existing measurement techniques with an eye toward their potential use in hyperthermia. Two types of measurements are important: first, determination of the responses of "large, thermally significant" blood vessels and, second, the actual tissue perfusion magnitudes. The former need to be measured for vessels supplying or passing through the tumor, preferably by a noninvasive technique such as Doppler ultrasound. To be useful, such measurements would need to be performed during the hyperthermia treatments for tumors for which it is known that the vessel supplies the tumor – a difficult task. As a step back from this, however, one can measure, before the treatment, the anatomy (size, location, and orientation) and blood flow rates in large vessels using imaging techniques such as X-ray subtraction angiography. This will at least give the location of the large vessels in the tumor and allow some best case/worst case studies to be performed. Such measurements are not made at present, but could become very necessary in the future.

The second set of measurements is needed for determining the actual perfusion levels in the tumor and the tissue. Here again, two types of measurements are available – those that give some perfusion measurements at a point, or for multiple sensors at a set of points, and those that give distributed values. The latter methods involve sophisticated imaging systems such as PET scanners, or MRI, SPECT, or CT systems, and again are useful for some pre-therapy measurements. However, their possible use during actual treatments is a long way in the future because of both financial and technical considerations. The use of point-measurement methods is much more promising for use during treatments, but the amount of information obtained is decreased considerably. That is, just as in the case of SAR values, the point information needs to be converted somehow into values for the complete distribution. Perhaps this can be done using simulations and the same general approach proposed in Fig. 3.74 for the SAR problem. Such an approch would use a procedure similar to that outlined in Fig. 3.75. Again, optimal sensor placement would be an important consideration. Such point measure-

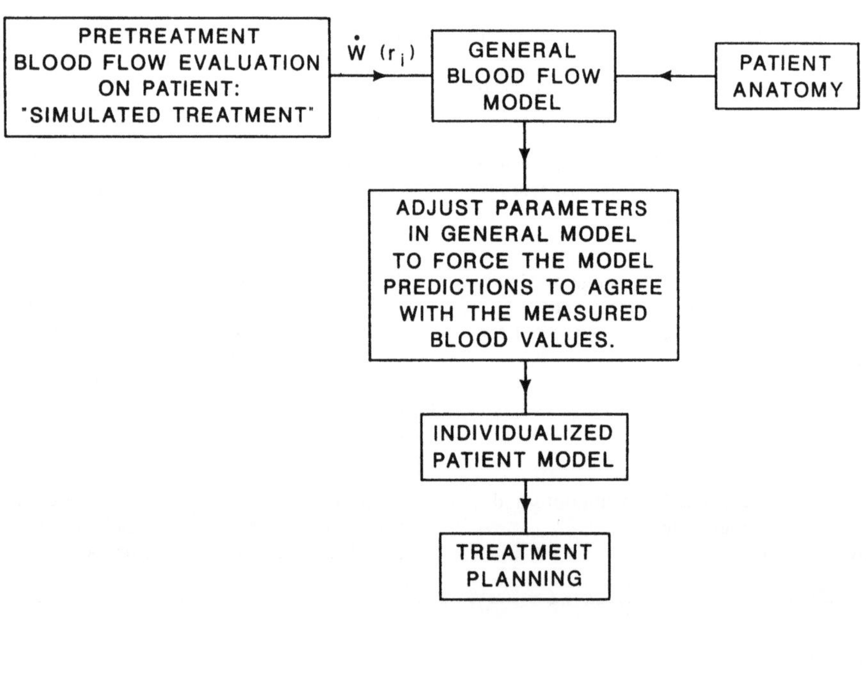

Fig. 3.75. Block diagram showing the proposed complementary use of blood perfusion magnitudes measured at a few points on patients and computer simulations to obtain complete maps of perfusion distributions

ments can be done using any of the thermal techniques previously described (see Chap. 1) and possibly done prior to, during and after a treatment.

Another method of measuring perfusion values in clinical situations that is very appealing at first glance (deceptively so) is to use existing thermometry and to measure the "thermal washout" of the decaying temperatures after power is turned off. This use of existing instrumentation and the ease of implementation give this approach its deceptive appeal. In theory, this technique takes the energy balance equation and assumes that all conduction and blood perfusion cooling effects can be put into an "effective perfusion" term, $\dot{W}_e$, which was defined previously (Eq. 3.26) as

$$\dot{W}_e = \frac{U_{tc}}{c_b} = \frac{\dot{Q}_a(\vec{r})}{c_b[T(\vec{r})-T_{ar}]} \quad . \qquad (3.64)$$

This method is important to discuss here because of its deceitful nature – it is so easy to implement but yields so very little useful information. To understand the basis and limitations of this technique fully, one must first understand its origin through a thorough look at its derivation. This starts by noting that an energy balance at any time (t) during a treatment gives (for negligible metabolism)

$$\dot{Q}_a(t) - \varrho c \frac{dT(t)}{dt} = \dot{Q}_c(t) + \dot{Q}_b(t) \quad . \qquad (3.65)$$

If the conduction ($\dot{Q}_c$) and blood convection ($\dot{Q}_b$) terms are combined into a single (net) "loss" term

$$\dot{Q}_{loss}(t) = \dot{Q}_c(t) + \dot{Q}_b(t) \qquad (3.66)$$

and this loss term is further defined to be the product of an effective tissue perfusion rate ($\dot{W}_e$), c_b, and the temperature difference ($T-T_{ar}$), then we have

$$\dot{Q}_{loss}(t) = \dot{W}_e c_b [T(t) - T_{ar}(t)] \quad . \qquad (3.67)$$

Combining Eq. 3.65, which is an energy balance, and Eq. 3.67, which is a definition, gives

$$\dot{W}_e(t) = \frac{\dot{Q}_a(t) - \varrho c \, (dT(t)/dt)}{c_b[T(t) - T_{ar}(t)]} \quad , \qquad (3.68)$$

as has been proposed by Guy et al. [46] and used by others, although never with the notation of an "effective" perfusion.

Two commonly encountered special cases bear consideration. First, consider the situation for which power $\dot{Q}_a$ is applied to a subject and a steady-state condition at temperature T_0 is maintained. Then, Eq. 3.68 reduces to

$$\dot{W}_e = \frac{\dot{Q}_a}{c_b(T_0 - T_{ar})} \quad . \qquad (3.69)$$

For the second situation, assume that the applied power is suddenly decreased to zero so that the temperature begins to fall, yielding a "thermal washout" curve. Since $\dot{Q}_a(t) = 0$, Eq. 3.68 becomes a differential equation in the unknown temperature T

$$\varrho c \frac{dT}{dt} + \dot{W}_e c_b (T - T_{ar}) = 0 \quad . \qquad (3.70)$$

If it is further assumed that $\dot{W}_e$ and T_{ar} remain constant during the short time of interest, this has the commonly encountered exponential solution

$$T - T_{ar} = (T_0 - T_{ar}) \exp[-(\dot{W}_e c_b/\varrho c)t] \qquad (3.71)$$

where T_0 is the initial probe temperature. To apply this equation to experimental data, the transient experimental temperature data are fit to Eq. 3.71 using measured values for T_0 and T_{ar} to obtain the time constant, $\tau = \varrho c/\dot{W}_e c_b$. The effective perfusion, $\dot{W}_e$, can then be calculated using published values for the tissue properties, c_b, ϱ, and c. The value of perfusion calculated by previous investigators from either the steady-state Eq. 3.69 or the transient Eq. 3.71 is an "effective" value because it is dependent on the values of conduction and the actual perfusion present, as indicated by Eqs. 3.66 and 3.67. [As can be seen from their common source (Eq. 68), both the steady-state and transient approaches calculate exactly the same quantity ($\dot{W}_e$) using different methods, as discussed later.]

Two additional special cases are of interest here: First, the situation of a power-on-transient at the beginning of a heating and, second, the case where the applied power is held constant and the blood perfusion changes for either normal physiological reasons or due to some biophysical/biochemical experimental or clinical manipulation. At the beginning of a power-on transient (step function), an energy balance gives

$$\varrho c \frac{dT}{dt} + \dot{W}_e c_b (T - T_{ar}) = \dot{Q}_a \qquad (3.72)$$

which, assuming $\dot{W}_e$ and T_{ar} are constant [as in the derivation of Eq. 3.71], has the solution

$$T(t) - T_{ar} = \frac{\dot{Q}_a}{\dot{W}_e c_b} + \left[T_0 - T_{ar} - \frac{\dot{Q}_a}{\dot{W}_e c_b} \right] \exp[-(\dot{W}_e c_b/\varrho c)t] \quad . \qquad (3.73)$$

Thus, for a power-on transient, the initial effective perfusion value could be obtained from the time constant of the exponential temperature growth.

Second, for the constant applied power case, consider an experiment where tissue is heated to elevated temperatures at constant power and then suddenly a vasoactive drug is administered. If the drug is assumed to act instantaneously in a step-function manner, then it is known that the tissue metabolism and the thermal conduction terms just before ($t = t^-$) and just after ($t = t^+$) the step function are equal

$$\dot{Q}_m(t^-) = \dot{Q}_m(t^+) \ , \quad \dot{Q}_c(t^-) = \dot{Q}_c(t^+) \ .$$

Thus, from the energy balances at times t^- and t^+ we have since $\dot{Q}_a(t^+) = \dot{Q}_a(t^-)$,

$$\dot{Q}_b(t^-) + \varrho c \frac{dT(t^-)}{dt} = \dot{Q}_b(t^+) + \varrho c \frac{dT(t^+)}{dt} \ . \quad (3.74)$$

If the blood cooling term ($\dot{Q}_b$) is expressed as

$$\dot{Q}_b = \dot{W} c_b (T - T_{ar}) \quad (3.75)$$

then the change in perfusion is

$$\dot{W}(t^+) - \dot{W}(t^-) = \frac{-\varrho c[(dT(t^+)/dt) - (dT(t^-)/dt)]}{c_b(T - T_{ar})} \quad (3.76)$$

where t^- and t^+ are assumed close enough so that $[T(t^-) - T_{ar}(t^-)] \cong [T(t^+) - T_{ar}(t^+)]$. This is an extended version of the equation of Babbs et al. [4]. Note that the above analysis gives perfusion values as defined by Eq. 3.75, which is the bioheat transfer equation definition of perfusion. This is not an effective perfusion value since conduction effects are not included.

However, if the drug acts slowly such that the maximum perfusion change does not occur until later, at a time (t_2) when the temperatures have changed (so $\dot{Q}_c$ and $\dot{Q}_m$ have changed), the above equation does not hold. In this case, the effective perfusion concept can again be employed to obtain a qualitative indication of the perfusion change; that is, Eq. 3.69 can be applied before (t_1) and after (t_2) the drug administration to evaluate the change in perfusion caused by the drug. This gives a relative ratio of the two effective blood perfusions

$$\frac{W_{e_2}}{W_{e_1}} = \frac{T_1 - T_{ar}}{T_2 - T_{ar}} \quad (3.77\,a)$$

in which SAR does not need to be known; or a relative change in the tissue cooling coefficient can be obtained

$$\frac{U_{tc_2}}{U_{tc_1}} = \frac{W_{e_2}}{W_{e_1}} \ . \quad (3.77\,b)$$

The above theoretical derivation showing that both the traditional thermal washout technique (Eq. 3.71) and the steady-state technique (Eq. 3.69) are equivalent was tested experimentally using the experimental approach just described for the SAR evaluation (see Figs. 3.69, 3.70). For any given experiment, the effective perfusion at the end of region II of Fig. 3.70 should, theoretically, be identical to that just at the beginning of region III. Thus, calculations of $\dot{W}_e$ from Eqs. 3.69 and 3.71 at these two respective times should give the same results. To demonstrate this, the steady-state Eq. 3.69 was applied to the data at the end of region II by using the known tissue and arterial temperatures along with the known value of $\dot{Q}_a$ obtained from the previously described linear fits. If temperatures were still slowly changing at the end of region II, then Eq. 3.68 was used in place of Eq. 3.69. To calculate effective perfusions from the transient Eq. 3.71, the first 40 s of data from the beginning of region III were used in a least squares fit for the exponential decay given by Eq. 3.71, as previously discussed. Figure 3.76 compares the results of these steady-state Eq. 3.69 calculations ($\dot{W}_{e,ss}$) with the results of the transient Eq. 3.71 calculations ($\dot{W}_{e,tr}$). Each data point represents a pair of such calculations for a given experiment. The straight line drawn at 45° indicates the equality between the two methods of calculation, as predicted by theory. In all calculations, values of $\varrho = 1000\ kg/m^3$ and $c_b = c = 4186\ j/kg/°C$ were used. From the definition (Eqs. 3.66 and 3.67), the value of effective perfusion at the end of region II and at the beginning of region III must be equal since

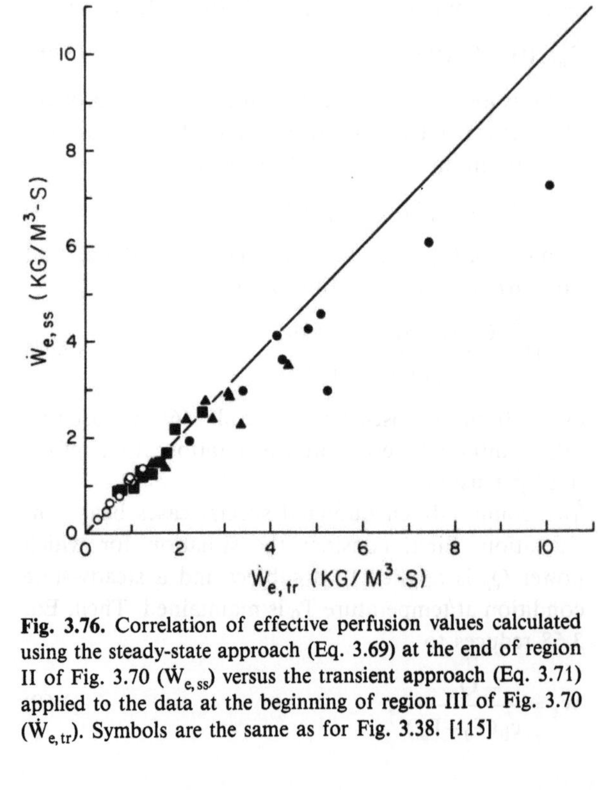

Fig. 3.76. Correlation of effective perfusion values calculated using the steady-state approach (Eq. 3.69) at the end of region II of Fig. 3.70 ($\dot{W}_{e,ss}$) versus the transient approach (Eq. 3.71) applied to the data at the beginning of region III of Fig. 3.70 ($\dot{W}_{e,tr}$). Symbols are the same as for Fig. 3.38. [115]

the values of T, T_{ar}, $\dot{Q}_c$, $\dot{Q}_b$, and $\dot{Q}_m$ are equal at those two points. It can be seen from Fig. 3.76 that the two calculation methods give the same results (as predicted by the theory) for low effective perfusion levels. However, at the higher effective perfusion values, the results begin to differ, with the transient thermal washout method giving higher values than the steady-state method. It is believed that the reason for this difference in the presence of significant conduction effects that change in magnitude with time following the power-off step. For these experiments, this effect is seen more prominently in the results of the 0.5-cm- and 1.5-cm-deep sensors because these more superficial tissues have the highest power deposition values and they are closest to the cooled skin. When power is turned off, these locations drop in temperature more rapidly. This causes the conduction losses to increase, resulting in an increase in the effective perfusion – even if the actual perfusion value is constant.

The effects of including conduction in the effective perfusion can cause large errors in perfusion

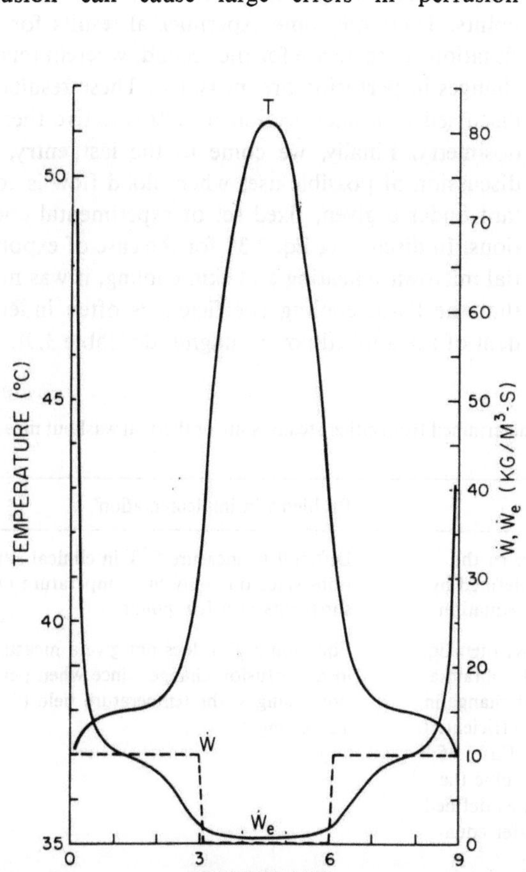

Fig. 3.77. Temperatures (T), blood perfusion ($\dot{W}$), and calculated effective blood perfusion ($\dot{W}_e$) versus position for a one-dimensional model of a tumor with a necrotic core and a highly perfused periphery. [115]

estimates, as was described earlier (e.g., see Fig. 3.45 and the accompanying discussion). That example was for a superficial heating application with skin cooling, which can give regions where conduction ($-k\nabla^2 T$) is dominant. Conduction effects may also be important for tumors with poorly perfused or necrotic regions and well-cooled peripheries. To illustrate this, a one-dimensional bioheat transfer analysis was done for the case shown in Fig. 3.77, where the tissue perfusion was set at 10 kg/m^3 per second for the left and right sides of the region, whereas the center third was modeled as a necrotic core with zero perfusion. The power deposition was set at a uniform value of 40 kw/m^3 for the whole region, and the outer boundaries were fixed at 37 °C. After the bioheat transfer equation was solved for the resultant steady-state temperature profiles, T(x), those values were used in the steady-state Eq. 3.69 to solve for the effective perfusion as a function of position. The results of this calculation (Fig. 3.77) show again that conduction effects are important in the calculation of the effective perfusion. Because of this dependence on conduction effects (i.e., on the temperature distribution in a particular situation), the effective blood perfusion is not a physiological measure of perfusion only, but rather a measure of both a physiological factor, blood perfusion, and the particular situation studied (i.e., conduction effects). Therefore, this concept has limited validity when results from different situations are being compared.

To analyze this problem further, Fig. 3.78 shows the curves of the percentage of the local absorbed power that is removed by conduction for the one-dimensional tumor that was modeled in Fig. 3.77. Results are shown for three perfusion magnitudes (W = 1, 5, and 10 kg/m^3 per second). For each of those values, the power (uniform) was adjusted so that the maximum tissue temperature was 50 °C. The temperature profiles obtained had shapes similar to those of Fig. 3.77. For this situation, conduction again plays an important role in removing energy. (The negative values indicate that net energy is being conducted into a given position, as previously discussed.) Recently, Sandhu [121] analyzed other situations and reinforced the conclusions regarding potential errors introduced by conduction, errors which cause the effective perfusion to lose its value as a physiological measure and to be restricted in its use.

It is for these reasons that it is much more preferable to use the nomenclature "tissue cooling coefficient" (U_{tc}) rather than "effective perfusion", or "PERF", or any other nomenclature which implies direct knowledge of perfusion values. The connection between these quantities and the actual perfusion is too

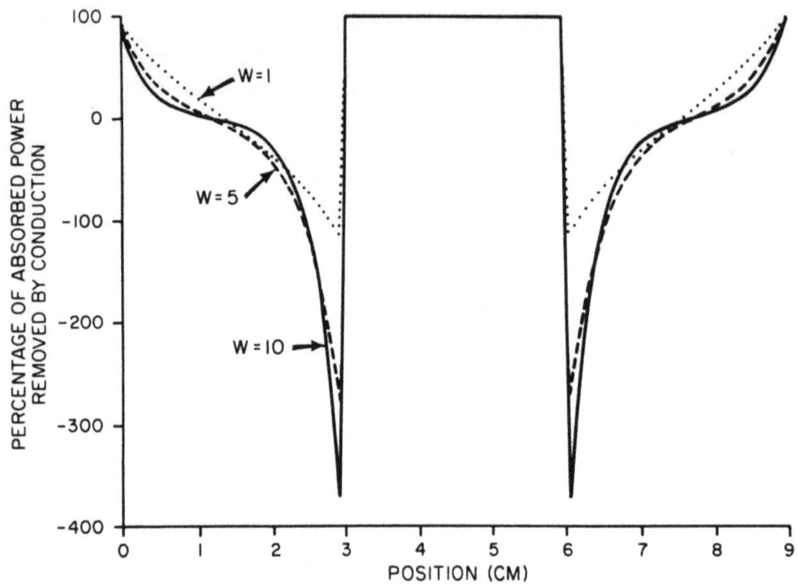

Fig. 3.78. Percentage of local energy absorbed that is removed by conduction versus position for the uniform power absorption simulation of Fig. 3.77. For each blood perfusion case shown, the power was adjusted so that the maximum tumor temperature was 50 °C

tenuous to be useful and can lead to significant misperceptions of what has actually been measured. Given this change in nomenclature, it is of interest to determine when and how this tissue-cooling coefficient [which is still easy to measure – Eq. 3.69 or 3.71 with $U_{tc} = \dot{W}_e/c_b$ – and thus tempting to use] can be used, and when (or if) it can be directly related to blood perfusion (Table 3.20). Of the three cases described in that table, the first (no conduction) can occur with very flat temperature profiles, which can happen, approximately, in some clinical situations. In practice, however, it will be difficult in an actual clinical situation to know if the temperature slopes are constant (∇T = constant, therefore $\nabla^2 T = 0$), since temperatures are generally measured at only a few points. There are some experimental results for this situation, as there are for the second, wherein relative changes in perfusion are measured. These results are discussed in a later section on retrospective thermal dosimetry. Finally, we come to the last entry, the discussion of possible uses when blood flow is constant under a given, fixed set of experimental conditions. In discussing Eq. 3.38 for the case of exponential microwave heating and skin cooling, it was noted that the tissue-cooling coefficient is often independent of the applied power magnitude (Table 3.9). It is

Table 3.20. Useful applications of the tissue-cooling coefficient as determined from either steady-state or thermal washout measurements

Situation	Usefulness	Problems in implementation
Conduction effects are negligible, i.e., $\nabla^2 T \cong 0$, or $\nabla^2 T$ = known; thus conduction effects can be subtracted out	To obtain a measure of the blood perfusion as defined by the bioheat transfer equation	Difficult to measure $\nabla^2 T$ in clinical situations since one only has temperature measurements at a few points
A fixed experimental or clinical situation at constant power and constant external cooling when spontaneous changes in temperature are caused by changes in tissue perfusion	If the change is slow, then Eq. 3.77b can be used to obtain a measure of the local change in the tissue-cooling coefficient. If the change is rapid, Eq. 3.76 can be used to determine the change in perfusion as defined by the bioheat transfer equation	Equation 3.77b does not give a measure of local perfusion changes since when perfusion changes, the temperature field ($\nabla^2 T$) also changes
Conduction effects are unknown but constant in a given, fixed experimental or clinical situation in which the blood perfusion is constant	To obtain a prediction of future temperatures at higher powers from patient "simulation treatments" at low power values	Limited to cases where perfusion remains constant

most significant to note that the independence of U_{tc} from applied power is much more general. That is, for the linear bioheat transfer equation, the temperature solution for the most general case can always be expressed as the superposition of the effect of boundary conditions (T_{bc}) and the effect of the applied power (T_p) (e.g., see Eq. 3.15b)

$$T(\vec{r}) = T_{bc}(\vec{r}) + T_p(\vec{r}) \tag{3.78}$$

where the particular solution due to the applied power will always be linearly related to the magnitude of the total applied power (P_a) as

$$T_p = P_a g[\vec{r}, \dot{W}(\vec{r})] \tag{3.79a}$$

where $g(\vec{r})$ gives the geometric variation of the temperature with position. Additionally, the solution for the boundary conditions will always be linearly related to the boundary temperature, T_{sk}

$$T_{bc} = T_{sk} h[\vec{r}, \dot{W}(\vec{r})] \tag{3.79b}$$

where h gives the geometric variation of the skin-cooling effect. Thus, for the tissue-cooling coefficient (Eq. 3.26) this gives, again for $T_{ar} \triangleq 0$ for convenience and using the fact that $SAR(\vec{r}) = P_a q(\vec{r})$, where $q(\vec{r})$ describes the geometric distribution of SAR in the tissue per unit of applied power and P_a is the total applied power in watts:

$$U_{tc} = \frac{\varrho SAR(\vec{r})}{T - T_{ar}} = \frac{\varrho P_a q(\vec{r})}{P_a g(\vec{r}, \dot{W}) + T_{bc}(\vec{r})} \tag{3.80}$$

or

$$U_{tc} = \frac{\varrho q(\vec{r})}{g(\vec{r}, \dot{W}) + [T_{sk} h(\vec{r})/P_a]} \; . \tag{3.81a}$$

Again, when there is a small effect of the boundary conditions, U_{tc} is not a function of the applied power and the second term in the denominator of Eq. 3.81a can be neglected – for any heating modality. In particular, the effect of boundary conditions at the deeper positions will be negligible for regional heating devices and thus the term T_{bc} drops from both Eqs. 3.80 and 3.81a. This condition gives

$$U_{tc} = \frac{\varrho SAR(\vec{r})}{T - T_{ar}} = \frac{\varrho P_a q(\vec{r})}{T - T_{ar}} \; . \tag{3.81b}$$

It should be noted that this general result (Eq. 3.81 and the independence of U_{tc} from the applied power) is not dependent on the bioheat transfer equation, but will be valid for any equation as long as it is linear in temperature so that superposition of solutions can be used.

F. Waterman (1987, personal communication) has also proposed using the absence of tissue-cooling coefficient dependence on applied power to help in predicting the total power required to reach a desired treatment temperature. To do this, a low power heating ("simulation treatment") could be run initially to obtain $U_{tc}(r_i)$ and $SAR(r_i)$ [and thus $q(r_i)$] for the sensor locations (r_i). Now, using these facts, if the tissue blood perfusion does not change during the treatment [so $U_{tc}(r)$ is constant], then Eq. 3.81b can be rearranged and used to predict the applied power needed to reach a specified temperature (e.g., 43 °C) at a given location

$$P_a = \frac{U_{tc}(r_i)\,[43 - T_{ar}]}{\varrho q(r_i)} \; . \tag{3.82}$$

Furthermore, for the above conditions in which the blood perfusion remains constant from the initial low-power test until the full-power treatment conditions are reached, the measurement location where the maximum temperature will be reached can be determined. That is, we know from Eq. 3.81b that

$$T(r_i) = T_{ar} + \frac{P_a \varrho q(r_i)}{U_{tc}(r_i)} \; . \tag{3.83}$$

Since $q(r_i)$ and $U_{tc}(r_i)$ can be determined from the low-power tests, the predicted temperatures at the measurement locations can be determined as a function of the applied power. Again, for deeper positions, and for homogeneous boundary conditions ($T_{sk} = T_{ar}$), the tissue-cooling coefficient is not a function of the applied power, and so the temperatures vary linearly with applied power (Eq. 3.79). For the more superficial locations, when inhomogeneous boundary conditions are present, U_{tc} is then a function of the applied power (Eq. 3.81a) and the temperatures are nonlinearly related to the applied power (P_a). It is this nonlinearity that makes predicting the location of the maximum therapeutic temperature difficult a priori. Although if h(r) were measured separately, Eq. 3.81a could be used as the basis for an extended analysis which included skin effects. All of these results are valid, of course, only when the actual blood perfusion remains constant, the power applicator geometry also remains constant [so that $q(\vec{r})$ and $g(\vec{r})$ remain fixed], and the skin-cooling parameters remain fixed [so that $h(\vec{r})$ remains constant for the superficial measurement locations]. The most significant general use of this result for patient treatment planning would be that if blood perfusion changed little during a treatment (or at least in the beginning of a treatment) – a consideration which should be checked experimentally with clinical results by calculating tissue-cooling coefficient values at different applied power magnitudes – then significantly more useful results could be obtained from experimental patient "treatment simulations", as discussed previously. These improved results would be possible since some temperature prediction capabilities would be possible – again dependent on the constancy of the actual blood perfusion during a treatment.

In summary, the tissue-cooling coefficient concept appears to be useful quantity to monitor changes in perfusion qualitatively when all other conditions are kept constant, or to predict temperature as a function of applied power (or skin temperature) when all other variables, including blood perfusion, are kept constant. But, if it is used in an attempt to "measure" blood perfusion, great caution is needed since in general it can contain a significant conduction component. This conclusion is further strenghened by the knowledge that there has never been a comprehensive experimental investigation comparing effective perfusion values calculated using these thermal methods (either steady state of thermal washout) to perfusion values measured using other, nonthermal methods, for example, radioisotope clearance. Thus, while this simple thermal method of calculating effective perfusion can give a very useful indicator of perfusion changes within any given experiment, the numbers so obtained have questionable value for comparison from experiment to experiment or from investigator to investigator because of their inclusion of conduction effects.

To correct for these effects, conduction processes must be properly included in a numerical model. Two such approaches exist: First, the use of heated probes, for example, those of Bowman and colleagues (e.g., [147]), and Chen and Holmes [19] who use a homogeneous, spherically symmetrical model for the tissue surrounding the tip of a heated thermistor probe. The local perfusion values are then calculated using a bioheat transfer equation model of the tissue thermal response to a heating pulse. This approach has the distinct advantage of containing a model for the conduction process so that a conduction-corrected (and not an effective) perfusion can be calculated, but it is more difficult and expensive to apply than the methods used to calculate $\dot{W}_e$. The second approach to account for conduction effects is to calculate perfusion values by using a bioheat transfer equation model which contains anatomical and physical information for the heated tissue of interest. Optimization techniques are used to find a set of blood perfusions which force the predicted model temperatures to match the experimentally obtained temperatures at several locations. The latter approach is still being developed, but it does have the advantage that it requires only temperature measurements and does not need separate perfusion probes. It will be discussed more extensively in the section on retrospective thermal dosimetry.

Temperature Predictions

Once the power deposition and blood flow information is available (at one of the levels previously described), then temperature calculations can be performed using the bioheat transfer equation, or an improved version thereof. In the interest of completeness, it should be noted that in actually an exact, physically correct equation exists which could, in principle, be used to determine the temperature distribution in tissues. This is simply the normal convective energy balance equation, which is, in terms of temperature

$$-\nabla \cdot k \nabla T + \varrho c \vec{V} \cdot \nabla T + \varrho c \frac{\partial T}{\partial t} = \dot{Q}_a(\vec{r}) + \dot{Q}_m(\vec{r}) \ . \tag{3.84}$$

To solve this exact equation would, however, require that the velocity vector $\vec{V}$ be known for all positions – i.e., inside all vessels from capillaries up to all larger vessels – and the location of those vessels (and of the adjacent tissue regions where $\vec{V} \equiv 0$) would also need to be known. This is an insurmountable task, and thus some approximations are needed. The traditional bioheat transfer equation makes this approximation by replacing $\varrho c \vec{V} \cdot \nabla T$ by $\dot{W} c_b (T - T_{ar})$. Other researchers, e.g., Chen and Holmes [18] and Weinbaum and Jiji [152], use different approximations. The important point to note is that all of these attempts are not attempts to find an exact equation, but to find a better approximation to a known, exact equation which is not solvable because of its overwhelming data input requirements.

From the blood perfusion discussion, we have noted the great difficulty in being able to predict absolutely, a priori, the actual distribution of perfusion *to be present* in the tumor and normal tissue *during the hyperthermia treatment.* Therefore, it is perhaps best at this stage of development of hyperthermia to take a less ambitious goal for patient treatment planning, that of the limiting case analysis (best case/worst case). This requires less knowledge and is within the scope of present systems. That is, since tumors can have a range of properties and blood flows, the designation of a single general model may be impossible. However, it is possible to conceive of one tumor perfusion model that is easy to heat and of one which has perfusion characteristics that make it difficult to heat. Thus, we can possibly construct limiting case tumor perfusion models that bracket the characteristics of real tumors. For many situations, the uniform blood flow model shown in Fig. 3.51 represents an easy-to-heat perfusion pattern, and the annular blood flow model is a hard-to-heat perfusion pattern. To verify the validity of this concept, Roemer et al. [112, 113] generated many tumor models in which the blood flow pattern was set randomly by computer (Fig. 3.51). Except in a few cases in which extreme blood flow patterns resulted, the results of the heating as characterized by their acceptable power range parameter (ΔP, Fig. 3.50) were intermediate between the limiting case models of uniform blood flow and annular blood flow, which indicates that these two tumor perfusion patterns may be able to be used as limiting or bracketing case models between which the results for most other tumor perfusion patterns will lie. This concept needs to be investigated further since it is a potential way of avoiding a very difficult problem.

In treatment planning, the actual blood flow in the tumor and normal tissues that will be present during the treatment is still a significant unknown, so it is presently impossible to compute the treatment isotherms. Nevertheless, it might be possible to use the bracketing case tumor model concept and hence establish if the heating technique in question has a reasonable chance of producing an acceptable heating of the tumor. Initially, both the uniform blood flow model and the annular blood flow model could be used to represent the tumor. If additional information is available on the location of major vessels, it could be incorporated into the models as well. If the computer simulation indicates that the most difficult-to-heat tumor perfusion model can be heated acceptably, then it is probable that the method will work on a real tumor located similarly in the patient. Conversely, if the easiest-to-heat tumor perfusion model cannot be heated by the method, then it is unlikely that the method would work in a real case. If the results of the model computations are mixed, then either further development of the models is necessary or the physician and physicist, together, must exercise their judgment as to the level of risk. While definite anwers cannot be given as in, radiation dosimetry, at least some basis for judgment is provided.

From calculations such as these, it will eventually be possible to optimize the treatment protocol prior to therapy so that the patient is likely to receive maximum benefit at minimal risk. One additional feature of this approach is that the methods may be able to help indicate the places where thermometer probes could be placed in order to monitor the treatment procedure properly. The risk of not measuring at points of high temperature in normal tissues or in cool locations within the tumor, such as near a major vessel, will be reduced. It is clear that advances in the area of prospective thermal dosimetry will require development of the ability to be able to predict (before a hyperthermia treatment) what each patient's tissue perfusion will be during the treatment. More light needs to be shed on this subject through continued experimentation.

Although the general problem of patient treatment planning is clearly difficult, it appears to be possible to make reasonably good predictions of hyperthermia treatment temperature distributions in tissues using the bioheat transfer equation. This is evident from some early work of Sekins and Emery [124] and Sekins et al. [125] for diathermy experiments on humans and, more recently, for a series of simulations by the Dartmouth group [142] of patient treatments performed by Oleson [90]. The simulations used two-dimensional inhomogeneous tissue models of the concentric coil and annular array devices similar to those described previously (e.g., see Figs. 3.52–3.56). The results of their analysis are given in Fig. 3.80 for the digitized CT scan of a lung tumor shown in Fig. 3.79. Temperature comparisons are made along the single track shown in Fig. 3.79 for the three different blood flow distributions given in Table 3.21. The patient was treated with, and simulations were run for, both of these devices. Good general agreement was

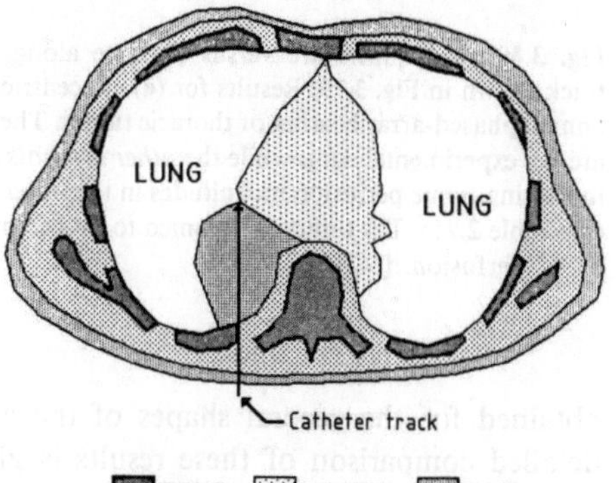

Fig. 3.79. Digitized CT scan of thoracic tumor heated by the concentric coil and annular phased array. [142]

Table 3.21. Blood perfusion levels used to obtain the results of Fig. 3.79

Marker	Perfusion rates (ml/100 g/min)				
	Fat	Muscle	Bone	Heart	Lung
*	0.03	2.7	0	84	433
+	5	15	5	84	433
Δ	10	27	10	84	433

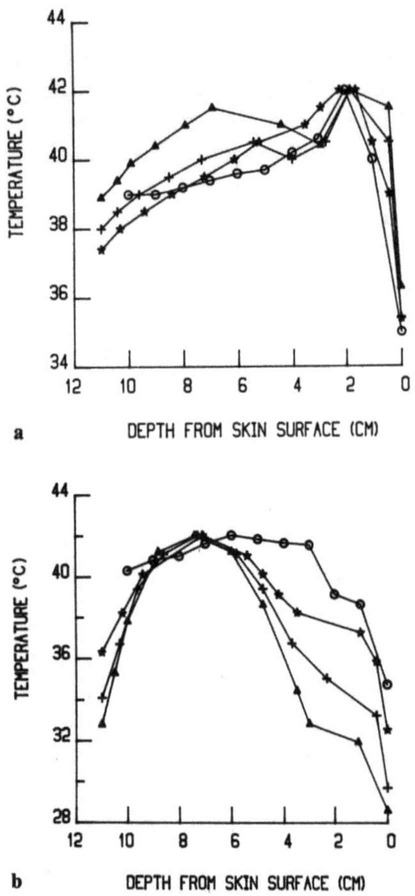

Fig. 3.80 a, b. Temperature versus distance along the catheter track shown in Fig. 3.79. Results for **(a)** concentric coil and **(b)** annual phased-array heating of thoracic tumor. The *open circles* are the experimental data, while the *other symbols* are for three increasing tissue perfusion magnitudes in the order *, +, and Δ (see Table 2.21). The tumor is assumed to be necrotic with zero blood perfusion. [142]

obtained for the general shapes of the curves. The detailed comparison of these results is given in the original reference. For our purposes, it is important to note that particular tumor/tissue models can be found that predict the temperatures *to be obtained* during a treatment, thus increasing the probability that patient treatment planning can become a useful tool.

3.3.2.3 Summary

Patient treatment planning plays a small role in hyperthermia treatments at present due to both a lack of need for such plans, since inflexible heating systems are generally used, and a lack of adequate predictive capabilities. The need is increasing as more flexible heating systems become available, and thus as the predictive abilities of simulations become more powerful, they will see a greatly increased use. The ready availability of sophisticated imaging modalities means that patient/tumor anatomies can be obtained, although exact tumor margins are not always readily defined and the locations (or presence) of thermally significant vessels are not always known. Also, the ability to simulate individual SAR patterns is increasing significantly, as expected, since this is primarily a difficult numerical mathematics problem once the patient's anatomy is known – i.e., there is no large unknown physiological factor. Unfortunately, this is not the case for calculating temperatures – which are affected by blood perfusion. Since the blood flow of a patient can vary significantly during a treatment, it is necessary to know the blood flow a priori in order to plan a treatment. This involves predicting a physiological response, always a difficult task. For this reason, it is suggested that the use of both low-power, preliminary "simulation treatments" and the limiting-case tumor models be encouraged since they seem to be approaches that can be practically implemented in the near future.

3.3.3 Concurrent Thermal Dosimetry

3.3.3.1 Introduction

Concurrent thermal dosimetry consists of the monitoring and control of temperatures during actual treatments. Ideally, one would prefer to control the complete temperature field, preferably using noninvasive tomographic thermometry. However, at present, all such tomographic systems are in the research stage, with unproven performance characteristics in terms of resolution and accuracy. In addition, a real difficulty with such noninvasive techniques is the necessity of adequate space around the patient for sophisticated multi-aperture-heating equipment, as well as for the noninvasive temperature-monitoring equipment. Finally, the noise rejection requirements of any tomographic thermometry system will be extremely high if it is to perform in the presence of intense heating fields. Thus, it seems that temperatures will have to be monitored with invasive probes for quite some time to come, resulting in the basic question of concurrent thermal dosimetry: How can one control the complete temperature field based on measurements at a finite number of points? This section will investigate this question and also see how close we

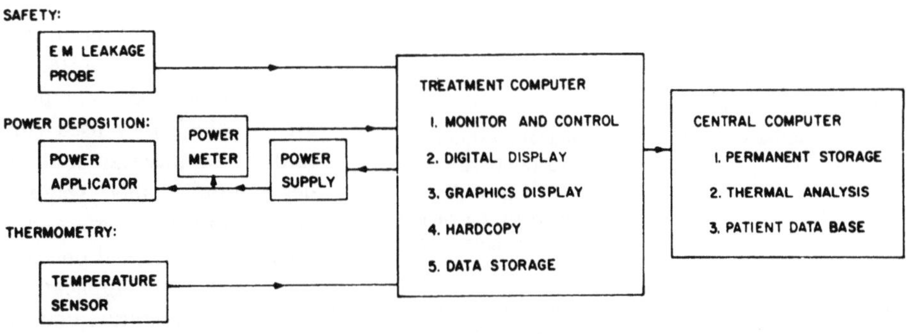

Fig. 3.81. System diagram indicating the characteristics required for a computerized data acquisition and control system for hyperthermia therapy which is coupled to a larger mainframe computer for data analysis and data base management. [110]

presently come to the ideal with present-day equipment.

Clinical systems are now inevitably based on a micro- or mini-computer, which allows great flexibility and opens many opportunities for using increasingly sophisticated feedback control schemes (Fig. 3.81). There are two main goals of these systems, as shown in Table 3.22. Most current clinical systems fulfill the first function of removing an attention-demanding task, that of constantly monitoring the temperatures and adjusting the power to keep the temperatures constant, a task which continues throughout the treatment. This frees the operator to perform other tasks, such as interacting with and observing the patient and intelligently observing the temperature patterns being produced – activities which can significantly improve the treatment and which are difficult for any automated system to perform. Therefore, just the automation of simple existing control schemes for single-point controllers is an improvement. These automated systems also allow improved control capabilities due to their more single-minded attentiveness and faster response times. Finally, computerized systems are able to perform control tasks which individual human operators could never do, in particular, to obtain multipoint control of temperatures at several locations within a tumor and to optimize such treatments.

A common, basic structure can be described for all such systems (Table 3.23, Fig. 3.82), where four regions are important: (I) the initial start-up phase at the beginning of the treatment where one uses an initial control strategy, (II) the region where one's basic control law is implemented (listed as a PID controller in the example of Table 3.23), (III) the region where excessive temperatures are reached, and (IV) the region were the controlled temperature is "far" below its desired condition. Regions I and II represent the normal, expected regions, whereas regions III and IV represent extremes in which some additional action must be taken. Different laws and numbers (e.g., T_{min}, T_{max}) will be implemented for particular systems, but the structure will remain. The above control laws are, of course, overridden by any patient safety considerations, some of which can also be automated.

The goal in all cases is to automatically get as close as possible to the ideal temperature distribution previously described. The ability to approach this goal closely is limited by both the hardware one is using and the feedback control system being used. That is, while flexible heating systems are needed to deposit power in variable geometric patterns in order to approach the ideal temperature goal, they will not be able to be optimally employed unless an intelligent, automated feedback control system is available to control them. This controllability implies detailed knowledge of the patient's temperature distribution, and the future development of improved feedback

Table 3.22. Goals of feedback control systems in hyperthermia treatments

1. *Automate* the tasks a human operator now performs: This reduces the requirements for the operator. If feedback control is performed manually, constant vigilance is needed for power control. If this task is taken over by the computer, the operator can concentrate on other jobs, such as interacting with the patient and/or optimizing the treatment
2. *Improve* the system response: computerized systems can respond more quickly and reliably to system disturbances, e.g., patient blood flow changes, that require adjustments in the applied power
3. *Extend* the control system capabilities beyond what a human operator can do: for example, automatic control over temperatures at multiple points and the optimization of the treatments can be performed using computers, tasks which are impossible to perform manually

Table 3.23. Control strategy region (see Fig. 3.82)

Region	Regional description	Goal
I	Initial start up	Control maximum rate of temperature rise to limit possible patient pain/tissue damage, yet obtain a short heat-up time
II	Normal operating range	Control of single or multiple points for temperature control (e.g., PID controller)
III	Excessively high temperatures	Power-off to provide the fastest possible cooling to prevent patient pain/tissue damage
IV	Excessively low temperatures	Rapidly return power to region I strategy

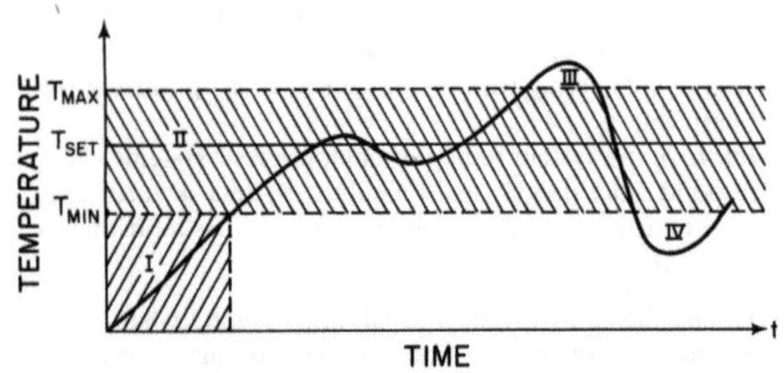

Fig. 3.82. Possible control regions during a hyperthermia treatment: *I*, initial start-up phase; *II*, normal operating region; *III*, excessively high temperature; *IV*, excessively low temperature (see Table 3.23)

control hinges crucially on our ability to increase our knowledge of this variable.

While current systems measure and control a single temperature, there are several experimental systems which control two or more points, and there have been proposals and attempts to control the complete temperature field. These three increasingly more useful and, of course, more difficult, approaches are outlined below.

3.3.3.2 Single-Point Control Systems

Single-point temperature controllers are in wide clinical use in a larger number of centers, with several commercial hyperthermia devices also providing automated single-point control systems. Some, but not all, of these systems have been described in detail in the open literature, including the modified PID controller of Salcman and Samaras [119] for interstitial microwave brain treatments and the work of Nilsson and Persson [85], who have described a single-temperature, computer-controlled microwave system which they used clinically on 80 superficial tumors. Sathiaseelan et al. [123] have given a similar description of their single-point controller. Of the many commercial systems now available, probably the most interesting and one of the most widely used is the French single-applicator microwave system which monitors temperature noninvasively using microwave radiometry (e.g., [102]). This is a noninvasive system which measures and controls an "average" temperature sensed by the radiometer. It essentially performs the automation and improvement tasks given in Table 3.22 and is not a tomographic system. These, and most other single-point control systems, are based on a standard PID (proportional-integral-derivative) controller, with variations to account for the particular nature of hyperthermia. In their usual computerized, digital form, these systems are modifications of the ideal PID control law [10]:

$$\dot{Q}_a(t_n) - \dot{Q}_{ave} = k_p e(t_n) + k_i \sum_{i=0}^{n} e(t_i)\tau_s + k_d \frac{e_n(t_n) - e(t_{n-1})}{\tau_s} \tag{3.85}$$

where the variation of the applied power about its average value, i.e., $\dot{Q}_a(t_n) - \dot{Q}_{ave}$, is given by the summation of three terms: one which is proportional to the error at time t_n, $e(t_n)$; one which is proportional to the numerical integral of all previous errors, $k_i \sum_{i=1}^{n} e(t_i)\tau_s$, and one which is proportional to the numerical derivative of the time rate of change of the system error, $k_d[e(t_n) - e(t_{n-1})]/\tau_s$. Here, τ_s is the time between successive samples of the system temperature; $e(t_n)$ is the system error at time t_n, $e(t_n) = T_{set} - T_m(t_n)$, where T_{set} is the set-point temperature and $T_m(t_n)$ is the measured system temperature at time t_n; and the three gain constants are given by k_p, k_i, and k_d – quantities which are all independent in the ideal, or noninteractive system. The proportional term immediately increases or decreases the amount of power being applied based on the present error signal, whereas the integral terms has a "memory" in order to adjust for the system's past performance and thus to avoid errors at steady state. The derivative term is proportional to the instantaneous time rate of change of the system error and is used to speed up the system response. PID controllers have mainly been used for industrial applications, and methods of choosing the systems gains have been developed in order to choose those gains which are most "robust", i.e., give the smallest errors over a wide range of disturbances. Also, a significant number of improvements have been made on these controllers in order to improve their performance. The interested reader should consult a standard feedback control text for further details (e.g., [3]). The best choice of gains for hyperthermia is yet to be determined. In practice, one always desires larger gains in order to have a rapid response to disturbances, primarily blood flow changes in hyperthermia applications. These increased gains give faster control, but are more susceptible to introducing unwanted oscillations into the system. Some work has been performed to investigate experimentally the effect of gain and blood flow on system performance, but the question has not been answered completely, especially for clinical situations where

1. the range of blood flows to be encountered remains unknown and
2. temperature sensors are generally placed at different depths so that their sensitivity to applied power is variable from patient to patient, a factor which must be calibrated for when comparing the gains used by different investigators.

All of the single-point controllers used to date have performed the function of providing automation (see Table 3.22) and performance improvement, and will continue to do so. They provide an automated way of adjusting power in response to some "thermal response" of the patient. For most controllers, this is the temperature for one of the sensors at some location in the tumor. For the noninvasive microwave radiometry temperature-monitoring system, the "measured temperature" is really an average temperature over a fairly large area parallel to the skin and for a centimeter or so deep. Therefore, the "thermal response" in these systems is the "average temperature", which is assumedly correlated with the tumor temperature magnitudes.

3.3.3.3 Multi-Point Control Systems

The next step toward improving the treatment temperature distributions involves controlling temperatures at more than one point. Controlling two points in a field presently has much appeal since most applications to treat superficial tumors involve

1. a heating system for which the amplitude of the applied power can be varied and
2. a skin-cooling system whose magnitude can be varied.

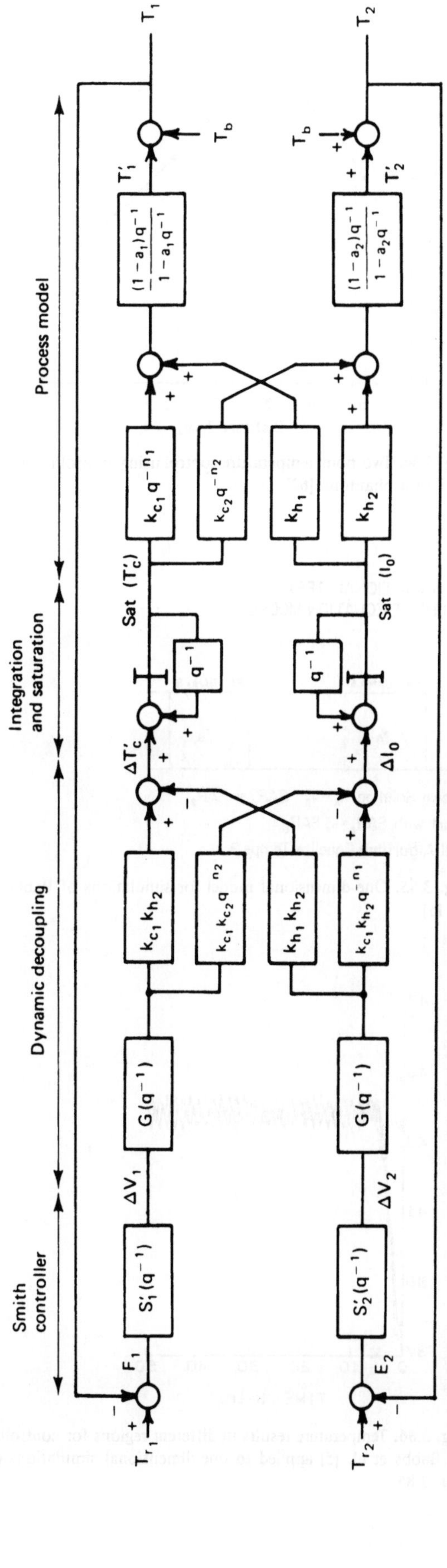

Fig. 3.83. Two-point controller to control temperatures at front and rear of tumor. [62]

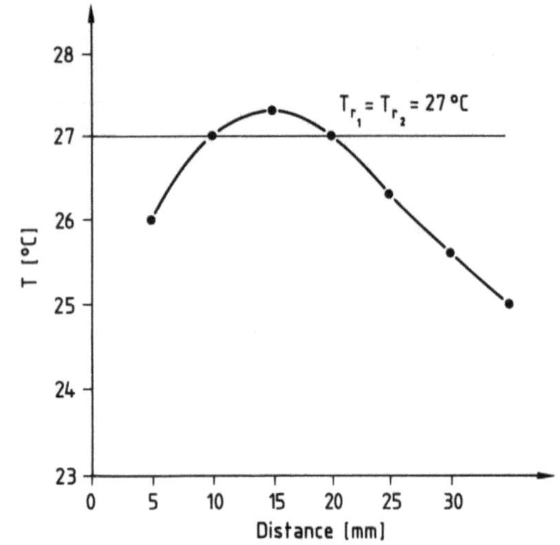

Fig. 3.84. Two-point temperature control using controller of Fig. 3.83 in a phantom. [62]

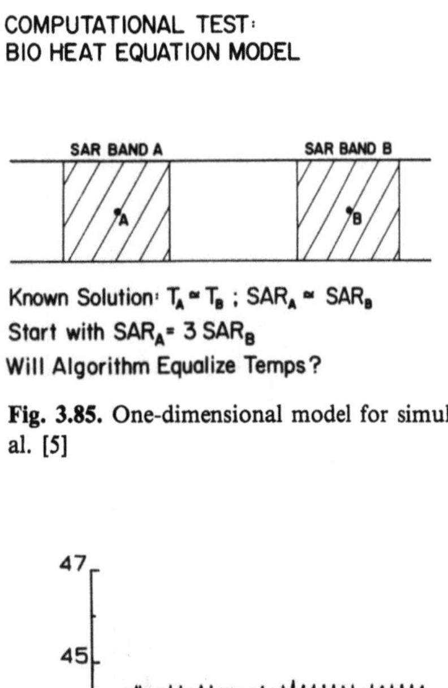

Fig. 3.85. One-dimensional model for simulations of Babbs et al. [5]

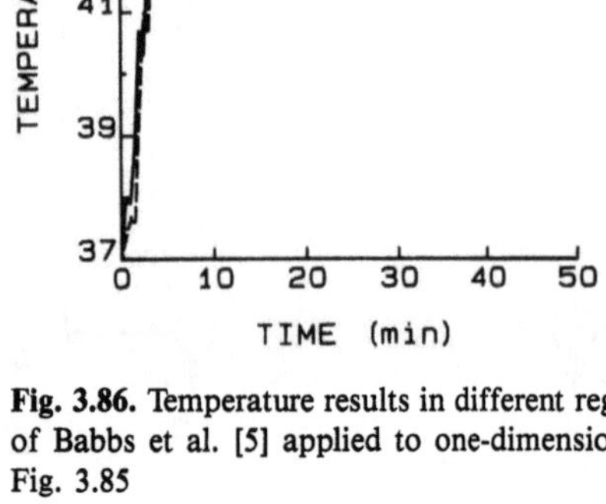

Fig. 3.86. Temperature results in different regions for controller of Babbs et al. [5] applied to one-dimensional simulations of Fig. 3.85

Thus, two independent variables are available, and two tumor temperatures can be controlled. This can be done at two depths, preferably for one sensor at the front and one at the rear of a tumor. This has been the proposed approach of Knudsen and Heinzl [62] and Knudsen and Overgaard [63], as illustrated in Figs. 3.83 and 3.84. Figure 3.83 shows the controller used, which included a modified Smith controller [128] in order to account for the time delay between the initiation of a surface temperature change and the effects of that change at the two depths. The effects of the two control actions have been separated using standard feedback control approaches, giving what appears to be a useful two-point controller. Figure 3.84 shows some experimental results for a phantom. No results were presented for any patient treatments.

Several other proposals for and implementation of sophisticated two-point feedback control systems have been reported recently, including a two-dimensional simulated interstitial RF controller by Doss [33] and a two-dimensional simulation of an optimal temperature controller for a phased-array RF hyperthermia system by Knudsen and Hartmann [61]. Nikawa et al. [84] present a controller which varies the applied power of a direct-contact converging applicator and the cooling water flow rate to vary the position of maximum temperature in the tissue. Also, De Wagter [29] presents simulation results for the control of transient temperatures of layered tissues using microwave heating plus skin cooling.

These controllers are, of course, limited to controlling two temperatures with the two available independent entities – skin temperature cooling and applied power amplitude. A more general approach would be to use many sensors to control the amplitude and phase of several applicators or the distributed power deposition field of a scanned system in order to achieve dynamic control of the power deposition field. Some studies have begun the investigation of this possibility. For example, Babbs et al. [5] have described a one-dimensional simulation of a proposed controller for localized hyperthermia. Their study was for a general control system in which the goal was to consider several measured temperatures and to reduce their variations while maintaining a given average setpoint temperature. Figure 3.85 shows the one-dimensional model used in their simulations, and Fig. 3.86 illustrates some of their results for that geometry given a hypothetical heating system which could deposit power at a constant value in any of the different blood perfusion regions, i.e., a highly conformable applicator.

Recently, experimental results for a multipoint control system have been presented for a scanned, focused

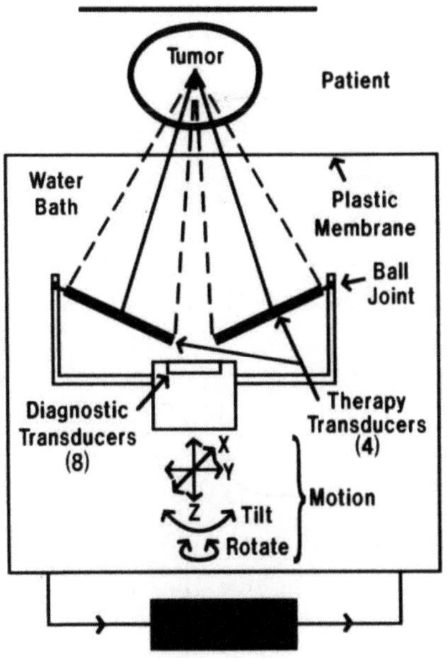

Fig. 3.87. Scanned, focused ultrasound system used for animal experiments of Figs. 3.88–3.91. [59]

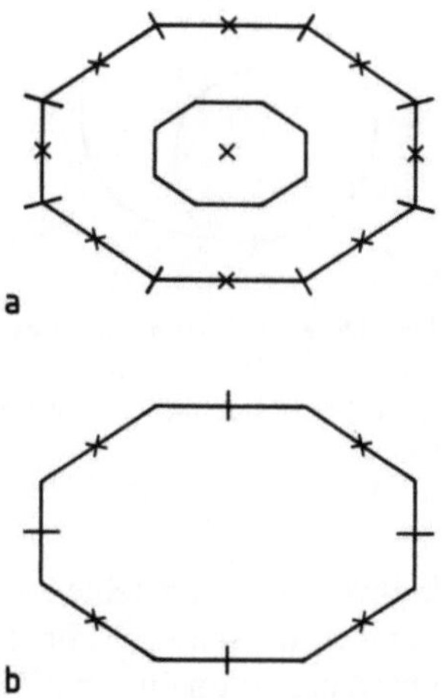

Fig. 3.88. Octagonal scanning pattern used for four- and nine-point controllers. [59]

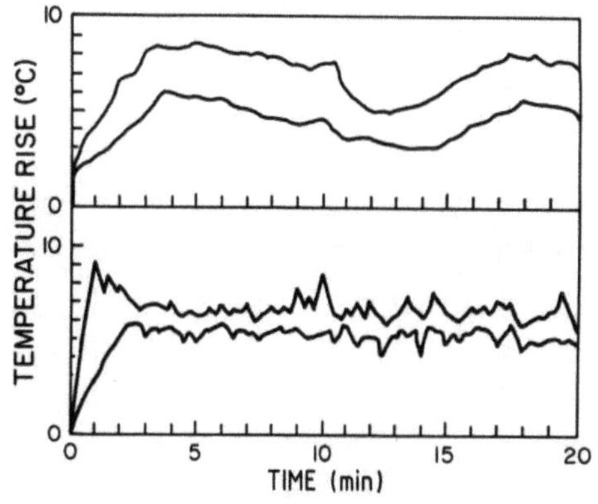

Fig. 3.89. Temperature versus time curves for multipoint control (*bottom curve*) in a dog thigh experiment which could not be controlled well manually (*top curve*) [59]. Only the highest and lowest temperature curves are shown

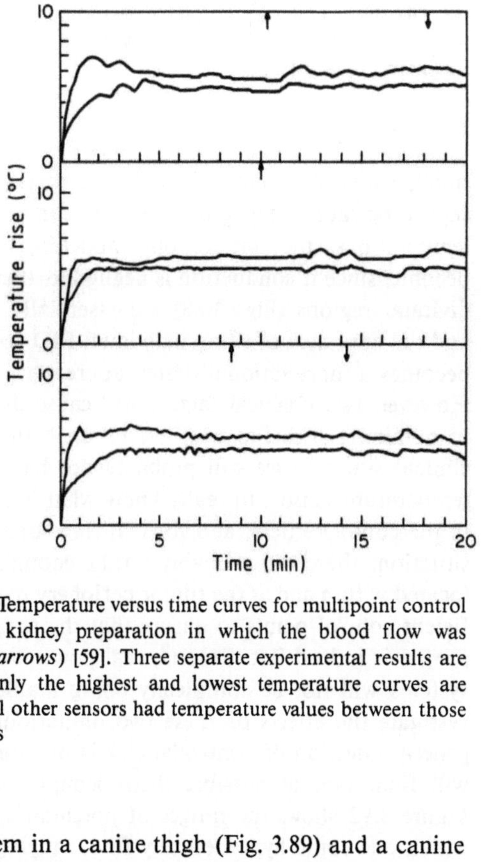

Fig. 3.90. Temperature versus time curves for multipoint control in a dog kidney preparation in which the blood flow was changed (*arrows*) [59]. Three separate experimental results are shown. Only the highest and lowest temperature curves are shown. All other sensors had temperature values between those two curves

ultrasound system [59] which structured the power deposition patterns to be constant within each of several regions. The scanning was done using the system shown in Fig. 3.87 with the ultrasonic focal point in a fixed plane. Figure 3.88 shows the octagonal pattern followed. Up to nine points were controlled, as per Fig. 3.88. The controller used a separate PID controller within each of the nine regions, and thus the whole system acted as a series of separate single-point controllers. The results of using this system in a canine thigh (Fig. 3.89) and a canine kidney preparation (Fig. 3.90) show that the system can work quite well, even in the presence of rather large blood perfusion changes (Fig. 3.90). This control scheme allowed the temperature to be preferentially raised within a fixed region of space delimited by the locations of the sensors (Fig. 3.91).

An interesting result from these experiments is that the temperature profile can be quite flat for a good controller, thus making conduction effects quite

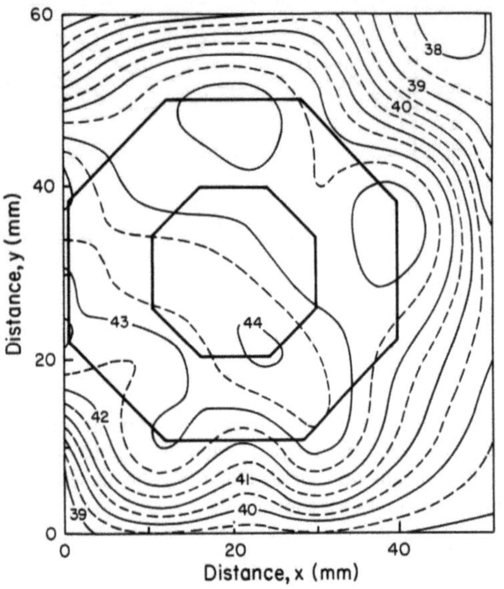

Fig. 3.91. Temperature distribution in the scanning plane for the canine thigh experiments of Fig. 3.89 with two concentric scan patterns as shown. [59]

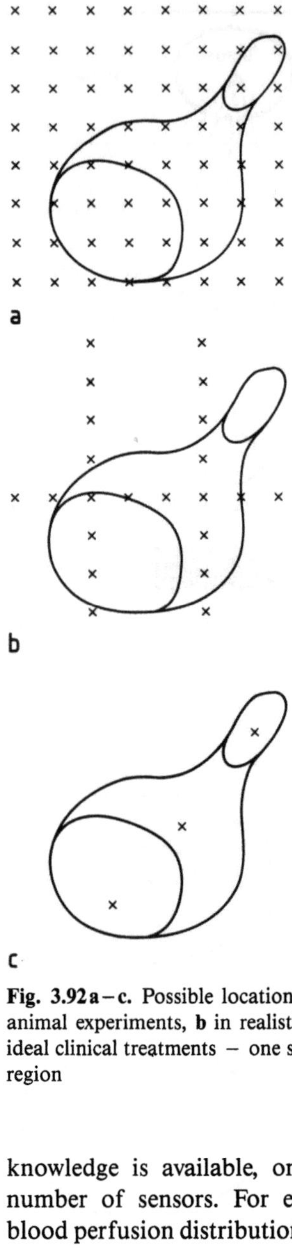

Fig. 3.92a–c. Possible locations of temperature sensors: **a** in animal experiments, **b** in realistic clinical treatments, and **c** in ideal clinical treatments – one sensor for each blood perfusion region

small, which may allow the effective perfusion concept to be valid. That is, the better we can control the temperatures, the simpler our modeling task may become, since if conduction is negligible, then the individual regions (Fig. 3.88) are essentially separate and the approach of using individual PID controllers becomes a more rational design approach.

However, two practical factors will cause difficulties in obtaining such flat profiles. First, in the general clinical situation we will probably not have enough temperature sensors to really know what is occurring in the complete field, and for real three-dimensional situations there will probably not be enough sensors located within and at the tumor periphery to give sufficient control points to ensure that the temperature profile is indeed flat. Second, real power deposition systems will not be completely conformable. To investigate the effects of these two limitations on the general question of controllability is of interest. We will first look at possible thermocouple positions. Figure 3.92 shows the ranges of potential situations which one could hypothetically find, ranging from a very dense array possible in an experimental situation (Fig. 3.92a) to a clinically realistic array (Fig. 3.92b) in which the sensor spacing is quite large. The experimental results of Fig. 3.91 were obtained for a situation closer to that of the dense spacing in Fig. 3.92a, and thus the validity of extrapolating their significance to clinical situations is problematic because of the significant change in the number of sensors available. On the other hand, if other knowledge is available, one need not have a large number of sensors. For example, if one knew the blood perfusion distribution pattern in the tumor, one could (in a simplistic sense) use just one temperature sensor per blood perfusion region (Fig. 3.92c) and deposit a constant power uniformly within each region of constant blood perfusion. That power magnitude would be equal to the power value needed to keep the sensor in that region at the set-point value; i.e., the problem would reduce to a series of single-point controllers.

Of course, attaining this ideal assumes that the power deposition is completely conformable (i.e., has an infinitely fine resolution), and unrealistic assumption whose consequences can be seen in Fig. 3.84, where a realistic power-deposition pattern (exponential with depth) is used with a limited number of sensors (two) to control a limited number of points (two). In this case, the temperature distribution at all other points is at the mercy of the unknown blood perfusions (equal to zero in this example) and the fixed, distributed power-deposition pattern – giving high temperatures between the two sensors in this phantom experiment. We have previously discussed the problems caused by a lack of conformability when trying to obtain the ideal temperature distributions, and now we will consider the general effects of the fixed, finite-sized, distributed nature of real power-deposition patterns on the feedback process. For a given heating system (e.g., a fixed modality, number and size of heating elements, and a choice of frequency) and a given geometric configuration of that system, $\vec{r}_s$ (e.g., a fixed position for a mechanical scanning system and a fixed set of phases for an electronic scanning system), there is a certain power-deposition pattern $\dot{Q}_a(\vec{r}_s)$. For any system, there is a large set (S) of possible geometric configurations ($\vec{r}_s$) into which the system can be put, and the basic control problem is how to select that set of configurations to reach some optimal goal. Given this formulation, we can examine the requirements for several different cases, with the recognition that the temperature profile will no longer be perfectly flat since $\dot{Q}_a(\vec{r}_s)$ is not a point source – and it thus may not be possible to force each sensor to the set point value. First, ideally, if one knows the temperatures at all locations, one can modify the power-deposition pattern to achieve some specified criteria, say to force all of the temperatures in the tumor to be equal to or above the set-point temperature and to minimize the average elevation above that set point. Mathematically, this problem would be to find the set of $\vec{r}_s$ (where $\vec{r}_s \in S$) that

$$\text{minimizes } \frac{1}{V_{\text{tumor}}} \int_{V_{\text{tumor}}} [T(\vec{r}) - T_{\text{set}}]\, d\vec{v} \tag{3.86}$$

subject to the

$$\text{constraint: } T(\vec{r}) - T_{\text{set}} \geq 0 \quad \text{for all } \vec{r} \in V_{\text{tumor}} \,.$$

For the more realistic case, we will have N sensor at the locations r_i, and our problem becomes: Find the set of $\vec{r}_s$ (again for all $\vec{r}_s \in S$) that will

$$\text{minimize } \frac{1}{N} \sum_{i=1}^{N} [T(r_i) - T_{\text{set}}] \tag{3.87}$$

subject to the

$$\text{constraint: } T(r_i) - T_{\text{set}} > 0 \quad \text{for all } r_i \in V_{\text{tumor}} \,.$$

Next, we need to note that the above process has neglected all normal tissue considerations – i.e., we have not put in any formal constraint on the allowable set of normal tissue temperatures being below some allowable values. For the case of all temperatures known, this would give the additional

$$\text{Constraint: } T(\vec{r}) - T_{\text{all}}(\vec{r}) < 0 \quad \text{for all } \vec{r} \in V_{\text{no}} \tag{3.88}$$

and for the nonideal case where normal tissue temperatures are measured at only a finite number of locations (r_i)

$$\text{Constraint: } T(\vec{r}_i) - T_{\text{all}}(\vec{r}_i) < 0 \quad \text{for all } \vec{r}_i \in V_{\text{no}} \,. \tag{3.89}$$

Further constraints could also be put on the maximum allowable measured tumor temperature in order to prevent potentially serious tumor necrosis and patient complications (e.g., see [112, 113] for examples of such limits).

Also, we have not solved the problem of the ideal placement of the temperature sensors, an issue which should be discussed further. If we know the tissue perfusion pattern, then we can optimally place one sensor in each such region. If we have fewer sensors than perfusion regions, then we need to fall back and choose the subset of those regions in which we will measure; subject to the clinical anatomical constraints and the geometric constraints placed on us by the physical construction of the sensors – i.e., they will be able to measure at points along several straight (at least before being pushed into the patient) lines. This is an unsolved problem at present. The only allowable advice would be to put them in locations such that, when those temperatures are controlled, one has the highest probability of maximizing the effect of the treatment. That is, if you do not know the blood perfusion, then you probably want to place your sensors in those locations where the lowest tumor temperatures are likely to occur – but this is a circular argument, since, if you are going to control these temperatures, they will be brought up to the set-point value and someplace else will have lower temperatures. Therefore, this advice needs to be refined to be: locate the sensors in such locations that, if the temperatures at those locations are controlled at the set-point temperature, then the volume of tissue at temperatures below the set-point value elsewhere in the tumor is minimized.

The actual minimization process outlined above will need to be iterative due to the lack of knowledge of a formal relationship between $T(\vec{r})$, or $T(\vec{r}_i)$, and the applied power patterns, $\dot{Q}_a(\vec{r}_s)$. Such formal relationships can be obtained from either experimental data or a treatment model, or from both. In all cases, the important consideration is really the system's sensitivity, i.e., the rate of change of temperature at location i with respect to the magnitude of the power at the different scan positions ($\vec{r}_s = r_j$)

$$S_{ij} \triangleq \frac{\partial T_i}{\partial |\dot{Q}_a(r_j)|} \quad . \tag{3.90}$$

In general, this sensitivity will be a function of the local blood perfusion and the surrounding temperature field, in addition to being a function of the applied power pattern. That is

$$S_{ij} = f[T(\vec{r}), \dot{W}(\vec{r}), \dot{Q}_a(r_j)] \tag{3.91}$$

making it a quantity which changes during a treatment. Thus, its calculation cannot be easily performed at the beginning of a treatment and used thereafter. To account for these changes, one needs to do a continuous series of such investigations, an effort which is impractical in a clinical setting, or one must use a model of the treatment. The use of models of treatments has an additionally strong role to play since they not only will allow us to adjust the sensitivity coefficients to account for changed circumstances, but a good model, if properly used, could possibly allow one to estimate the complete temperature field from a few measurements (see the next section on retrospective thermal dosimetry for a full development of this approach). Thus, attempts can be made to control the complete temperature field, rather than just the temperatures at a few locations. This could give much improved control, particularly as hyperthermia is being used increasingly in deeper and more critical locations (brain, abdomen, pelvis) where there are organs which are not only more sensitive to increased temperature, but may also lack (a) temperature/thermal pain sensors and (b) the thermoregulatory protective mechanisms of muscle tissue, and (c) are more crucial to the health and life of the patient. Thus, if tumors in these locations are to be treated in an optimal way using the flexibility of the newer heating systems, attempts must be made to more closely reach the goal of controlling the complete temperature field and not just the temperatures at a few measurement locations.

3.3.3.4 Control of the Complete Temperature Field

In order to reach this goal in practical cases where the number of temperature sensors is limited, the crucial task is to be able to estimate the temperature at unmeasured locations, a task which requires a good model of the treatment process. The development of such a model is described more fully in the next section on retrospective thermal dosimetry, while this section will assume the existence of such a model and will concentrate on its use during feedback control. At

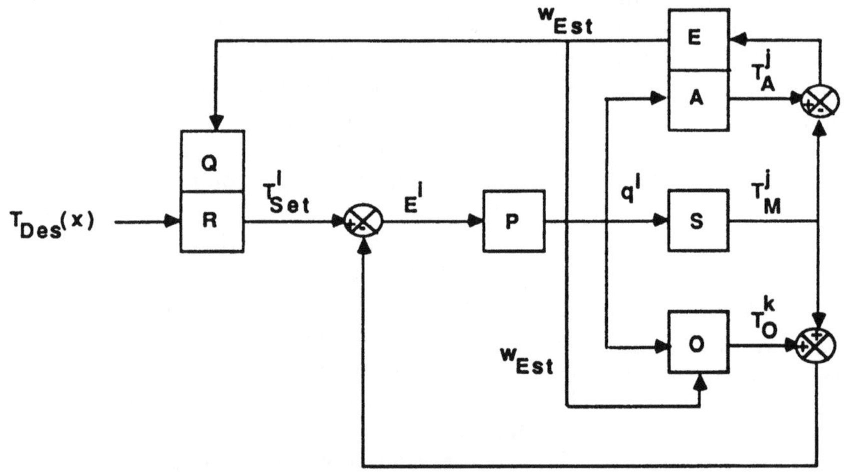

Fig. 3.93. Block diagram of model reference approach to controlling the complete temperature field from temperature measurements at a few locations in the tumor [64]. Block P is the PID control system with error inputs of E^i. These errors are the differences between **a** the desired set point temperatures T^i_{set} from block R and **b** the actual measured system (block S) temperatures T^M_j and/or the temperature predicted by an observer (a model of the system, block O). Block E uses a model of the system to estimate the blood perfusion distribution in the system W_{est}. These estimated perfusions are used in both the observer model and in block Q, which determines the optimal power deposition pattern needed to minimize the objective function – i.e., to minimize the difference between the desired input temperature profile, $T_{des}(x)$, and the predicted temperature profile for the optimal power deposition pattern and the estimated perfusion pattern. Block R then selects the set-point temperatures from this optimal, predicted temperature profile. The system can be operated with an observer but no power optimizer, the power optimizer but no observer, both the observer and the power optimizer, or neither (pure PID control)

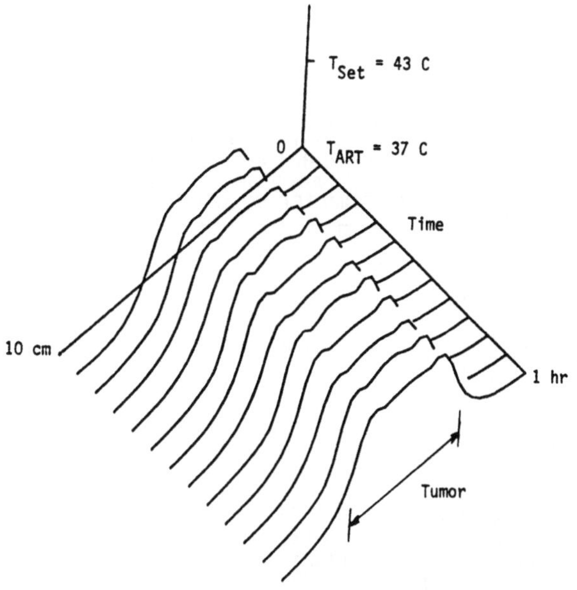

Fig. 3.94. Temperature versus position and time using the reference model approach shown in Fig. 3.93 for controlling one-dimensional, simulated hyperthermia treatments. A uniform temperature of 43 °C inside the tumor was desired. [64]

present, this technique is in its infancy, with only some preliminary parametric, one-dimensional, simulations studies and a few experiments on an in vitro kidney preparation available [64]. The basic scheme employed in that study is shown in Fig. 3.93 and is based on the model reference adaptive control approach. It uses a model of the treatment in two ways. First, the major unknown in the model is assumed to be the blood perfusion (for reasons that have been previously discussed) and thus the first step is to estimate the tissue blood perfusion a priori (block E). Then, these perfusions are used in a treatment model to obtain an optimal scanning pattern for the treatment (block Q), i.e., the minimization problem is solved to find the set of $\dot{Q}_a(r_j)$ that will minimize a form of Eq. 3.86 since all temperatures are assumed to be known. The resultant model predicts the optimal temperature field, including the temperatures at the measurement locations (block R) which would result from the optimal power deposition (note that these could be higher than the desired treatment temperature since the finite, distributed power source will not be able to give the perfect solution of a uniform temperature profile). These optimal set temperatures are then used in a standard PID controller (block P) for the temperature measurement locations. The controller is periodically interrupted to perform a power-off test so that the techniques of the next section can be used to reestimate the tumor perfusions from the transient temperature decays. The new estimates of perfusion are then used in the power optimization model to obtain the new set-point temperatures, and the cycle is repeated. (This interruption could also be performed when the applied power required to maintain those temperatures is significantly different from that predicted by the model.) The results of using this technique for simulations of one-dimensional treatments are given in Fig. 3.94. It is important to note in these results that not only is the complete temperature field well controlled, but that, so far, all of the results obtained have been stable, an encouraging sign for the clinical application of this technique. It is, however, a time-consuming task, both in terms of the need for transient, power-off temperature data during the treatments and the need for a good computer model of the treatment – a computationally intensive task which requires excessive times to be clinically useful at present. This was true even though attempts were made to reduce computation times by using spectral methods to compute the temperature fields [64].

3.3.3.5 Summary

The increased interest in automated, multipoint feedback control is a sign of the increased complexity and flexibility in the technology of the second generation of hyperthermia heating systems that are becoming available. It should be noted, however, that while increasing the number of measurement points that reach a set temperature is definitely a worthwile step forward, and it will give improved treatments, it is only a necessary, but not a sufficient, condition for acceptable clinical treatment control. To attain such complete control, one must, in principle, be able to control the complete temperature field, not just selected points. For present clinical systems, little control is available, and the current general practice can be summarized by noting that normal tissue pain usually limits the amount of power than can be applied with the existing heating technology, thus limiting the attainable tumor temperatures. This situation is changing rapidly to meet the demands of the improved heating systems, and much activity can be expected in the controls area in the near future. While indications of this have been given by the previously referenced feedback control papers, it should also be noted that other papers regarding treatment optimization are also beginning to appear that describe complex two-dimensional models [1, 30].

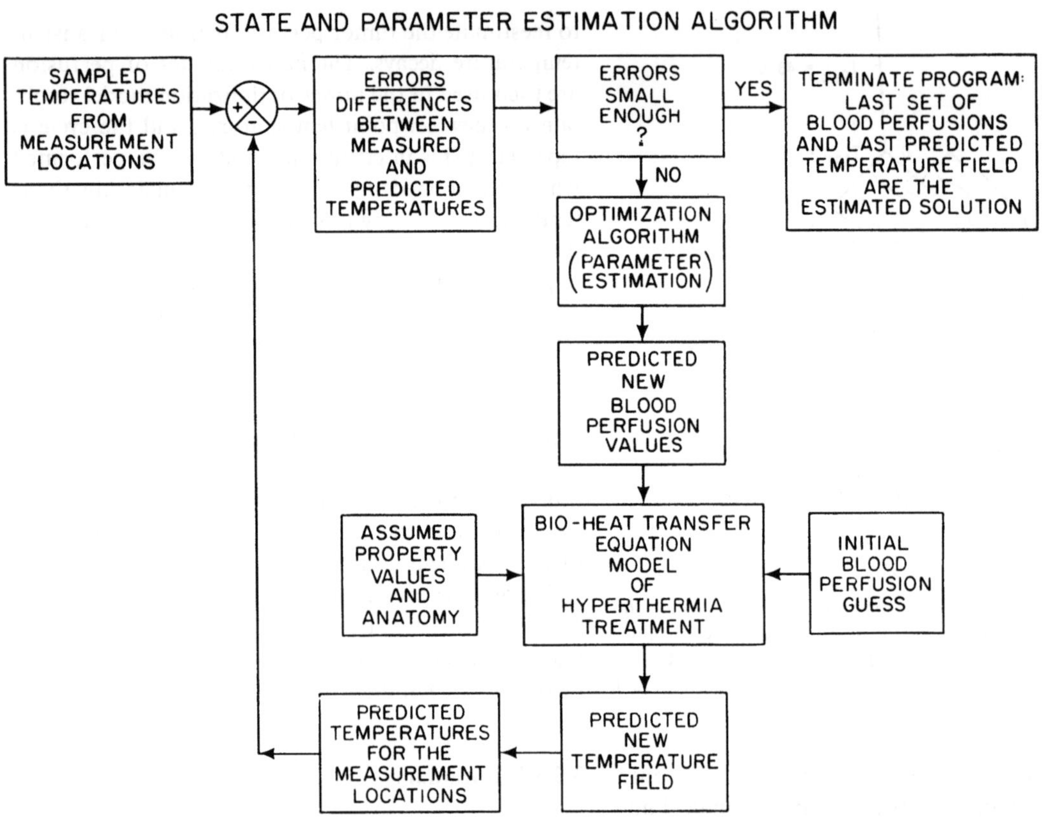

Fig. 3.95. State and parameter estimation technique used to estimate the complete temperature field from clinical temperatures measured at a limited number of points. [26]

3.3.4 Retrospective Thermal Dosimetry

3.3.4.1 Introduction

Since in practical hyperthermia treatments the temperatures are measured at only a few locations, the temperatures at most points in the tumor remain unknown. Solving this major problem is the goal of retrospective thermal dosimetry, which can be defined as the computation of the isothermal distributions that were attained during a completed treatment based on the actual measured treatment temperatures. These distributions can be used as the basis of dose calculations, against which response will be correlated. An additional application will be to use experimental data taken during a treatment to normalize the predictions of the model calculations in any subsequent treatment-planning phase. While these distributions may eventually be computed and displayed in real time during the treatment, in the immediate future they are more likely to be calculated after the treatment, due to the size and speed of the computer programs required. The general approach used (Fig. 3.95) is to adjust the major unknown parameter in a model of such treatments, i.e., the blood perfusion, until the model predictions agree well with the experimentally measured temperatures at discrete locations. If good agreement is reached, the model's prediction of blood perfusion and the complete temperature field are accepted as the best estimates of those values.

It should be noted that the above approach of using a model to manufacture estimated temperatures during a treatment has two end products – an estimate of the temperature field and, in order to be able accurately to do that, an estimate of the perfusion values during a treatment. While the temperatures are of immediate interest for evaluating a given treatment, estimation of the blood perfusion during the treatment will allow knowledge of that variable to be accrued for later use. As mentioned in the previous section on prospective thermal dosimetry, if one is to be able to perform accurate patient treatment planning and control, one must know, a priori, the blood perfusions to be present during the hyperthermia treatment. Thus, the blood perfusion estimates which

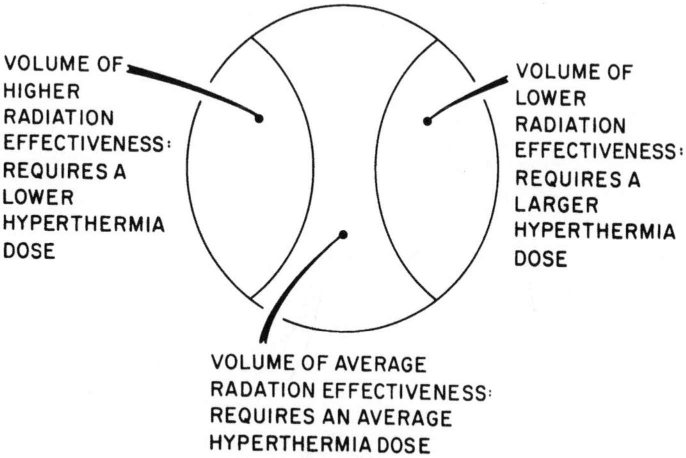

Fig. 3.96. The efficacy of a hyperthermia treatment depends on local physiological factors and on the efficacy of any complementary treatment modality (as shown in this figure for radiation therapy), as well as on the treatment temperature and time. Thus, in principle, the minimum tumor temperature is not strictly the proper measure of treatment efficacy, but, due to lack of knowledge of all of the above factors, it is the only practical (conservative) measure to use

are a by-product of the temperature estimation process will be most useful in all other thermal dosimetry applications. Indeed, Arkin et al. [2] have performed one simulation study using these general optimization technique approaches to estimate blood perfusion for general physiological evaluations.

It is also significant to note that the quantities one really wants to determine in these studies are limited to only a few temperatures. First, one is interested in knowing the minimum temperature in the tumor (and the location of that temperature) so that one can evaluate the thermal efficacy of the treatment. This is a useful measure since minimum tumor temperature seems, clinically, to be a reasonable measure of treatment efficacy [31, 92, 148] and is logically a good, simple measure of the thermal adequacy of the treatment. However, one should keep in mind the fact that other biochemical variables, plus the primary therapy modality, e.g., radiation, also have an effect on the treatment outcome. If, for example, the lowest tumor temperature occurs in a location where the radiation dose is very large and the cells will be killed by radiation, or if the lowest temperature occurs at a location where a sensitizing variable such as pH is also low so those cells are more sensitive to temperature, then the minimum tumor temperature is not the single crucial tumor temperature (Fig. 3.96). Thus, it is useful as a simplistic general measure, but there are qualifications that must be kept in mind. In any case, knowledge of the minimum tumor temperature gives one a conservative guide for estimating treatment effectiveness.

With these general considerations in mind, the goals of retrospective thermal dosimetry can be succinctly put, as in Table 3.24. To attain these goals, the technique shown in Fig. 3.95 must be developed, tested, and applied. Three major fundamental uncertainties exist when applying this technique (Table 3.25):

1. one is not guaranteed a priori that the process will converge to a solution at all, i.e., no solution may be found;
2. the solution may not be unique, i.e., many different blood flow distributions and magnitudes may give the same temperature estimates for the measurement locations; and

Table 3.24. Goals of retrospective thermal dosimetry

I. Primary goal:	(a)	Estimate the complete temperature distribution in the treatment volume and in any normal tissue at risk of being thermally damaged. Or, if this is not possible,
	(b)	Estimate the minimum temperature in the tumor and its location, and estimate the maximum temperature in the normal tissue and its location
II. Secondary goal:		Estimate the blood perfusion distribution in the tumor and surrounding normal tissue – both the perfusion pattern and magnitude, and the flow in and location of any large blood vessels

Table 3.25. Retrospective thermal dosimetry: major questions

I. Existence	Do solutions to the inverse problem outlined in Fig. 3.95 exist, or will that process tend to diverge?
II. Uniqueness	Will many different solutions to a given inverse problem exist – solutions which give the same temperature at the measurement locations, but different temperatures in the rest of the field?
III. Accuracy	How accurately can the process estimate the temperatures at the unmeasured locations?

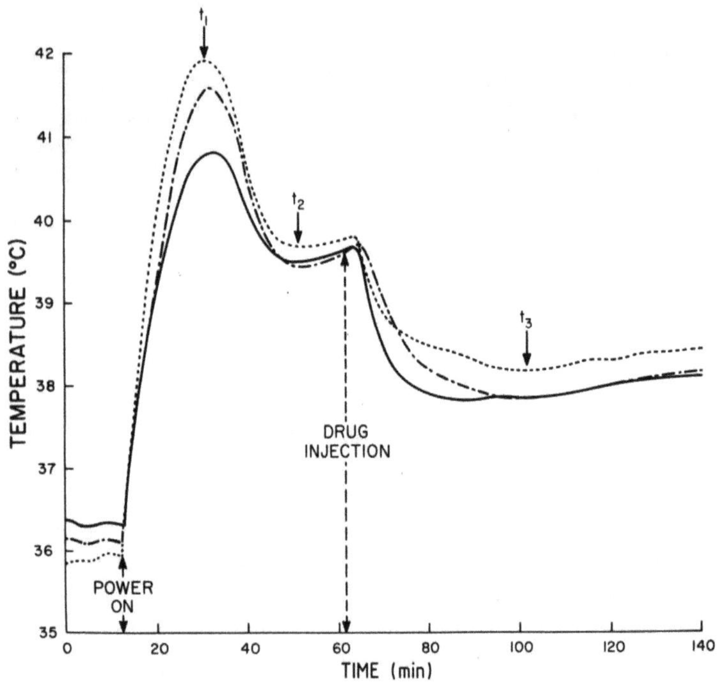

Fig. 3.97. Typical temperature versus time curve for a step input of microwave power into a dog thigh (see Fig. 3.69). Thermally induced vasodilation is shown to begin at point t_1, while a vasodilator (hydralazine) is injected as shown. The data are analyzed at the steady-state times t_1, t_2, and t_3 using the algorithm of Fig. 3.95. [117]

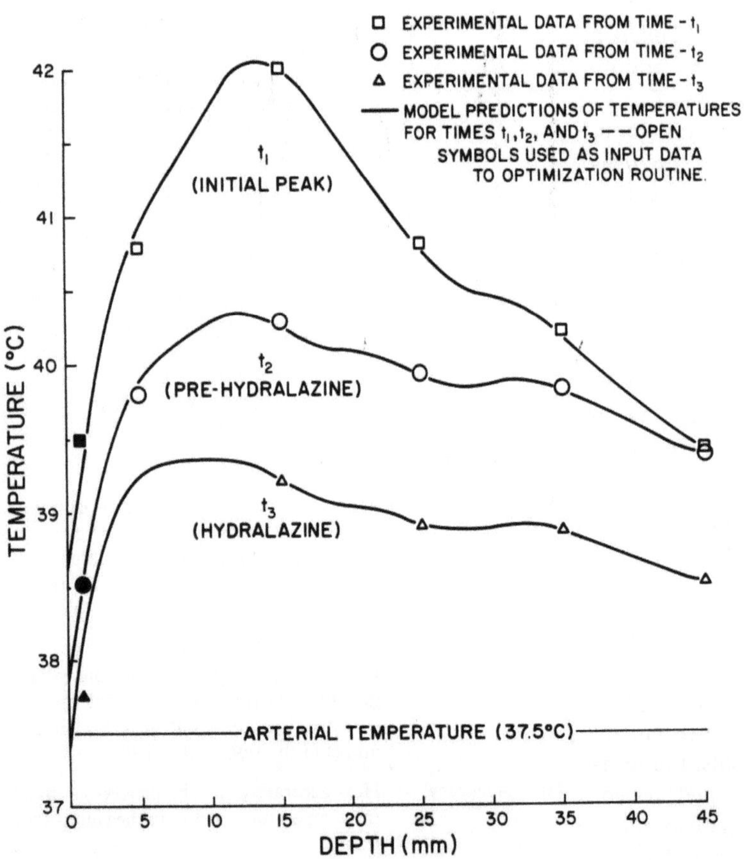

Fig. 3.98. The measured and estimated temperatures versus depth for times t_1, t_2, and t_3 of Fig. 3.97. [117]

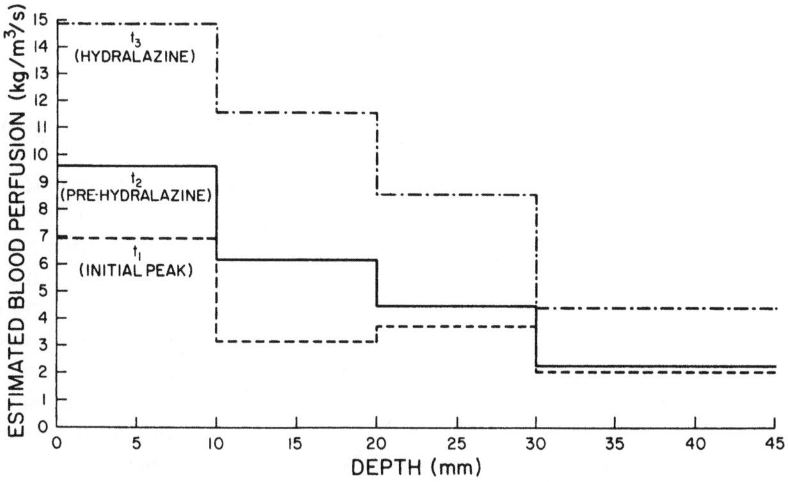

Fig. 3.99. The perfusions estimated by the treatment model as a function of depth for times t_1, t_2, and t_3 of Fig. 3.97. The perfusion was assumed to be uniform in regions centered on the subcutaneous measurement locations of Fig. 3.69

3. the solution may not be accurate, i.e., the measured temperatures may be accurately predicted but the complete temperature field may be inacurately estimated.

To date, it has been our experience (see results described below) that the first two major concerns are not valid for this application; i.e., we have generally found that solutions exist and are unique. Thus, the question of accuracy, or sensitivity, is the question of main concern. To illustrate and demonstrate these results, examples will be given for both steady-state and transient techniques.

This general problem of determining complete temperature distributions, either from calculations based on measured temperatures at a few locations or from non-invasive thermometry, remains a fundamental problem in hyperthermia research. It is a difficult problem which will require considerable effort to solve regardless of which approach is taken. Work done in this area includes the steady-state analysis of such problems [23, 24, 32, 102, 156] and the extension of those techniques to transient situations [22, 25, 26] for which more information is available. The steady-state approach will be discussed first.

3.3.4.2 Steady-State Approach

In a series of theoretical studies [23, 24, 32], it has been shown that the steady-state technique works and that it seems to give unique solutions for simulated treatments. These studies have all been one dimensional and have also included parametric evaluations of sensitivity to sensor number and placement and a comparative study of optimization algorithms.

In a related clinical study, Plancot et al. [102] successfully used noninvasive thermometry plus a one-dimensional patient treatment model to estimate the temperature distribution in a tumor by adjusting the skin heat transfer coefficient and a blood flow scale factor. Winget et al. [156] have also presented similar two-dimensional results from a clinical teatment.

The steady-state technique has also been successfully applied to a series of experiments using a vasoactive drug, hydralazine, to induce increases in blood perfusion in dog's thighs [117]. The experimental arrangement is illustrated in Fig. 3.69, where the thermocouples at different depths are shown. In the model, each subcutaneous thermocouple is assumed to be surrounded by a region of constant blood perfusion. Figure 3.97 illustrates a typical experimental temperature response; Fig. 3.98 shows the typical temperature-versus-depth curves for times t_1, t_2 and t_3; and Fig. 3.99 shows the estimated blood perfusions for this case.

While these results are quite promising (in that the measured temperatures were accurately predicted and the expected trends in the predicted perfusion were seen) and clearly illustrate that a solution exists and that, under some circumstances, the technique can automatically and accurately reproduce experimental temperatures, there are two major points which must be made regarding the use of the steady-state technique. The first is that the number of unknown blood perfusions exactly equals the number of temperature measurement locations (which, for the steady-state case, equals the number of measured temperatures). That is, the problem is fully determined [26] with the number of unknowns (N blood flows) exactly equating the number of knowns (N steady-state temperatures). Therefore, this steady-state technique cannot predict more blood perfusions that the number of steady-state measurement locations since, in that case,

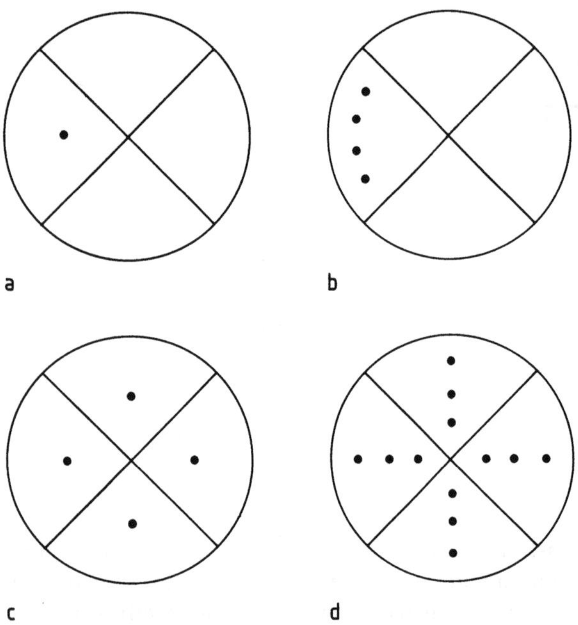

Fig. 3.100 a–d. Possible spatial distributions of temperature sensors (●) in a tumor with four blood perfusion regions: **a** an underdetermined problem with fewer sensors than perfusion regions; **b** a fully determined problem with an equal number of temperature measurements and unknown blood perfusions, but a nonoptimal sensor placement; **c** a fully determined problem with optimal sensor locations; **d** an overdetermined problem with optimal sensor locations

the problem becomes underdetermined (more unknowns than equations). Second, since the measured temperatures are centered in the regions of unknown blood perfusions, this process is really one of interpolating temperatures between the measurement points. This could also be done with some simple (nonphysical) curve-fitting routine, such as B-splines, but those techniques would not give any estimates of the blood perfusion – one of the important goals of this process as outlined in Table 3.24.

Thus, the steady-state technique has great potential value in hyperthermia in terms of fulfilling the objective of estimating blood perfusions during a treatment. It is also relatively easy to obtain data for this application since the steady-state temperatures are naturally measured during the treatments. The major problems that remain, clinically, are

1. to have good knowledge of the number of unknown perfusions needed to model the tumor;
2. to have enough temperature sensors to solve for those perfusions, i.e., to make the problem fully determined; and
3. to obtain these measurements in the best, or at least good, positions for the estimation process.

However, in order to fulfill all of the goals of retrospective hyperthermia (i.e., not only to estimate blood perfusion distributions but also to estimate the complete temperature distribution in a manner which provides an accurate method of both interpolating *and* extrapolating the temperature profile data – to be able to predict *unmeasured maximum* and *minimum* temperatures in a field), we must have at least a fully determined problem and preferably an overdetermined problem. That is, to overcome the effects of noise and measurement error, we would like to have as many temperature data as possible during a treatment (as long as those data are giving us new information, as discussed later). Figures 3.100 and 3.101, respectively, illustrate the two ways by which one is able to obtain more temperature data – spatially and temporally:

1. measure data at more points (either through the use of multiple-junction probes or pullback techniques and
2. obtain more data from a given number of probes by changing the treatment conditions so that transient temperatures can be obtained.

In the examples given in Figs. 3.100 and 3.101, it is assumed that there are, in reality, four separate blood perfusion regions with known boundaries; Fig. 3.100 illustrates the process of increasing the spatial data base and Fig. 3.101 does this for the temporal data base.

Thus, for the steady-state situation of Fig. 3.100a, we have four unknown blood perfusion values and only one data point, so the problem is underdetermined and unsolvable. Figures 3.100b, c shows a case with four sensors, so the problem is fully determined, with increasingly better sensor locations portrayed in going from case b to c; i.e., the sensors are placed closer to the locations of the unknowns they are trying to predict. Figure 3.100d shows the overdetermined problem with close to optimal spacing. The best spatial solution would be to have an overdetermined problem with optimal spatial resolution. Clinically, this is not possible, of course, since

1. one does not generally know the distribution of perfusions in a tumor a priori (and they will not be nice, neat divisions as shown in Fig. 3.100) and
2. the placement of thermocouples is often severely limited by clinical considerations.

The ideal is therefore not possible, and it is necessary to consider using temporal data, as illustrated in Fig. 3.101a for the underdetermined spatial case of Fig. 3.100a with one sensor and four regions. Of course, in the best of all possible worlds, we would choose

Fig. 3.100d, the optimally placed, overdetermined spatial solution, and also use overdetermined transient data to maximize our data base. However, the important general principles can be developed using the geometry of Fig. 3.100a for a simulated transient test in which power is suddenly turned off. (Other temporal changes are also possible; for example, since clinicians have one main independent variable at their disposal, the applied power, it is this variable which can be most readily used – by changing either the magnitude or, in some cases where more flexible power-distribution systems are available, by changing the distribution of power. Surface-cooling changes can also be used, but these have limited penetration depths, as noted previously.) First, it is important to note that the transient problem can be made a fully determined problem by, in this case, taking temperatures at just four times (Fig. 3.101a) so that, again, we have four unknown blood perfusions and four data points. This is an approach investigated previously [60] for a different application, giving results which are quite sensitive to measurement noise. Second, it is important to note that, just as in the spatial case, there exists an optimal solution to the data-gathering process – if all of the temperature data are taken at either very short or very long times (Fig. 3.101a), then all of the data are essentially the same and the solution becomes very sensitive to noise. Thus, some optimal selection of time intervals is important (Fig. 3.101b). Finally, if temperatures are taken at more than four times, the temporal problem becomes overdetermined and thus less susceptible to noise and measurement errors (Fig. 3.101c).

In practice, of course, the blood perfusion is probably a continuous variable in space, as shown in Fig. 3.102 for the classical, idealized tumor perfusion model based on results from implanted tumors in animals. Thus, for any accurate simulations, one must use some distribution of perfusions. For example, if one digitizes the curve of Fig. 3.102, one gets the results given in Fig. 3.103. This digitization, or zonal, approach can be extended to two (Fig. 3.104) or three dimensions. In all cases, one must make the decision of how large a spatial step size to take and, for the two- and three-dimensional problems, the problem becomes quite large numerically as we are plagued by the "curse of dimensionality" [9]. Thus, for numerical reasons alone, we are restricted to describing the tumor blood perfusion by a limited number of zones of constant blood perfusion, whose boundaries must be found and whose magnitudes must be determined. Alternatively, one can describe the blood perfusion distributions by curve-fitting routines (see Fig. 3.105) using any standard approach from simple straight

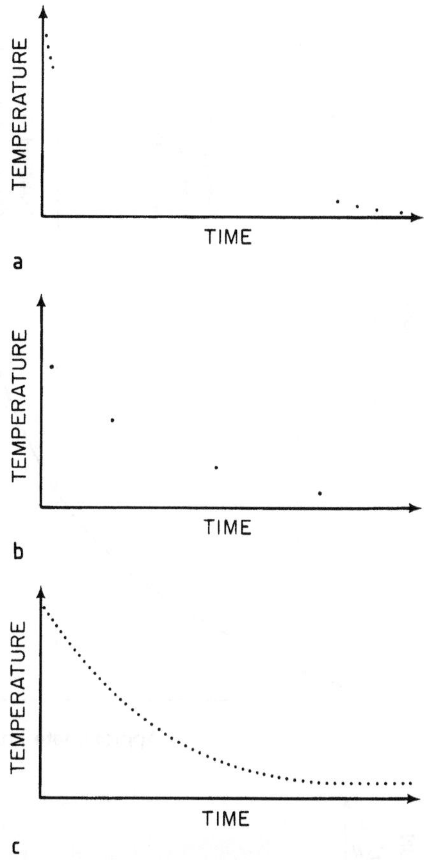

Fig. 3.101a–c. The transient temperature resulting from a power-off transient for the spatially underdetermined problem of Fig. 3.100a: **a** fully determined nonoptimal time samples since, if the four time samples are taken either too early or too late, the data are all essentially the same and the solution is ill posed and very susceptible to noise; **b** fully determined optimal time samples; **c** overdetermined optimal time samples

lines to three-dimensional B-splines [78], but always one faces the question of resolution. One cannot have too many regions due to both a potential numerical overload and because the addition of more regions may not add much more to the problem solution – and, indeed, many even make it more ill posed, as the simulated temperatures at the measurement locations may become less sensitive to the perfusions of each region. Thus, there will inevitably be some mismatch between the actual tumor perfusion's and the simulated tumor perfusion's boundaries. A significant question is then, how sensitive are the temperature and blood perfusion estimates to the spatial resolution of the blood perfusion zones (or the resolution of the curve-fitting routine). This model mismatch problem is one which is now being investigated, but for which no good answers are available, except for the simple one-dimensional studies of

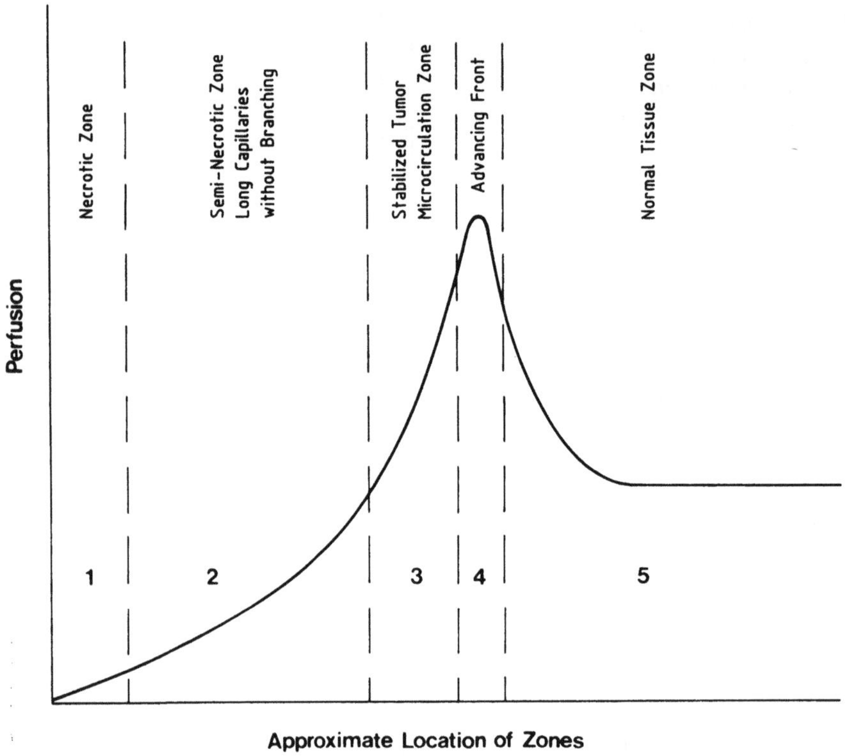

Fig. 3.102. Distribution of perfusion in an experimental animal tumor volume. [36]

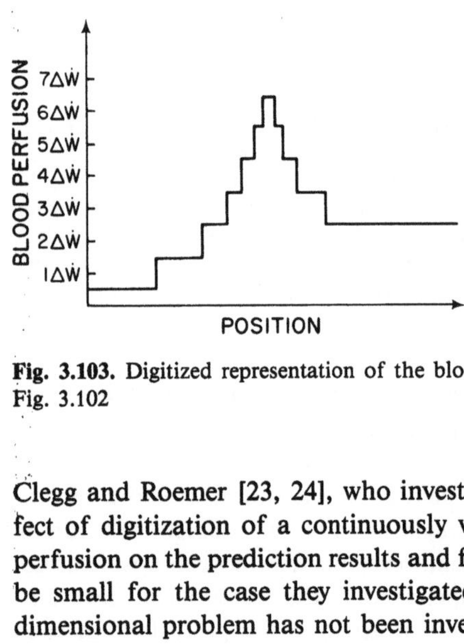

Fig. 3.103. Digitized representation of the blood perfusion of Fig. 3.102

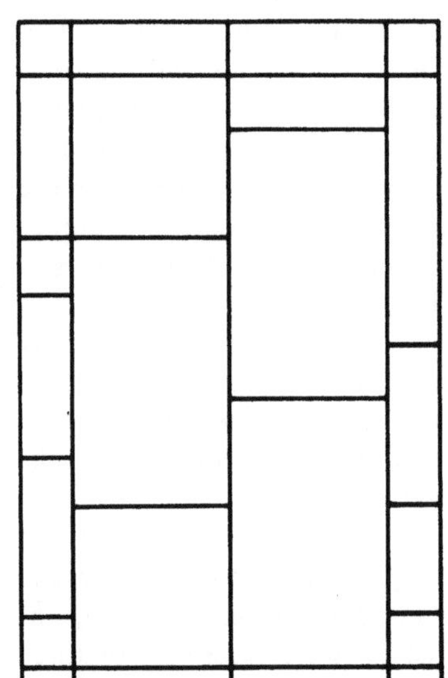

Fig. 3.104. A two-dimensional digitized blood perfusion pattern with each rectangular region having a different blood perfusion magnitude than its neighbors

Clegg and Roemer [23, 24], who investigated the effect of digitization of a continuously varying blood perfusion on the prediction results and found them to be small for the case they investigated. The three-dimensional problem has not been investigated yet.

3.3.4.3 Transient Approach

It is highly probable that the number of unknown blood perfusion regions in a tumor or, more generally, the number of unknown parameters needed to characterize the tumor's perfusion distribution accurately, is a variable which one will not know in advance and which will need to be determined during the analysis. Thus, one has a strong motivation to develop solutions to the transient problem, with fewer sensors than perfusion regions (or unknown parameters) and with nonoptimal sensor placement. This has been the approach of Clegg and Roemer [25], who have performed extensive analyses of the three-dimensinal problem for simulated treatments in which there are fewer sensors than unknown blood perfusions with, usually, seven unknown blood perfusions. For the simulated three-dimensional results, the basic scheme of Fig. 3.95 is used with the transient temperature data coming from a power-off transient which is introduced solely to gather transient temperature data for the estimation process. The three-dimensional problem which has been solved is illustrated in Fig. 3.106, with the parameters used given in Table 3.26. This problem was studied by taking data from only a few select locations and trying to reconstruct the complete temperature field, i.e., first using all seven sensors, then only six sensors (ignore measured temperatures in the central region), then only four sensors (ignore measured temperatures in even-numbered regions), and, finally, three sensors (ignore measured temperatures in odd-numbered regions). The general problem studied here is quite ill posed, and thus Tikhonov regularization [45] was used to damp out oscillations in the perfusion estimation. This signifi-

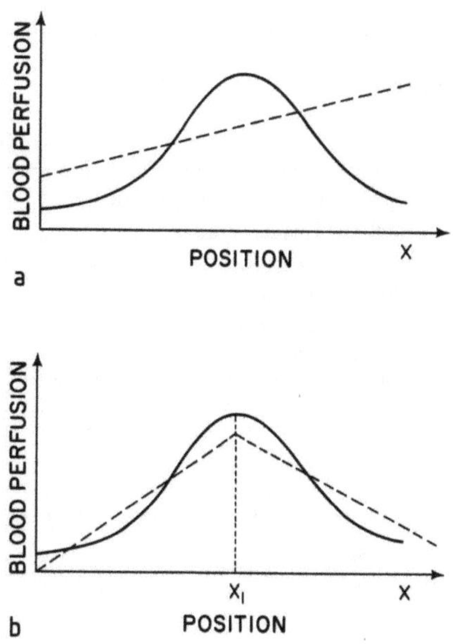

Fig. 3.105 a, b. Possible linear curve fits to spatially varying tumor perfusions: **a** a single (bad) linear fit and **b** separate (better) linear fits in two spatial zones

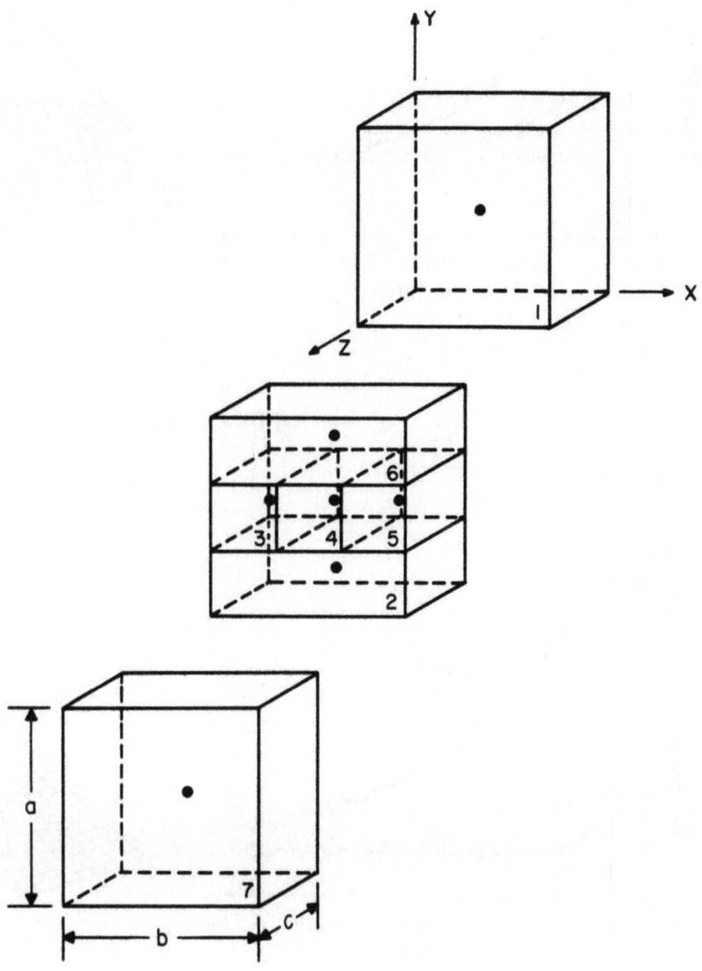

Fig. 3.106. Schematic of the simulated three-dimensional treatment model. Each zone represents a different region of perfusion and the center of each zone (●) is a temperature measurement location. The perfusion zone numbers are indicated within each zone. [25]

Table 3.26. Perfusion (kg/m^3-s) distributions for the cases studied using the model of Fig. 3.106

Model name	Perfusion region						
	$\dot{W}_1$	$\dot{W}_2$	$\dot{W}_3$	$\dot{W}_4$	$\dot{W}_5$	$\dot{W}_6$	$\dot{W}_7$
Low peripheral perfusion, necrotic center (LPPNC)	0.5	0.5	0.5	0.0	0.5	0.5	0.5
High peripheral perfusion, necrotic center (HPPNC)	8.0	8.0	8.0	0.0	8.0	8.0	8.0
Low peripheral perfusion, high-center perfusion (LPPHC)	0.5	0.5	0.5	8.0	0.5	0.5	0.5

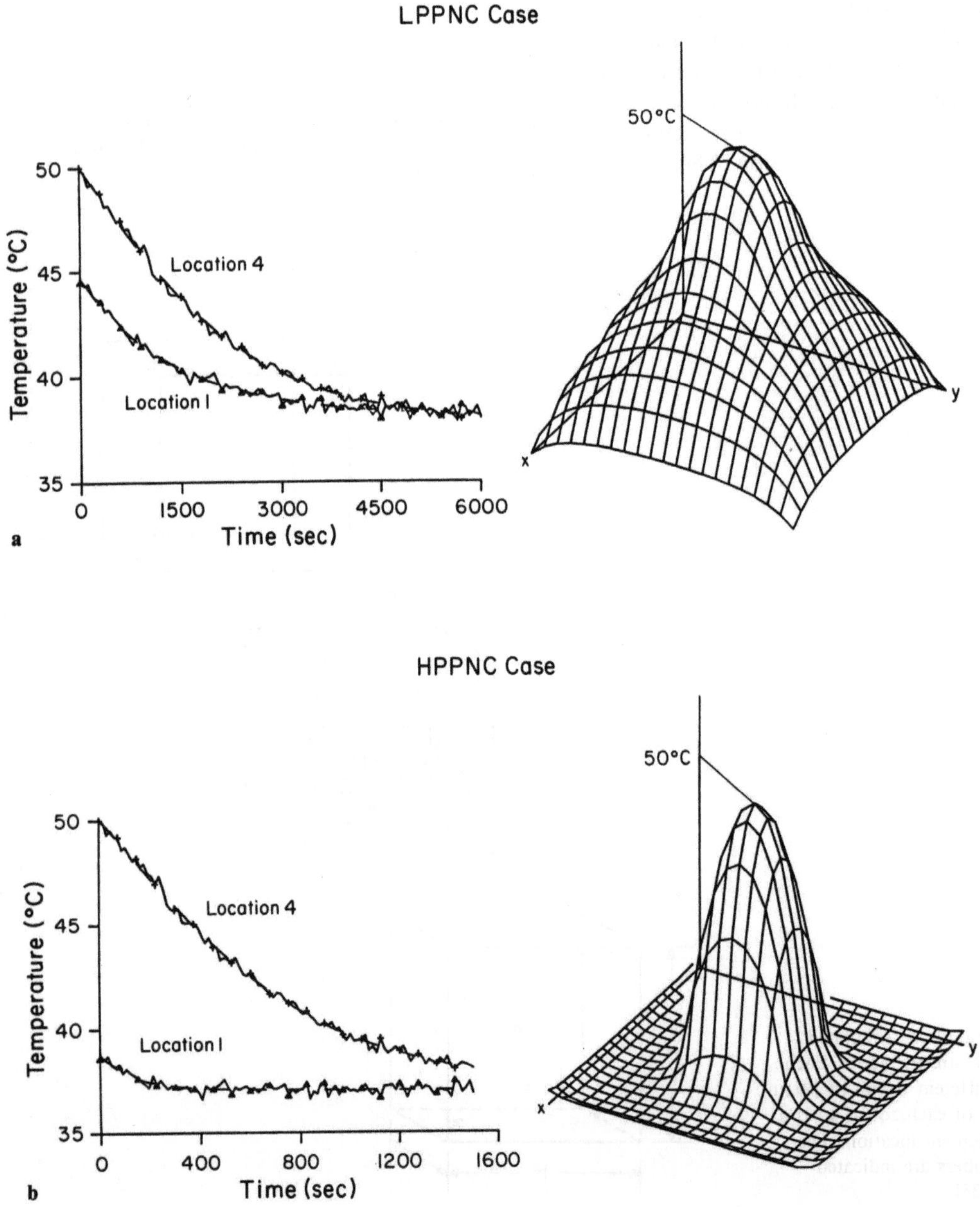

Fig. 3.107 a, b

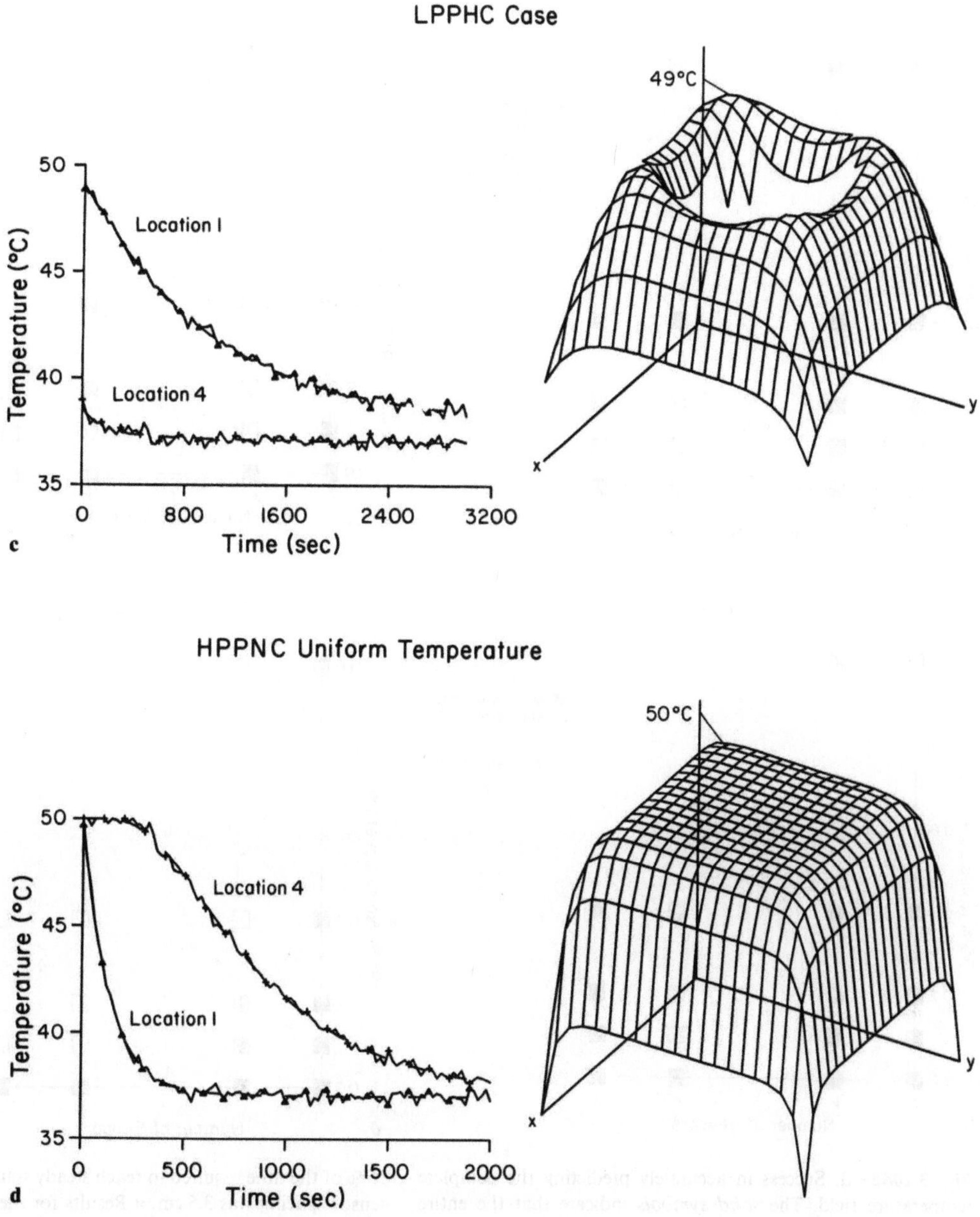

Fig. 3.107a–d. The transient temperature decay at the central measurement location and at one of the exterior locations, and the steady-state temperature distribution through the center plane: **a** low-periphery perfusion, necrotic center case (see Table 3.26); **b** high-periphery perfusion, necrotic center case; **c** low-periphery perfusion, high central perfusion case; **d** same as **b** but with a uniform initial temperature [25]. The cube studied measured 10.5 cm along its sides (a = b = c = 10.5 cm)

cantly improved the algorithm's performance. The temperature decay data used as input to the optimization algorithm included noise of various magnitudes (Fig. 3.107). A set of typical results is given in Fig. 3.108. The results from this study indicated that the complete three-dimensional temperature field could be reproduced within 1 °C for a variety of three-dimensional situations in which the problem was spatially underdetermined and the transient temperature data were noisy. This is an encouraging result which has motivated an investigation of three-dimensional animal experiments [22].

3.3.4.4 Summary

The fundamental problem of how to determine the complete temperature field that was present during a hyperthermia treatment remains unsolved. Because of

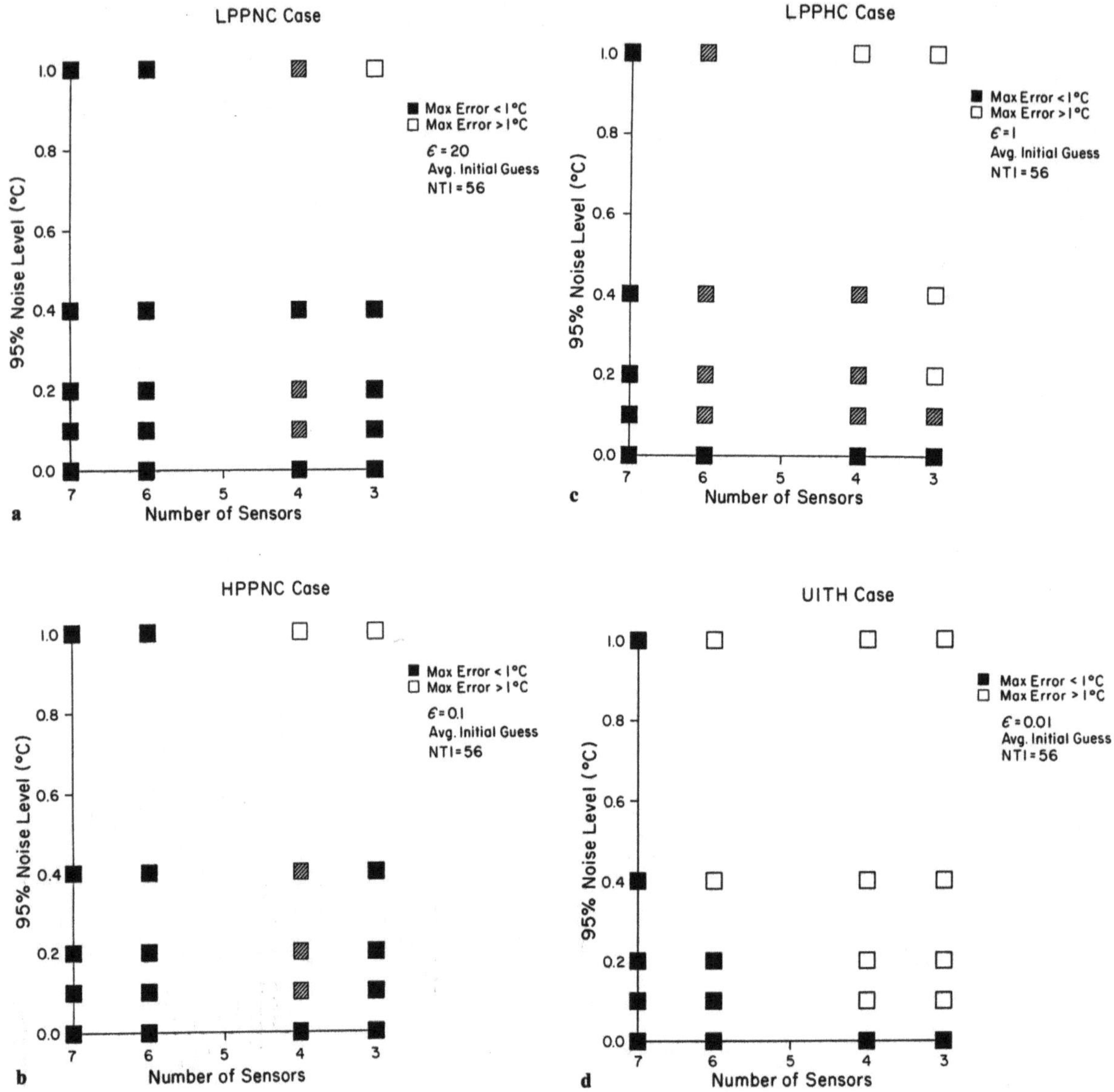

Fig. 3.108 a–d. Success in accurately predicting the complete temperature field. The *solid symbols* indicate that the entire three-dimensional steady-state temperature field was predicted within 1 °C of the actual values when the algorithm terminated. The *cross-hatched* symbols mean that the perfusion estimates were slowly and steadily convering to the correct values when the algorithm was terminated to save computer time. The *open symbols* mean that the temperature field was not predicted within 1 °C and the perfusion estimates were not converging to their true values. The number of time increments was 56, i.e., about 56% of the time required to reach steady state for each case. The sensor spacing was 3.5 cm. **a** Results for the low-periphery perfusion necrotic center case; the regularization parameter was 20.0. **b** Results fo the high-periphery perfusion necrotic center case; the regularization parameter was 0.1. **c** Results for the low-periphery perfusion high-center case; the regularization parameter was 1.0. **d** Results for the same perfusion patterns as **b** but with an initial uniform temperature distribution; the regularization parameter was 0.01. [25]

its basic importance, several research groups are attempting to answer this question by using various noninvasive thermometry approaches, the above state and parameter estimation techniques, or combinations of the two. To date, the state and parameter estimation approach continues to look promising; that is, even though the problem is ill posed, solutions seem to generally exist that are unique, and accurate predictions can be obtained. However, in order to become clinically practical, much difficult and basic research remains to be done on this technique, including the development of improved

1. heat transfer equation formulations for tumor simulations,
2. power deposition models,
3. estimation algorithms, plus
4. extensive research into the nature of the blood perfusion patterns and magnitudes present during hyperthermia treatments.

Most of these tasks are fundamental to all aspects of hyperthermia simulations, and thus, considerable progress can be made by investigators working in parallel on all different aspects of treatment modeling.

Acknowledgments. Connie Spencer's invaluable assistance in preparing and editing this manuscript is gratefully acknowledged, as is Allison Habel's preparation of the figures. Dr. Michel Gautherie is thanked for his encouragement and financial support during the lengthy process of writing this chapter. NCI Grant 36428 and the Association pour la Recherche sur le Cancer (ARC) provided financial support for portions of this work, without which it would not have been performed.

Nomenclature

A	Area
A_c	Cross-sectional area of blood vessel
AP	Applied power (W)
c	Specific heat
D	Diameter
$g(\vec{r})$	Geometric variation of temperature
h	Heat transfer coefficient
$h(\vec{r})$	Geometric variation of skin-cooling effect
k	Thermal conductivity
K_0	Bessel function
L	Length
L*	Normal vessel length
$\dot{M}$	Mass flow rate (kg/s)
Nu	Nusselt number
P	Power (W); perimeter (M)
$\dot{Q}$	Power density (W/m^3)
q	SAR per unit of applied power
$\dot{q}$	Energy flux (w/m^2)
$\vec{r}$	Position
R	Radius
R_M	$\dfrac{\dot{M}/A_c L}{\dot{W}}$
S	Set of possible heating system configurations ($\vec{r}_s$)
SAR	Specific absorption rate of power (w/kg)
T	Temperature
U	Overall heat transfer coefficient
V	Velocity; volume
$\dot{W}$	Blood perfusion rate ($kg/m^3/s$)
x	x-position

Greek

α	$UPL/\dot{M}c$
Δ	Change
ϱ	Density
μ	Exponential penetration depth of microwaves
τ	Time constant

Subscripts

a	Applied
acc	Acceptable
air	Air
all	Allowable
aph	Amount of preheating (of arterial blood)
an	Arterial to normal tissue
ar	Arterial
ave	Average
b	Blood; blood flow
ba	Basal
bc	Boundary conditions
bn	Blood flow in normal tissue
bt	Blood flow in tumor tissue
c	Conduction
cc	Countercurrent
conv	Convection
e	Effective
env	Environment
eq	Equilibrium
hn	Heated normal
hp	Highly perfused
m	Metabolism; measured
no	Normal
ne	Necrotic
nv	Normal tissue to venous
o	Tumor boundary/interface boundary; initial condition
p	Applied power
ph	Preheated
pn	Penetration
R	Radial position R
rad	Radiation
SAR	Specific absorption rate
set	Set point
sk	Skin
ss	Steady state
tc	Tissue cooling
th	Therapeutic
tu	Tumor
tumor	Complete tumor
tr	Transient; treatment
v	Venous
wa	Wall of artery
wv	Wall of vein
x	x-direction

References

1. Arcangeli G, Lombardini PP, Lovisolo GA, Marsiglia G, Piattelli L (1984) Focusing of 915 MHz electromagnetic power on deep human tissues; a mathematical model study. IEEE Trans Biomed Eng 31:47–52
2. Arkin H, Chen MM, Holmes KR (1986) Adaptive thermal modeling: a concept for measurement of local blood perfusion in heated tissues. ASME J Biomech Eng 108:306–311
3. Åström K, Wittenmark B (1984) Computer controlled systems: theory and design. Prentice-Hall, Englewood Cliffs
4. Babbs CF, Dewitt DP, Voorhees WD, McCaw JS, Chan RC (1982) Theoretical feasibility of vasodilator-enhanced local tumor heating. Eur J Cancer Clin Oncol 18:1137–1146
5. Babbs CF, Vaguine VA, Jones JT (1986) A predictive-adaptive, multipoint feedback controller for local heat therapy of solid tumors. IEEE Trans Microwave Theory Tech MTT 34:604–611
6. Baish JW, Ayyaswamy PS, Foster KR (1988) Heat transport mechanisms in vascular tissues: a model comparison. Trans ASME 108:324–331
7. Baish JW, Ayyaswamy PS, Foster KR (1986) Small-scale temperature fluctuations in perfused tissue during local hyperthermia. Trans ASME 108:246–250
8. Baish JW, Foster KR, Ayyaswamy PS (1986) Perfused phantom models of microwave irradiated tissue. ASME J Biomech Eng 108:239–245
9. Bellman RE (1960) Introduction to matrix analysis. McGraw-Hill, New York
10. Bibbero R (1977) Microprocessors in instruments and control. Wiley, New York
11. Brezovich IA, Atkinson WJ, Chakroborty DP (1984) Temperature distributions in tumor models heated by self-regulating nickel-copper alloy thermoseeds. Med Phys 11:145–152
12. Brezovich IA, Atkinson WJ, Lilly MB (1984) Local hyperthermia with interstitial techniques. Cancer Res. (Suppl) 44:4752s–4756s
13. Burger PC (1983) Pathologic anatomy and CT correlations in the glioblastoma multiforme. Appl Neurophysiol 46:180–187
14. Cetas TC (1982) Thermal dosimetry during hyperthermia. In: Gautherie M (ed) Biomedical thermology. Liss, New York, pp 561–583
15. Cetas TC, Kimball W, Roemer R, Hynynen K (1988) Comparative clinical evaluation of SAR patterns for regional power deposition systems (to be published)
16. Charny CK, Hagmann MJ, Levin RL (1987) A whole body thermal model of man during hyperthermia. IEEE Trans Biomed Eng BME 34:375–387
17. Chato J (1980) Heat transfer to blood vessels. ASME J Biomech Eng 102:110–118
18. Chen MM, Holmes KR (1980) Microvascular contributions in tissue heat transfer. Ann NY Acad Sci 335:137–150
19. Chen MM, Holmes KR (1980) The thermal pulse-decay method for simultaneous measurement of thermal conductivity and local blood perfusion rate of living tissues. Adv Bioeng, ASME 115–115
20. Chen ZP, Cetas TC, Haider SA, Roemer RB (1988) Three-dimensional analysis of ferromagnetic seed temperature distributions (in preparation)
21. Chen ZP, Miller WH, Roemer RB, Cetas TC (1990) Three-dimensional computer simulation for hyperthermia treatment planning (accepted, Int J Hyper)
22. Clegg S (1988) Estimation of three-dimensional temperature fields from a limited number of temperature sensors during hyperthermia. Dissertation, University of Arizona, Tucson
23. Clegg ST, Roemer RB (1985) A comparative evaluation of unconstrained optimization methods applied to the thermal tomography problem. ASME J Biomech Eng 107:228–233
24. Clegg ST, Roemer RB (1985) A study of the effect of sensor placement and perfusion pattern variation on thermal tomography problems in hyperthermia. IEEE Trans Biomed Eng BME 32:677–683
25. Clegg ST, Roemer RB (1989) Estimation of three-dimensional temperature fields from noisy data during hyperthermia. Int J Hyper. Vol 5, 9:967–989
26. Clegg ST, Roemer RB, Cetas TC (1985) Estimation of complete temperature fields from measured transient temperatures. Int J Hyperthermia 1:265–286
27. Dagan Z, Weinbaum S, Jiji LM (1986) Parametric studies on the three-layer microcirculatory model for surface tissue energy exchange. ASME, J Biochem Eng 108:89–96
28. deLeeuw AAC, Lagendijk JJW (1987) Design of a deep-body hyperthermia system based on the "Coaxial Tem" applicator. Int J Hyperthermia 3:413–423
29. DeWagter C (1985) Computer simulation for local temperature control during microwave-induced hyperthermia. J Microwave Power 20:31–42
30. De Wagter C (1986) Optimization of simulated two-dimensional temperature distributions induced by multiple electromagnetic applicators. IEEE Trans Microwave Theory Tech MTT 34:589–596
31. Dewhirst MW, Sim DA, Sapereto S, Connor WG (1984) Importance of minimum tumor temperature in determining early and long-term responses of spontaneous canine and feline tumors to heat and radiation. Cancer Res 44:43
32. Divrik AM, Roemer RB, Cetas TC (1984) Inference of complete tissue temperature fields from a few measured temperatures: an unconstrained optimization method. IEEE Trans Biomed Eng BME 31:150–160
33. Doss JD (1985) Simulation of automatic temperature control in tissue hyperthermia calculations. Med Phys 12:693–697
34. Durney CH (1987) Electromagnetic field generation and propagation. In: Field SB, Franconi C (eds) Physics and technology of hyperthermia. Nijhoff, Dordrecht, pp 123–151
35. Emami B, Song CW (1984) Physiological mechanisms in hyperthermia: a review. Int J Radiat Oncol Biol Phys 10:289–295
36. Endrich B, Reinhold HS, Gross JF, Intaglietta M (1979) Tissue perfusion inhomogeneity during early tumor growth in rats. J Natl Cancer Inst 62:387–395
37. Fessenden P, Lee ER, Anderson TL, Strohbehn JW, Meyer JL, Samulski TV, Marmor JB (1984) Experience with a multitransducer ultrasound system for localized hyperthermia of deep tissues. IEEE Trans Biomed Eng BME 31:126–135
38. Field SB (1987) Biological aspects of hyperthermia. In: Field SB, Franconi C (eds) Physics and technology of hyperthermia. Nijhoff, Dordrecht, pp 19–53
39. Fletcher GH (1980) Textbook of radiotherapy, 3rd edn. Lea and Febiger, Philadelphia
40. Gerweck LE (1985a) Environmental and vascular effects. In: Overgaard J (ed) Hyperthermic oncology 1984, vol 2 (review lectures, symposium summaries and workshop summaries). Taylor and Francis, London, pp 253–262
41. Gerweck LE (1985b) Hyperthermia in cancer therapy: the biological basis and unresolved problems. Cancer Res 45:3408–3414

42. Gibbs FA (1984) Regional hyperthermia: a clinical appraisal of noninvasive deep-heating methods. Cancer Res (Suppl) 44:4765s–4770s
43. Gordon RG, Roemer RB, Horvath SM (1976) A mathematical model of the human temperature regulatory system-transient cold exposure response. IEEE Trans Biomed Eng BME 23:434–444
44. Griffiths H, Ahmed A, Smith CW, Moore JL, Kerb IJ, Davies RME (1987) Specific absorption rate and tissue temperature in local hyperthermia. Int J Radiat Oncol Biol Phys 12:1997–2002
45. Groetsch CW (1977) Generalized inverses of linear operators. Dekker, New York, pp 73–75
46. Guy AW, Lehmann JF, Stonebridge JB (1974) Therapeutic applications of electromagnetic power. Proc IEEE 62:55–75
47. Hagmann MJ, Levin RL (1986) Aberrant heating: a problem in regional hyperthermia. IEEE Trans Biomed Eng 33:405–411
48. Hahn GM (1982) Hyperthermia and cancer. Plenum, New York
49. Haider SA, Chen ZP, Roemer RB, Cetas TC (1988) Ferromagnetic seed hyperthermia: treatment planning and evaluation (to be published)
50. Halac S, Roemer RB, Cetas TC (1983) Uniform regional heating of the lower trunk: numerical evaluation of tumor temperature distribution. Int J Radiat Oncol Biol Phys 9:1883–1890
51. Halac S, Roemer RB, Oleson JR, Cetas TC (1983) Magnetic induction heating of tissue: numerical evaluation of tumor temperature distributions. Int J Radiat Oncol Biol Phys 9:881–891
52. Hand JW, Cheetham JL, Hind AJ (1986) Absorbed power distributions from coherent microwave arrays for localized hyperthermia. IEEE Trans Microwave Theory Tech MTT 34:484–489
53. Handl-Zeller L, Kärcher KH, Lesnicar H, Budihna M, Schreier K (1987) Newly developed liquid heated interstitial hyperthermia system KHS-9/W18. Int J Hyperthermia 3:567
54. Hugander A, Robins HI, Martin P, Schmitt C (1987) Temperature distribution during radiant heat whole-body hyperthermia: experimental studies in the dog. Int J Hyperthermia 3:199–208
55. Hynynen K (1986) Generation of ultrasonic fields and the acoustic properties of tissues. In: Watmough D, Ross W (eds) Hyperthermia. Blackie, Glasgow, pp 76–98
56. Hynynen K, Roemer R, Anhalt D, Johnson C, Xu ZX, Swindelll W, Cetas T (1987) A scanned, focused, multiple transducer ultrasonic system for localized hyperthermia treatments. Int J Hyperthermia 3:21–35
57. Jain RK, Wart-Hartley K (1984) Tumor blood flow – characterization, modifications and role in hyperthermia. IEEE Trans Sonics and Ultrason 31:504–526
58. Jiji LM, Weinbaum S, Lemons DE (1984) Theory and experiment for the effect of vascular microstructure on surface tissue heat transfer. Part I. Model formulation and solution. ASME J Biomech Eng 106:331–341
59. Johnson C, Roemer R, Kress R, Hynynen K (1988) Multipoint feedback control system for scanned, focussed ultrasound hyperthermia (to be published)
60. Kleinman AM, Roemer RB (1983) A direct substitution equation error technique for solving the thermographic tomography problem. ASME J Biomech Eng 105:237
61. Knudsen M, Hartmann U (1986) Optimal temperature control with phased array hyperthermia system. IEEE Trans Microwave Theory Tech MTT 34:597–603
62. Knudsen M, Heinzl L (1986) Two-point control of temperature profile in tissue. Int J Hyperthermia 2:21–38
63. Knudsen M, Overgaard J (1986) Identification of thermal model for human tissue. IEEE Trans Biomed Eng BME 33:477–485
64. Kress R (1988) Adaptive model-following control system for hyperthermia treatments. PhD Dissertation, University of Arizona, Tucson
65. Kress R, Roemer R (1987) A comparative analysis of thermal blood perfusion measurement techniques. ASME J Biomech Eng 109:218–225
66. Lagendijk JJW (1982) The influence of bloodflow in large vessels on the temperature distribution in hyperthermia. Phys Med Biol 27:17–23
67. Lagendijk JJW (1983) A new coaxial TEM radiofrequency/microwave applicator for non-invasive deep-body hyperthermia. J Microwave Power 18:367–376
68. Lagendijk JJW (1987) Heat transfer in tissues. In: Field S, Franconi C (eds) Physics and technology of hyperthermia. Nijhoff, Drodrecht, pp 517–552
69. Lagendijk J, Mooibroek J (1986) Hyperthermia treatment planning. In: Bruggmoser G, Hinkelbein W, Enggelhardt R, Wannenmacher M (eds) Locoregional high-frequency hyperthermia and temperature measurement. Springer, Berlin Heidelberg New York pp 119–131 (Recent results in cancer research, vol 101)
70. Lagendijk J, Schipper J (1986) Clinical hyperthermia systems. In: Hand J, James J (eds) Physical techniques in clinical hyperthermia. Research Studies, Letchworth, pp 452–506
71. Lagendijk JJW, Schellekens M, Schipper J, van der Linden PM (1984) A three-dimensional description of heating patterns in vascularized tissues during hyperthermic treatment. Phys Med Biol 29:495–507
72. Lagendijk JJW, Hofman P, Schipper J (1988) Perfusion analysis in advanced breast carcinoma during hyperthermia. Int J Hyperthermia, vol 9, 5:979–996
73. Lamouri M (1988) Microwave power deposition in bounded and inhomogeneous lossy, media. PhD Dissertation, University of Arizona, Tucson
74. Lee ER, Samulski TV, Fessenden P, Kapp DS (1986) Controlled scan surface heating. 6th annual North American Hyperthermia Group meeting, Las Vegas, NV
75. Lele PP (1983) Physical aspects and clinical studies with ultrasound hyperthermia. In: Storm FC (ed) Hyperthermia in cancer therapy. Hall Medical, Boston, pp 333–367
76. LeVeen HH, Ahmed N, Picconne VA, Shugaar S, Falk G (1981) Radio-frequency therapy: clinical experience. Ann NY Acad Sci 335:362–371
77. Lin J (ed) (1986) IEEE trans on microwave theory and techniques. Special issue on phased arrays for hyperthermia treatment of cancer. Institute Electrical and Electronics Engineering, New York
78. Lin WL, Clegg ST, Roemer RB (1988) Application of tricubic splines for interpolation between irregularly spaced 3-D SAR data (to be published)
79. Matloubieh AY, Roemer RB, Cetas TC (1984) Numerical simulation of magnetic induction heating of tumors with ferromagnetic seed implants. IEEE Trans Biomed Eng BME 31:227–234
80. Mechling JA, Strohbehn JW (1987) A theoretical comparison of the temperature distributions produced by three interstitial hyperthermia systems. Int J Radiat Oncol Biol Phys 12:2137–2149
81. Mitchell JW, Myers GE (1968) An analytical model of the countercurrent heat exchange phenomena. Biophys J 8:897–911

82. Mori S, Sakakibara M, Tanimoto A (1974) Steady heat transfer to laminar flow in a circular tube with conduction in the tube wall. Heat Transfer Jpn Res 3:37–46
83. Moros EG, Roemer RB, Hynynen K (1988) Simulation of scanned focussed ultrasound hyperthermia: the effects of scanning speed and pattern on the temperature fluctuations at the focal depth. IEEE Trans vol 35, 5:552–560
84. Nikawa Y, Watanabe H, Kikuchi M, Mori S (1986) A direct-contact microwave lens applicator with a microcomputer-controlled heating system for local hyperthermia. IEEE Trans Microwave Theory Tech MTT 34:626–630
85. Nilsson P, Persson B (1985) Computer controlled microwave system for clinical hyperthermia. Phys Med Biol 30: 283–292
86. Nussbaum GH, Babbs CF, Mintum MA (1986) Results of a preliminary study of the potential of vasodilators for improving thermotherapy of deep seated tumors. Int J Hyperthermia 2:61–64
87. Nussbaum GH, Sidi J, Rouhanizadeh N, Morel P, Jasmin C, Convert G, Mabire JP, Azam G (1986) Manipulation of central axis heating patterns with a prototype, three-electrode capacitive device for deep-tumor hyperthermia. IEEE Trans Microwave Theory Tech MTT 34:620–625
88. Ocheltree KB, Frizzell LA (1987) Determination of power deposition patterns for localized hyperthermia: a steady state analysis. Int J Hyperthermia 3:269–279
89. Ocheltree KB, Frizzell LA (1988) Determination of power deposition patterns for localized hyperthermia: a transient analysis. Int J Hyperthermia, vol 4, 3:281–296
90. Oleson JR (1984) Comparison of intratumoral temperature distributions achieved with magnetic induction vs. annular microwave array methods. Presented at 32nd annual meeting of the Radiation Research Society, Orlando, FL
91. Oleson JR, Cetas TC, Corry PM (1983) Hyperthermia by magnetic induction: experimental and theoretical results for coaxial coil pairs. Radiat Res 95:175
92. Oleson JR, Sim DA, Manning MR (1984) Analysis of prognostic variable in hyperthermia treatment of 161 patients. Int J Radiat Oncol Biol Phys 10:2231–2239
93. Oleson J, Dewhirst M, Duncan D, Engler M, Thall D (1985) Temperature gradients: prognostic and dosimetric implications. In: Proceedings of the 1985 IEEE conference on engineering in medicine and biology, Lin JC, Feinberg BN (eds) Chicago, pp 335–340
94. Oleson JR, Sim DA, Conrad J, Fletcher AM, Gross EJ (1986) Results of a phase I regional hyperthermia device evaluation: microwave annular array versus radiofrequency induction coil. Int J Hyperthermia 2:327–336
95. Overgaard J, Nielsen OS (1980) The role of tissue environmental factors on the kinetics and morphology of tumor cells exposed to hyperthermia. An NY Acad Sci 35:254–279
96. Overgaard J, Nielsen OS, Lindegaard JC (1987) Biological basis for rational design of clinical treatments with combined hyperthermia and radiation. In: Field SB, Franconi C (eds) Physics and technology of hyperthermia. Nijhoff, Dordrecht, pp 54–79
97. Parks LC, Minaberry D, Smith DP, Neely WH (1979) Treatment of far advanced bronchogenic carcinoma by extracorporeally induced systemic hyperthermia. Cardiovasc Surg 28:467–477
98. Paulsen KD, Strohbehn JW, Hill SC, Lynch DR, Kennedy FE (1984) Theoretical temperature profiles for concentric coil induction heating devices in a two-dimensional, axi-asymmetric, inhomogeneous patient model. Int J Radiat Oncol Biol Phys 10:1095–1107
99. Paulsen KD, Strohbehn JW, Lynch DR (1984) Theoretical temperature distributions produced by an annular phased array-type system in CT-based patient models. Radiat Res 100:536–552
100. Paulsen KD, Strohbehn JW, Lynch DR (1985) Comparative theoretical performance for two types of regional hyperthermia systems. Int J Radiat Oncol Biol Phys 11:1659–1671
101. Pennes HH (1948) Analysis of tissue and arterial blood temperatures in the resting human forearm. J Appl Physiol 1:93–122
102. Plancot M, Prevost B, Chive M, Fabre JJ, Ledee R, Giaux G (1987) A new method for thermal dosimetry in microwave hyperthermia using microwave radiometry for temperature control. Int J Hyperthermia 3:9–20
103. Reinhold H (1987) Tumor microcirculation. In: Field S, Franconi E (eds) Proceedings of 1986 NATO advanced study institute on the physics and technology of hyperthermia. Nijhoff, Dordrecht, pp 448–457
104. Reinhold HS, Endrich B (1986) Invited review: tumour microcirculation as a target for hyperthermia. Int J Hyperthermia 2:111–137
105. Reinhold HS, Berg-Blok AE van den (1984) Heat-induced microcirculatory stoppage strongly enhances tumour control by radiation. In: Overgaard J (ed) Hyperthermic oncology 1984, vol 1 (summary papers). Taylor and Francis, London, pp 149–152
106. Roemer RB (1983) Thermal dosimetry. Presented at Radiation Research Society meeting, Orlando, FL
107. Roemer R (1988) Heat transfer in hyperthermia treatments: basic principles and applications. In Biological, Physical and Clinical Aspects of Hyperthermia. Paliwal B, Hetzel F, Dewhirst M (eds) Amer Ass of Phys in Med, 210–293, New York
108. Roemer R (1988) Heat transfer processes in hyperthermia. Ann Rev Hyperthermia (in press)
109. Roemer R (1988) Optimal power deposition in hyperthermia. I. The treatment goal; the role of large blood vessels (to be published)
110. Roemer RB, Cetas TC (1984) Applications of bioheat transfer simulations in hyperthermia. Cancer Res 44:4788s–4798s
111. Roemer RB, Tharp H (1988) Optimal power deposition patterns for practical hyperthermia systems (to be published)
112. Roemer RB, Cetas TC, Oleson JR, Halac S, Matloubieh AY (1984) Comparative evaluation of hyperthermia heating modalities. I. Numerical analysis of thermal dosimetry bracketing cases. Radiat Res 100:450–472
113. Roemer RB, Cetas TC, Oleson JR, Halac S, Matloubieh AY (1984) Comparative evaluation of hyperthermia heating modalities. II. Application of the acceptable power range technique. Radiat Res 100:473–486
114. Roemer RB, Swindell W, Clegg ST, Kress RL (1984) Simulation of focused, scanned ultrasonic heating of deep-seated tumors: the effect of blood perfusion. IEEE Trans Sonics Ultrason SU-31:457–466
115. Roemer RB, Fletcher AM, Cetas TC (1985) Obtaining local SAR and blood perfusion data from temperature measurements: steady-state and transient techniques compared. Int J Radiat Oncol Biol Phys 11:1539–1550
116. Roemer RB, Oleson JR, Cetas TC (1985) Oscillatory temperature response to constant power applied to canine muscle. Am J Physiol 249:R153–R158
117. Roemer RB, Forsyth KA, Oleson JR, Clegg ST, Sim DA (1988) The effect of hydralazine dose on blood perfusion

changes during hyperthermia. Int J Hyperthermia, vol 9, 4:901–916
118. Ruggera PS, Kantor G (1984) Development of a family of optimized RF helical coil applicators which produce transversely uniform axially distributed heating in cyclindrical fat-muscle phantoms. IEEE Trans Biomed Eng BME 31:98–106
119. Salcman M, Samaras CM (1983) Interstitial microwave hyperthermia for brain tumors. J Neurooncol 1:225–236
120. Samulski T, Kapp D, Fessenden P, Lohrbach A (1987) Heating deep seated eccentrically located tumors with an annular phased array system: a comparative clinical study using two annular array operating configurations. Int J Radiat Oncol Biol Phys 13:83–94
121. Sandhu TS (1986) Measurement of blood flow using temperature decay: effect of thermal conduction. Int J Radiat Oncol Biol Phys 12:373–378
122. Sapozink MD, Gibbs FS, Thomson JW, Stewart JR (1985) A comparison of deep regional hyperthermia from an annular phased array and a concentric coil in the same patients. Int J Radiat Oncol Biol Phys 11:179–190
123. Sathiaseelan V, Howard GCW, Kedar IH, Bleehen NM (1985) A clinical microwave hyperthermia system with multipoint real-time thermal dosimetry. Br J Radiol 58:1187–1195
124. Sekins KM, Emery A (1982) Thermal science for physical medicine. In: Lehmann J (ed) Therapeutic heat and cold. Williams and Wilkens, Baltimore, pp 70–132
125. Sekins KM, Lehmann JF, Esselmann P, Dundore D, Emery AF, deLateur BJ, Nelp WB (1984) Local muscle blood flow and temperature responses to 915 MHz diathermy as simultaneously measured and numerically predicted. Arch Phys Med Rehabil 65:1–7
126. Sidi J, Jasmin C, Convert G, Dufour J, Azam G, Huber H, Leger G (1982) Short-wave regional hyperthermia on the pelvis. In: Liss AR (ed) Biomedical thermology. Liss, New York, pp 739–744
127. Sidi J, Convert G, Dufour J, Azam G, Mabire JP, Oweidat L, Taffare G, Jasmin C (1985) Hyperthermie profonde de la région pelvienne par le Jasmin 3-1000. J Biophys Biomech 9:45–48
128. Smith OJM (1957) Closed control of loops with deadtime. Chem Eng Prog 53:217–219
129. Song CW (1984) Effect of local hyperthermia on blood flow and microenvironment: a review. Cancer Res 44:47215–47305
130. Song CW, Rhee JG, Lee CKK, Levitt SH (1986) Capacitive heating of phantom and human tumors with an 8 MHz radiofrequency applicator (thermotron RF-8). Int J Radiat Oncol Biol Phys 12:365–372
131. Song WJ, Weinbaum S, Jiji LM (1987) A theoretical model for peripheral tissue heat transfer using the bioheat equation of Weinbaum and Jiji. ASME J Biomech Eng 109:72–78
132. Stauffer PR, Cetas TC, Fletcher AM, DeYoung DW, Dewhirst MW, Oleson JR, Roemer RB (1984) Observations in the use of ferromagnetic implants for inducing hyperthermia. IEEE Trans Biomed Eng 31:76–90
133. Stauffer PR, Cetas TC, Jones RC (1984) Magnetic induction heating of ferromagnetic implants for inducing localized hyperthermia in deep-seated tumors. IEEE Trans Biomed Eng 31:235–251
134. Stolwijk JAJ (1980) Mathematical models of thermal regulation. Ann NY Acad Sci 335:98–106
135. Stolwijk JAJ, Hardy JD (1977) Control of body temperature. In: Lee DHK (ed) Handbook of physiology – reactions to environment. American Physiological Society, Bethesda, pp 45–67
136. Storm FK, Elliot RS, Harrison WH, Morton DL (1982) Clinical RF hyperthermia by magnetic-loop induction, a new approach to human cancer therapy. IEEE Trans Microwave Theory Tech 30:1149–1158
137. Strohbehn JW (1982) Theoretical temperature distributions for solenoidal-type hyperthermia systems. Med Phys 9:673–682
138. Strohbehn JW (1983) Temperature distributions from interstitial RF electrode hyperthermia systems: theoretical predictions. Int J Radiat Oncol Biol Phys 9:1655–1667
139. Strohbehn J, Mechling J (1987) Interstitial techniques for clinical hyperthermia. In: Hand J, James J (eds) Physical techniques in clinical hyperthermia. Research Studies Press, Letchworth, pp 210–287
140. Strohbehn JW, Trembly BS, Douple EB (1982) Blood flow effects on the temperature distributions from an invasive microwave antenna array used in cancer therapy. IEEE Trans Biomed Eng 29:649–661
141. Strohbehn JW, Trembly BS, Douple EB, de Sieyes DC (1982) Evaluation of an invasive microwave antenna system for heating deep-seated tumors. J Natl Cancer Inst Monogr 61:489–491
142. Strohbehn J, Paulson K, Lynch D (1987) Use of the finite element method in computerized thermal dosimetry. In: Hand J, James J (eds) Physical techniques in clinical hyperthermia. Research Studies Press, Letchworth, pp 383–445
143. ter Haar G, Hopewell JW (1985) The induction of hyperthermia by ultrasound; its value and associated problems. II. Scanned-plane transducer. Phys Med Biol 30:1327–1333
144. Turner PF (1984) Hyperthermia and inhomogeneous tissue effects using an annular phased array. IEEE Trans Microwave Theory Tech MTT 32:874–882
145. Turner PF (1984) Regional hyperthermia with an annular phased array. IEEE Trans Biomed Eng BME 31:106
146. Underwood HR, Burdette EC, Ocheltree KB, Magin RL (1987) A multi-element ultrasonic hyperthermia applicator with independent element control. Int J Hyperthermia 3:257–268
147. Valvano JW, Allen JT, Bowman HF (1984) The simultaneous measurement of thermal conductivity, thermal diffusivity, and perfusion in small volumes of tissue. J Biomech Eng 106:192–197
148. van der Zee J, van Putten WLJ, van den Berg AP, van Rhoon GC, Wike Hooley JL, Broekmeyer-Reurink MP, Reinhold HS (1986) Retrospective analysis of the response of tumors in patients treated with a combination of radiotherapy and hyperthermia. Int J Hyperthermia 2:337–350
149. van der Zee J, Faithfull NS, van Rhoon GC, Reinhold HS (1987) Whole body hyperthermia as a treatment modality. In: Field SB, Franconi C (eds) Physics and technology of hyperthermia. Nijhoff, Dordrecht, pp 420–440
150. van Rhoon GC, Visser AG, van den Berg PM, Reinhold HS (1988) Regional deep heating with a field shaping device. Int J Hyperthermia, vol 4, 2:133–142
151. von Ardenne M (1986) The present developmental state of cancer multistep therapy. In: Anghileri L, Robert J (eds) Hyperthermia in cancer treatment. CRC Press, Boca Raton, pp 1–24
152. Weinbaum S, Jiji LM (1985) A new simplified bioheat equation for the effect of blood flow on local average tissue temperature. ASME J Biomech Eng 107:131–139

153. Weinbaum S, Jiji LM, Lemons DE (1984) Theory and experiment for the effect of vascular microstructure on surface tissue heat transfer. Part I. Anatomical foundation and model conceptualization. ASME J Biomech Eng 106:321–330
154. Whitmore RL (1968) Rheology of the circulation. Pergamon, Oxford
155. Williams W (1990) A structured model for heat transfer in living tissue. PhD Dissertation, University of Arizona, Tucson
156. Winget JM, Dewhirst MW, Engler MJ, Oleson JR (1986) The use of limited temperature observations to predict complete temperature fields. IEEE 8th annual conference of Engineering in Medicine and Biology Society. IEEE, Piscataway, pp 1507–1511
157. Wissler EH (1985) Mathematical simulation of human thermal behavior using whole-body models. In: Shitzer A, Eberhart RC (eds) Heat transfer in medicine and biology. Plenum, New York, pp 325–373

Subject Index

Clinical Thermology

Subseries Thermotherapy

Series Editor: M. Gautherie

Biological Basis of Oncologic Thermotherapy

Methods of External Heating

Methods of Hyperthermia Control

Thermal Dosimetry and Treatment Planning

Whole-Body Hyperthermia in Clinical Oncology

Interstitial, Endocavitary and Perfusional Hyperthermia – Methods and Clinical Trials

Subseries Diagnosis

Series Editor: M. Gautherie

Thermal Measuring, Recording and Imaging Techniques

Chronobiology and Thermophysiology

Clinical Thermology of Breast Diseases

Clinical Thermology of Rheumatic and Bone Diseases

MIX
Papier aus verantwortungsvollen Quellen
Paper from responsible sources
FSC® C105338
FSC
www.fsc.org

If you have any concerns about our products,
you can contact us on
ProductSafety@springernature.com

In case Publisher is established outside the EU,
the EU authorized representative is:
Springer Nature Customer Service Center GmbH
Europaplatz 3, 69115 Heidelberg, Germany

Printed by Libri Plureos GmbH
in Hamburg, Germany